SECOND EDITION

Audiology and Communication Disorders

AN OVERVIEW

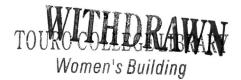

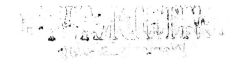

SECOND EDITION

Audiology **and** Communication Disorders

AN OVERVIEW

Larry E. Humes, PhD

Distinguished Professor and Chair
Department of Speech and Hearing Sciences
Indiana University
Bloomington, Indiana

Fred H. Bess, PhD

Professor, Department of Hearing and Speech Sciences
Director, National Center for Childhood and Family Communication
Vanderbilt Bill Wilkerson Center for Otolaryngology and
  Communication Sciences
Vanderbilt University School of Medicine
Nashville, Tennessee

WITHDRAWN
TOWRO-CHILDELAWRRY
Women's Building

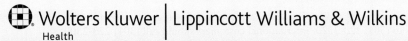
Wolters Kluwer | Lippincott Williams & Wilkins
Health

Philadelphia · Baltimore · New York · London
Buenos Aires · Hong Kong · Sydney · Tokyo

Acquisitions Editor: Michael Nobel
Product Development Editor: Michael Egolf
Marketing Manager: Leah Thomson
Art Director: Jennifer Clements
Designer: Stephen Druding
Compositor: SPi Global

Library of Congress Cataloging-in-Publication Data
Humes, Larry, author.
  [Audiology & communication disorders]
  Audiology and communication disorders : an overview / Larry E. Humes, Fred H. Bess. — Second edition.
       p. ; cm.
  Preceded by Audiology & communication disorders / Larry E. Humes, Fred H. Bess. 2008.
  Includes bibliographical references and index.
  ISBN 978-1-4511-3213-7 (paperback)
  I. Bess, Fred H., author. II. Title.
  [DNLM: 1. Communication Disorders. 2. Hearing—physiology. 3. Hearing Disorders. 4. Hearing Impaired Persons—rehabilitation.   WV 270]
  RF290
  617.8—dc23
                                                                                          2013021882

To our wives, Susie and Marty

Our children, Danny, Jenny, Amy, and Rick, and Andy, Lauren, and Adam

Our grandchildren, Matthew, Molly, Jack, Mary Helen, and Sam, and Noah, Sam, and Grace

and

To the undergraduate and graduate students with whom

we have had the pleasure to work

over the past few decades

CONTENTS

We have coauthored an introductory textbook in audiology, *Audiology: The Fundamentals*, that ran for four editions when we introduced the first edition of this textbook. The simultaneous offering of the first edition of *Audiology and Communication Disorders: An Overview* and the more advanced fourth edition of *Fundamentals* was an attempt to better serve two types of readership: those wishing for a more basic version of the material (*Overview*) and those desiring a more advanced version (*Fundamentals*). In preparation for this edition of the text, the authors, publishers, and reviewers agreed that potential adopters of the text would be better served by one textbook with the framework patterned after than that of *Overview* and the level of difficulty targeting a middle ground between the two texts. With this objective in mind, we are pleased to offer the second edition of *Audiology and Communication Disorders: An Overview*. From the authors' perspective, we feel as though we "got it right" this time around and hope the reader agrees.

ORGANIZATION

This book is divided into four main sections. In the first section, Chapters 1 to 3, a very broad overview of "normal" or typical human communication is provided. This overview is framed around the "communication chain," an extension of the "speech chain" popularized many years ago by Denes and Pinson (1963, 1994). The communication chain is used to demonstrate the central role that hearing plays in everyday communication and in its development. This helps one to better understand the impact of hearing loss experienced at different ages on the development of the communication chain.

After demonstrating the critical importance of sound and hearing in communication (especially spoken communication) in the first section, the next section of the text (Chapters 4 and 5) is devoted to descriptions of the two key professions involved in addressing breaks in the communication chain: audiologists and speech-language pathologists. For speech-language pathologists, the most likely future profession for the majority of the readers of this book, the emphasis is placed on the role of the speech-language pathologist working in concert with audiologists to manage children and adults with auditory disorders.

The next section (Chapters 6 to 8) is devoted to the description of various disorders that result in hearing loss and the impact of this hearing loss on communication. The point is made that it is important to identify hearing loss as early as possible to minimize its negative impact on communication. Because this text is primarily directed toward those planning to be in professions other than audiology, the focus is placed on screening procedures for the detection of hearing loss, rather than procedures for detailed diagnostic procedures. However, it is still likely that such professionals will need to understand audiologic information for the children and adults with whom they will be working. As a result, information on the interpretation of basic diagnostic measures, including pure-tone audiometry, speech audiometry, and immittance measurements, is also presented in this section.

The final section of this book (Chapters 9 and 10) discusses approaches to the treatment of hearing loss once it has been identified. Here, it is assumed that the child or adult with impaired hearing is a part of the hearing world (as opposed to the Deaf world) and wishes to remain a part of "hearing culture." As such, the main treatment alternatives are hearing aids and cochlear implants, depending primarily on the severity of the hearing loss. Again, the assumption is that the reader of this text will not likely become an audiologist in the future but will be interacting with adults and children with impaired hearing who have been seen by an audiologist. As a result, the focus will not be on the procedural details of selecting, fitting, and evaluating hearing aids or cochlear implants on patients. Rather, the focus is on understanding the processes and the results from these processes to better manage the hearing-impaired person's communication.

TEACH AUDIOLOGY YOUR WAY

Audiology and Communication Disorders: An Overview, second edition, makes use of an innovative learning system designed to make important audiology concepts accessible to new students while also providing instructors with the depth of coverage required for more advanced students. Using the innovative communication chain model, we have combined a concise book with assignable online articles, case studies, and multimedia activities that enable instructors to adapt the content to the needs of their students.

Innovative System for Linking Hearing and Communication

The communication chain approach is an innovative, yet easy-to-understand, model of the interactive network of processes in auditory-oral communication. We use this model to demonstrate the central role that hearing plays in everyday communication and help students better understand how hearing loss can impact the development of communication. The communication chain model is introduced as the organizing theme of the text in the first chapter, and subsequent chapters cover the detection and repair of breaks in the chain, as well as the professionals tasked with detecting and repairing those breaks. By relating even the most complex topics in audiology to the communication chain model, the authors have created an accessible program that effectively aids students and professionals in learning the principles of audiology.

Concise and Accessible Reference

Audiology and Communication Disorders: An Overview, second edition, is designed for students who need a foundation in the principles of audiology. Anyone who works with children or adults with impaired hearing, including audiologists, speech-language pathologists, psychologists, and educators, will find that this text helps them better appreciate and understand the impact of hearing loss, its detection, and its treatment. Concise and accessible, the book enables instructors to cover key audiology concepts effectively in a limited amount of time.

Flexible Online Articles and Multimedia Activities

The online article library was developed to integrate seamlessly with the main text, making it easy for instructors to present an advanced course without sacrificing the benefits of teaching from a text designed solely for undergraduate students, the majority of whom are unlikely to be future audiologists. In addition, the accessibility of the main text gives students a firm foundation to tackle the advanced online materials without feeling lost or overwhelmed.

FEATURES

This text makes use of several pedagogic features to enhance learning. Each chapter, for example, begins with a set of chapter objectives and concludes with a brief summary. Chapter review questions are at the end of each chapter to facilitate integration of the material. Five different types of vignettes— Experiments, Conceptual Demos, Further Discussion, Clinical Applications, and Historical Notes—are used throughout the text to drive home key points or to elaborate on them to facilitate understanding. In addition, Key Terms are identified at the beginning of each chapter, then highlighted, and defined at first use in that chapter. These, and other terms, are defined as well in the Glossary at the end of the text.

ADDITIONAL RESOURCES

Audiology and Communication Disorders: An Overview, second edition, includes additional resources for both instructors and students that are available on thePoint at http://thepoint.lww.com.

Instructors

Approved adopting instructors will be given access to the following additional resources:

- PowerPoint presentations, including multiple-choice questions for use with interactive clicker technology
- Test generator
- Image bank

Students

Students who have purchased *Audiology and Communication Disorders: An Overview*, second edition, have access to the following additional resources:

- A glossary with audio pronunciation
- Interactive screening tests
- Labeling exercises to reinforce terms and concepts from the text
- Chapter quizzes
- Case studies
- Animations of the anatomical structures
- Audio and video demonstrations (these are marked in the margins with audio or video icons to direct the reader to the companion site on thePoint. Additional details indicate exactly which clip coincides with the icon.)

In addition, purchasers of the text can access the searchable full-text version online by going to the *Audiology and Communication Disorders: An Overview*, second edition, Web site at http://thepoint.lww.com. See the inside front cover of this text for more details, including the passcode you will need to gain access to the Web site.

We hope that this text meets the needs of those teaching undergraduates in need of a broad understanding of audiology, but who do not envision themselves to be "future audiologists." Perhaps, with this text and some luck, we will be able to change the minds of at least some of them!

LARRY E. HUMES, PhD
FRED H. BESS, PhD

REVIEWERS

Mathieu Hotton, AuD
Université du Québec à
  Trois-Rivières
Trois-Rivières, Quebec, Canada

Richard Hurtig, PhD
The University of Iowa
Iowa City, Iowa

Charissa Lansing, PhD
University of Illinois at
  Urbana-Champaign
Champaign, Illinois

Torrey Loucks, PhD
University of Illinois at Urbana-
  Champaign
Champaign, Illinois

Colleen McAleer, PhD
Clarion University
Clarion, Pennsylvania

Lori Pakulski, PhD
University of Toledo
Toledo, Ohio

Vishkha Rawool, PhD
West Virginia University
Morgantown, West Virginia

Yula Serpanos, PhD
Adelphi University
Garden City, New York

Lu-Feng Shi, PhD
Long Island University, Brooklyn
Brooklyn, New York

Deborah Welling, AuD
Seton Hall University
South Orange, New Jersey

Susan Wortsman, AuD
Hunter College
New York, New York

The Communication Chain

1

The Communication Chain

Chapter Objectives

- To understand the basic components of the communication chain as the framework that facilitates the exchange of information, ideas, and emotions between two human beings;
- To identify key benchmarks in the typical development of the communication chain; and
- To appreciate the potential consequences of breaks in the communication brought about by impaired hearing.

Key Terms and Definitions

- **Communication chain:** The chain of events that is initiated by a person (the talker or sender) who wishes to share information, ideas, or emotions with another person (the listener or receiver). In typical auditory-oral communication, this begins with the talker's conceptualization of the information or ideas to be exchanged and the initiation of speech production, which sends an acoustic signal to the listener. The listener's auditory system converts the arriving acoustical information to neural signals; these neural signals are processed by the listener's brain to decipher the speaker's message.

- **Language:** The code used by members of the same culture or group to decipher or produce sequences of sounds or signs capable of communicating thoughts, ideas, and actions to other members of the same culture or group. Two key components are the lexicon (mental dictionary), which matches sound or sign sequences to objects or actions, and syntax (grammar), which contains the rules by which words are sequenced in a language to form meaningful phrases and sentences.

- **Hearing impairment:** A loss of hearing that results in a need to have sounds increased in intensity to levels greater than those normally heard by young adults so as to be heard by the individual. The need for greater intensity to hear the sound is typically due to a disorder of some type located in the auditory system somewhere between the outer ear and the auditory portions of the brain.

3

It has been argued that communication of abstract concepts, thoughts, and ideas is a truly unique human experience, part of what distinguishes humans from other animals. This is not limited to communication about complex ideas or notions such as philosophical, religious, or political viewpoints, but includes many everyday aspects of communication as well. For example, consider the following simple scenario. You are planning a trip with a friend in which a map is consulted and costs are estimated for travel and accommodations—a very "concrete" exchange. Yet, this simple everyday dialogue between two friends involves the use and exchange of considerable abstract information. In this example, the exchange might include the processing of visual information on a map, perhaps a small, two-dimensional (e.g., 6-inch piece of paper) abstract representation of a much larger area, such as the Midwestern United States, including the roads running through that area. It might also include the exchange of numerical monetary information relating to the costs involved, which is also an abstract system. Finally, such a dialogue might include statements of opinion by either party as to whether potential sites along the journey would be interesting or expensive. Typically, these ideas are exchanged between you and your friend rapidly and effortlessly through auditory-oral communication. Of course, the words used in the communication of thoughts and ideas are themselves abstract concepts—sound sequences that individuals in a shared culture have learned to associate with various objects, actions, descriptors, or modifiers.

Figure 1.1 provides a simplified overview of the various processes and systems involved in human communication. For clarity, only two individuals are depicted here: the talker and the listener or, more generally, the sender and the receiver of information. The sender has a thought or idea formulated in his or her mind and would like to convey this information to the mind of the receiver. This interactive network of the processes supporting such mind-to-mind communication is referred to here as the **communication chain**. This concept borrows heavily from the concept of the "speech chain," first introduced to the authors many years ago and still popular today (Denes & Pinson, 1963, 1993). The primary changes made to the original speech chain were to broaden it to include the exchange of visual information between the sender and the receiver. This visual information might be in the form of facial gestures that accompany speech production by the sender or the use of alternative modalities for communication, including manual forms of communication such as American Sign Language (ASL).

One important concept in Figure 1.1 is that there is a desire for the sender to send some information to the receiver, that is, to communicate some thoughts, ideas, or information. In typical auditory-oral communication, the exchange is initiated by the sender's brain, organizing his or her thoughts to be communicated in the sender's acquired **language**. Then, the sender directs the speech mechanism to produce a sequence of sounds associated with the words and

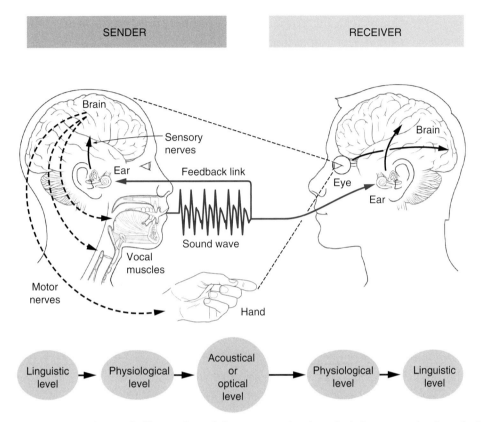

FIGURE 1.1 A schematic illustration of the communication chain between the "sender" and the "receiver." In typical auditory-oral communication, the sender is a talker and the receiver is a listener.

grammar used in that language to communicate the intended message. In this case of typical auditory-oral communication, the primary link between the sender and receiver is the acoustic information generated by the sender. At this stage, hearing plays a critical role in the communication chain. The receiver's sensory system for hearing is used to encode the sound sequence spoken by the sender. This information from the hearing system is then sent via the nervous system to the brain of the receiver and decoded, assuming the receiver knows the language used by the sender. If the auditory system of the receiver is damaged, then the information may not be delivered intact to the brain of the receiver, and the message may not be understood correctly. Of course, this is not the only place where there may be a break in the communication chain. For example, the sender may have impaired speech such that the acoustic stimulus sent to the receiver is degraded, which can hinder communication. Also, either the sender or the receiver may have higher-level cognitive or linguistic deficits that can degrade the message sent or the interpretation of the message received.

In this text, however, the primary breaks in the communication chain under consideration are those impacting the hearing of the sender or the receiver. In this regard, from the depiction of the communication chain in Figure 1.1, it is apparent that the receiver is not the only one who may be impacted negatively by impaired hearing. The sender's hearing system also encodes the spoken message as a way of monitoring the accuracy of the message and the sound sequence representing it. If the sender has impaired hearing, the way in which the sound sequence comprising the spoken message is produced may be impacted. Thus, hearing plays a critical role in deciphering the spoken message for the receiver and in the monitoring of the spoken message produced by the sender. An individual with impaired hearing not only may have difficulty hearing others but also may contribute to a breakdown in communication through poorly articulated speech owing to the inability to monitor the quality of the speech generated.

Note that visual information from the sender is also available to the receiver, even in typical auditory-oral communication. That is, as the sender is moving the articulators to produce speech, visible cues for the identity of the sounds spoken are also provided to the receiver. The bilabial speech sounds, /b/, /p/, and /m/, for example, are very visible and characterized by the rapid parting of the talker's lips. Similarly, the position of the lower teeth against the upper lip is a strong visual cue for the labiodental speech sounds /f/ and /v/. Not all speech sounds are readily visible—for example, the velar sounds /k/ and /g/ provide few, if any, visible cues. In addition, nonspeech visual information such as gestures and facial expressions can enhance auditory-oral communication. Some individuals are very adept at using additional visual information from the sender to help understand the spoken message so that they can understand the message. This may enable them to understand the message even when little acoustic energy from the spoken message is perceived by the receiver. Examples of conditions that require greater reliance on visible speech cues include high levels of background sound (noises, music, or other people talking), great distances between the sender and the receiver (perhaps even requiring devices such as binoculars to see the person speaking), or severely impaired hearing.

For some individuals, however, visual communication might be the primary means of communication between the sender and the receiver, rather than a supplement to the auditory information. This may again apply to persons with severe **hearing impairments** who use speechreading (also referred to as "lipreading") to perceive the message spoken by the sender. Some individuals with impaired hearing, especially many of those who developed the hearing impairment after spoken language had been acquired, can make good use of the visual cues in speech to enable very good "auditory-oral" communication. Speechreading ability is known to vary widely among individuals, however, and the factors that make one person a good speechreader and another seemingly similar person a poor speechreader are not well understood.

In other cases, communication between sender and receiver may make exclusive use of visual stimuli. An example of such a communication system in the United States is ASL. In this system, as illustrated schematically in Figure 1.1, sequences of finger, hand, and arm gestures constitute the primary link between the sender and the receiver. These hand gestures may be complemented by other visual or spatial cues, such as the spatial location of the hand gesture relative to the sender's location or accompanying facial gestures. As in typical auditory-oral communication, the communication sequence in manual communication is initiated in the mind of the sender. As noted in Figure 1.1, this, in turn, leads to signals from the brain of the sender to the motor nerves of the fingers, hands, arms, and face; this process then leads to a sequence of gestures conveying the message using the rules of the sender's language. These stimuli result in patterns seen by the receiver's visual system, which encodes the optical information and then sends it via the nervous system to the brain of the receiver. If the receiver knows the language used by the sender, this sequence of neural events is decoded by the receiver, and the sent message is understood. Note here that mind-to-mind communication has taken place between the sender and the receiver while completely bypassing the auditory systems of both the sender and the receiver. Thus, manual communication in this fashion would be unaffected by hearing loss of any severity.

Of course, just as with typical auditory-oral communication, there are factors that might restrict the ability to communicate manually. It is critical, for instance, that the sender and receiver be able to see one another. Thus, manual communication with the sender in one room and the receiver in another is not possible without a direct visual link. Modern technology, however, such as the use of videophones or webcams, has made a visual link between the sender and receiver much less problematic when each is separated by great distances from the other (just as telephones have enabled auditory-oral communication over great distances).

Perhaps, the most critical requirement for the successful use of manual communication, however, is that both the sender and receiver must have knowledge of the specific manual language being used. In contemporary cultures worldwide, auditory-oral communication is used by the overwhelming majority of people. In these same cultures, the use of manual communication is primarily restricted to situations or circumstances in which auditory-oral communication is not readily accessible without the intervention of others. One such circumstance for which manual communication systems have been developed involves communication with and by profoundly hearing-impaired or deaf individuals. Historically, the development of manual communication systems for deaf individuals preceded the development of modern technologies, such as hearing aids

#22

and cochlear implants, designed to provide the deaf with access to auditory-oral communication. Manual languages developed for and by deaf individuals serve a limited segment of society and are not the "default" system in a specific society, societies dominated by hearing people. This is not to imply, however, that manual languages like ASL are impoverished or otherwise incapable of supporting the communication chain. To the contrary, ASL has been demonstrated to be a rich language capable of supporting the highest levels of abstract mind-to-mind communication (see Vignette 1.1.). For such communication to take place, however,

VIGNETTE 1.1 • FURTHER DISCUSSION

The Language Centers of the Brain

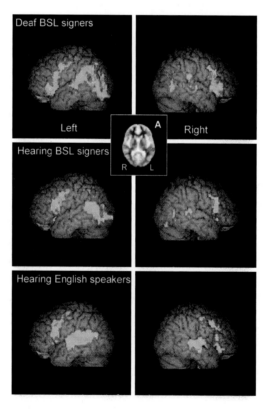

The images shown above are functional magnetic resonance images (fMRI) of the human brain showing areas of maximum brain activity under three conditions: (a) manually signed (British Sign Language, BSL) sentences presented to deaf individuals for whom BSL was the first language learned (left two images); (b) manually signed BSL sentences presented to normal-hearing individuals for whom BSL was the first language learned (middle two images); and (c) spoken sentences in British English presented to normal-hearing individuals for whom spoken British English was the first language learned (right two images). The top image of each vertical pair shows the left half (hemisphere) of each brain, and the bottom image of each pair shows the right hemisphere. Two observations can be made easily from this series of six fMRI images: the left hemisphere responds more to language input whether it is manual sign language or spoken speech, and there is quite a bit of overlap in the regions of the brain activated for the processing of the signed or spoken sentences. This is emphasized in the images shown below from the same study, but now illustrating only those areas of the brain that were activated for both signed and spoken sentences. This area can be thought of as a language-processing region of the brain. The same language-processing centers are stimulated for both signed and spoken languages. The primary difference in these two cases is how the stimuli carrying each language are delivered to the language-processing centers of the brain: via the eyes and the visual portions of the central nervous system for signs and through the ears and auditory portions of the central nervous system for spoken sentences. (Images from Mac-Sweeney M, Woll B, Campbell R. et al. Neural systems underlying British Sign Language and audio-visual English processing in native users. *Brain* 2002;125:1583–1593.)

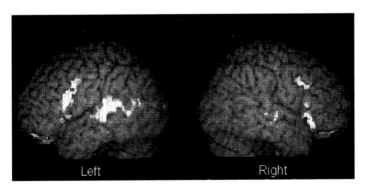

Left   Right

the sender and the receiver must be reasonably fluent in the language supporting mind-to-mind communication and, by sheer numbers alone, the overwhelming majority of individuals encountered in a given society are likely to be conversant in one of many spoken languages, rather than a manual language. This severely constrains the utility of manual languages, such as ASL, in broader society.

DEVELOPMENT OF THE COMMUNICATION CHAIN

Another key feature of the language system used for communication between the sender and the receiver is the manner in which language is usually acquired. Typically, language is acquired "naturally" through repeated exposures to the language early in life. Evidence suggests that the language-learning process itself is innate, and early experience with language determines the specific language system that will be developed. Thus, most children born and raised in France learn French as their first language and, likewise, most of those born and raised in Italy learn Italian as their native language. The learning of a first language is usually a process in which the infant and toddler capitalize on the prewired, innate, language-learning capabilities through repetitive exposures to language samples from members of the same language community, primarily the child's family, especially the mother. Within the context of the communication chain in Figure 1.1, the parent is the sender and knows the sequence of sound patterns associated with spoken words having various meanings and, through repetition of these same sound sequences in a variety of contexts, the child, as the receiver, begins to extract the code and develop an expanding vocabulary or lexicon, mapping sound patterns to various objects, actions, descriptors, or modifiers. Through frequent exposures, the child also learns the rules in the language that govern the order of such sound sequences in meaningful phrases or sentences (syntax). For communication to take place between the sender (parent) and the receiver (child), the receiver must develop the same code for deciphering the stream of sounds spoken by the sender. Otherwise, even with all other aspects of the communication chain functioning properly, communication between sender and receiver is not likely to take place.

Another aspect of this remarkable language-learning process is that it is a relatively rapid process. Table 1.1 lists some common language benchmarks for the development of typical auditory-oral communication. In general, the same developmental milestones have been observed for the development of ASL, at least for the case of deaf children raised by deaf parents. Clearly, language develops rapidly over the first 4 to 5 years of life when the young receiver is

TABLE

1.1

Some General Milestones for Typical Speech and Language Development

Age (In Years)	Milestone
1 y	Should have produced "first word"
2 y	Two-word phrases ("Daddy go") Expressive vocabulary of at least 40 words Receptive vocabulary of at least 50 words
4 y	Uses grammatically correct sentences Expressive vocabulary of at least 200 words Receptive vocabulary of at least 400 words 95% of speech is adult-like and readily understood by others (including strangers)

immersed in language produced by experienced senders (again, typically, the immediate family and primarily the mother).

Evidence supports the existence of a sensitive period for the development of a child's first language. As an upper bound for the limits to acquisition of typical language skills, it is generally believed that a child should know at least 50 to 100 words by the age of 5 to 7 years to have an opportunity to subsequently develop typical speech and language skills. Again, this is an upper age limit, and most children typically acquire this minimum proficiency *well before* the age of 5 years (typically, within the first year or two of life), as illustrated in Table 1.1. Again, they do so primarily through repetitive exposure to the language spoken by family members and members of the surrounding community. Once the child acquires a sufficient number of words in his or her lexicon or vocabulary, then the rules of grammar are developed to generate appropriate sequences of these words. For example, a young child acquiring spoken English will typically develop subject-verb or subject-verb-object word orders early in the use of sentences. Examples of such word orders include "Daddy go," "Baby cry," and "Puppy drink water." The key developmental trigger for the generation of meaningful strings of words in sentences appears to be the acquisition of a vocabulary of 50 to 100 words. If such a vocabulary size is not attained by an age of about 5 to 7 years, then future ability to generate meaningful sentences may be irreversibly impaired. In fact, there is some evidence from children raised in dire circumstances that indicates that failure to acquire this minimum vocabulary size of 50 to 100 words by 11 to 12 years of age may result in a total inability to generate meaningful sentences as an adult (Vignette 1.2).

 HEARING LOSS AND BREAKS IN THE COMMUNICATION CHAIN

For about 90% of the deaf children born in the United States, both parents have normal hearing, and their communication system is auditory-oral. This creates an immediate break in the communication chain between parents and the child. Figure 1.2 schematically illustrates this break in the communication chain when the child is the receiver and the parent is the sender of information. This is the most common direction of information exchange for the developing child and is discussed further below. Note here that the hearing-impaired child may not be able to monitor the quality of the vocal output being produced and that this may ultimately have a negative impact on the clarity of the child's speech. Deaf babies actually go through some of the same early stages of speech production (e.g., babbling) as typically developing auditory-oral babies. Without early intervention with hearing aids or cochlear implants, these early stages of speech production are not reinforced auditorily through

VIGNETTE 1.2 • FURTHER DISCUSSION

Forbidden Experiments

How do scientists confirm the existence of possible sensitive periods for language development? One approach, the "forbidden experiment," would be to raise a child in complete isolation, without any language input or contact from others. One child could be isolated at 6 months of age, another child at 12 months of age, another at 18 months of age, and so on. The impact of isolation for various periods on speech and language development could then be studied. It is obvious why such an experiment is forbidden and could not be performed by scientists.

Unfortunately, from time to time, there have been naturally occurring "experiments" such as these where, through a terrible set of circumstances, children are raised in isolation for various periods of time. Perhaps, two of the most well-known cases are Victor and Genie. Victor was the initial "wild child," apparently raised in isolation in the woods of France in the 1800s and not discovered by others until the age of about 12 years. Victor's story, and the attempts to restore speech and language, was popularized in the Francois Truffaut film, "The Wild Child [L'Enfant Sauvage]," released in 1970.

Coincidentally, at about the time this movie was being released, the case of Genie emerged in Los Angeles. Genie was discovered at the age of 13 years, having spent most of her life, since the age of about 18 months, raised by elderly parents who isolated her day and night in a small locked room, often tying her to a potty chair. The father, who was believed to be schizophrenic, apparently beat her whenever she vocalized, and she did not gain her freedom from these dire circumstances until her father's death. Genie's story was popularized in a variety of ways too, including a Public Broadcasting Service NOVA presentation in 1997 entitled, "Secret of the Wild Child." Although Genie could learn to communicate with a restricted vocabulary using isolated words or phrases, she never gained the ability to produce sentences and her language skills, despite extensive intervention, never approached "normal" levels.

Case studies of children, such as Victor and Genie, raised in dire circumstances and deprived of typical language input, have provided some of the evidence in support of the existence for a sensitive period for language acquisition. Because these "natural experiments" were not coordinated or conducted as empirical research, they offer only some general guidelines as to the nature and extent of the sensitive period.

subsequent imitation by the parent because the parent's mimicry "falls on deaf ears." As a result, the spontaneous vocal productions of profoundly hearing-impaired infants diminish in frequency and do not lead to the next stages of speech development observed in normal-hearing infants.

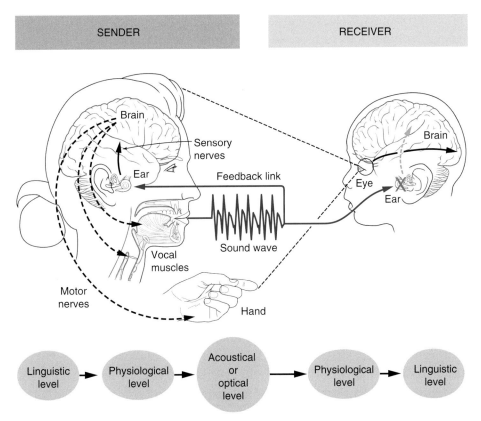

FIGURE 1.2 Illustration of a break in the communication chain resulting from hearing loss. The break is illustrated in the auditory periphery of the receiver (listener), who is a hearing-impaired child.

As noted, in the right portion of Figure 1.2, the receiver (the child) has a nonfunctional auditory pathway incapable of encoding the acoustic signals being generated by the senders (the parents), who are relying exclusively on an auditory-oral communication system. For communication to take place, and, in this case, for language to develop from repetitive communication, there are two choices. The break in the communication chain at the auditory system of the receiver must be repaired (e.g., through medical treatment, a hearing aid, or a cochlear implant), or the sender must switch to a communication mode that does not rely on hearing (e.g., ASL). The parents, however, as the language models for their deaf child, are not fluent in ASL or other forms of manual communication. Rather, in the United States, the parents are most likely to be fluent in spoken English or Spanish. The child, on the other hand, cannot hear the spoken English or Spanish messages being sent by the parents or other family members. As a result, there is a breakdown in communication, and the child is not learning the language of the parents, or any language for that matter. Moreover, as noted previously, there is a critical period for the development of sufficient language proficiency to support adequate mind-to-mind communication. Thus, the clock is ticking for the resolution of this dilemma. Either the impaired auditory system of the child must be identified quickly and treated to enable the development of typical auditory-oral communication, or the child must be immersed in ASL. The latter solution typically involves the parents learning ASL as a second language and frequently turning over their language-modeling roles to members of the deaf community who are fluent in ASL.

Debates about the most effective resolution to this dilemma have raged for well over a century. Our perspective on this debate is as follows. First, regardless of the communication system to be used, the early identification of hearing impairment is critical. Without knowing the status of the child's hearing, it is not possible to intervene effectively, regardless of the path chosen. Second, for the overwhelming majority of profoundly hearing-impaired children, the 90% born to two normal-hearing parents, the default intervention should be restoration of hearing and reliance on auditory-oral communication rather than reliance on manual communication, although manual communication can be used as a supplement to auditory-oral communication as needed.

Our rationale for this stance is based on a number of practical circumstances rather than a clear superiority of auditory-oral language systems over manual language systems. For example, as indicated previously, the overwhelming majority of members in our society rely on auditory-oral forms of communication and, as noted in the discussion of the communication chain, effective communication requires knowledge of a common language by both the sender and the receiver. Thus, in most daily activities and encounters, a profoundly hearing-impaired person is more likely to encounter users of auditory-oral communication systems than manual communication systems. In addition, written languages for manual communication systems, such as ASL, do not exist at present. Consequently, the hearing-impaired person who learns ASL as the primary form of communication must learn a second language (e.g., English) for written communication and literacy. This is not the case, of course, when English is the choice for both written and spoken communication. In this case, there is greater redundancy between the acquisition of spoken and written language skills.

In addition, there is considerable evidence that communication, in either written or oral form, is less effective in a person's second language than in his or her first language. One way in which this has probably manifested itself has been in the long-standing observations of less than satisfactory reading and mathematics achievement scores for the deaf population in the United States. Statistics from a national research institute at the only liberal arts college in the United States for the deaf (Gallaudet Research Institute, 2005), for example, indicate that the average deaf high school graduate (Grade 12, or an age of 18 years) reads at a fourth-grade level on the Stanford Achievement Test (SAT), actually, on a special version of the test adapted for use with individuals having impaired hearing (SAT-HI). Average mathematics scores on the SAT-HI are at the sixth-grade level for the same age group of deaf individuals nationwide. Because the SAT-HI is administered in written English, at least part of the poor average performance may be due to a mismatch between the first language (ASL) of many of the test takers and the language of the test (written English). Nonetheless, to the extent that the test captures proficiency in reading and math when using written English, the written language in which the deaf were educated and on which they will need to rely in daily life, it suggests that performance in written English is less than satisfactory. It is acknowledged that the presumption made here is that similar large-scale data from hearing-impaired children with early auditory-oral intervention and exposure to oral English at an early age will exceed these reading and mathematics competencies for the SAT-HI. Although there is encouraging research with profoundly hearing-impaired children who received cochlear implants at an early age to support this supposition, the data available from such children, especially for those who have now reached an age of 18 years, are too sparse to clearly substantiate this argument.

Finally, there are other beneficial by-products of the child's reliance on auditory-oral communication that we consider to be beneficial to the person with impaired hearing. These include the ability to communicate with unseen senders and receivers (over the telephone, in other rooms, etc.), to simultaneously monitor multiple senders (talkers) in the same or different locations (while concurrently using the other modality, vision, to monitor yet another object or location), to hear a wide variety of audible warning and alerting sounds designed for safety and protection, and to appreciate other auditory stimuli involved in the communication of mood or other types of messages, such as instrumental and vocal music.

SUMMARY

The communication chain provides a general framework for the communication between a sender and a receiver and enables the ultimate human experience: mind-to-mind communication of feelings, thoughts, and ideas. For typical auditory-oral communication, the predominant modality for communication throughout the world, hearing plays a central role. Impaired hearing can have a negative impact on both the sender and the receiver in the communication chain. Breakdowns in communication may result. To minimize the impact of the hearing impairment on communication and its development, the hearing loss must first be detected as soon as possible after its onset (regardless of the individual's age). The best option for the overwhelming majority of children with impaired hearing is to restore communication by improving the individual's hearing as soon as possible so as to acquire or sustain typical auditory-oral communication abilities.

Given the foregoing, the subsequent chapters of this text assume the primacy of auditory-oral communication for the majority of hearing-impaired persons—the primary exception being deaf children raised by deaf parents and immersed in ASL and deaf culture. As such, for the remainder of this book, it is assumed that the primary link between sender and receiver is the acoustic signal generated by the sender. The acoustic signal is the topic of Chapter 2. Subsequent chapters deal with the encoding of the acoustic stimulus within the auditory system by both the receiver and the sender, the impact of various hearing disorders on communication, methods to identify the presence of hearing problems, and options for treatment of hearing disorders to improve auditory-oral communication.

CHAPTER REVIEW QUESTIONS

1. The communication chain illustrated in Figure 1.1 shows two separate auditory systems, one for the sender or talker and one for the receiver or listener. Figure 1.2 illustrates a break in the communication chain arising from a disorder in the auditory system. How would communication be impacted if the auditory system of the receiver was damaged so that it was completely nonfunctional? What if it was only the auditory system of the sender that had been damaged or destroyed? What if the auditory systems of both the sender and receiver are completely damaged?

2. What differences in speech-language development might you expect between the following two cases, assuming no intervention has taken place to repair the breaks in their respective communication chains? Both individuals have a complete loss of hearing in both ears, but one person has been like this since birth and the other since an age of 4 years. Both individuals are 6 years old at the time of examination. What differences would you expect and why?

3. The authors have adopted the viewpoint in this text that for persons with profound hearing loss who are considered deaf, auditory-oral communication is preferred over manual forms of communication, like ASL, in the overwhelming majority of cases. How do they support this position? Do you agree or disagree? Why?

REFERENCES AND SUGGESTED READINGS

Denes PB, Pinson EN. *The Speech Chain*. Edison, NJ: Bell Telephone Laboratories; 1963.

Denes PB, Pinson EN. *The Speech Chain*. 2nd ed. New York: W.H. Freeman; 1993.

Gallaudet Research Institute. *Stanford Achievement Test, 10th edition. Form A, Norms Booklet for Deaf and Hard of Hearing Students*. Washington, DC: Gallaudet University, Gallaudet Research Institute; 2005.

2

Sound: The Typical Link between Sender and Receiver in the Communication Chain

Chapter Objectives

- To appreciate the importance of sound as the primary link between the talker and the listener in the communication chain;
- To understand how sound waves are represented in the time domain;
- To see that the same sound can also be described in the frequency domain to emphasize the specific frequencies that are included in sound; and
- To understand the representation of a sound wave's magnitude or amplitude in terms of a sound level expressed in decibels.

Key Terms and Definitions

- **Sound wave:** A disturbance created in a medium, such as air, by a source of vibration.
- **Waveform:** A graphical description of the variation in a sound wave's amplitude as a function of time.
- **Spectrum:** A graphical description of the variation in a sound wave's amplitude and phase as a function of frequency.
- **Decibel:** The unit of measure used to describe the level or magnitude of a sound wave.

As noted in Chapter 1, the typical link between the sender and the receiver in the communication chain is via spoken speech—an acoustic signal. To better understand the impact of impaired hearing on communication, it is critical to obtain a basic understanding of sound, including speech sounds. This chapter begins with a discussion of selected characteristics of sound waves, which is followed by a section on the representation of sound in the time domain (its waveform) and the frequency domain (its spectrum). This chapter concludes with a brief description of the measurement of sound level in decibels (dB).

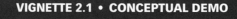

SOUND WAVES AND THEIR CHARACTERISTICS

The air we breathe is composed of millions of tiny air particles. The presence of these particles makes the production of a **sound wave** possible. This is made clear by the simple, yet elegant, experiment described in Vignette 2.1. The experiment demonstrates that air particles are needed for the production and transmission of sound in the atmosphere. There are approximately 400 billion air particles in every cubic inch of the atmosphere. The billions of

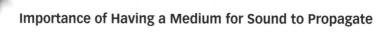

VIGNETTE 2.1 • CONCEPTUAL DEMO

Importance of Having a Medium for Sound to Propagate

The equipment shown in the accompanying figure can be used to demonstrate the importance of air particles, or some other medium, to the generalization of sound waves. An electric buzzer is placed within the jar. The jar is filled with air. When the buzzer is connected to the battery, one hears a buzzing sound originating from within the jar. Next, a vacuum is created within the jar by pumping out the air particles. When the buzzer is again connected to the battery, no sound is heard. One can see the metal components of the buzzer striking one another, yet no sound is heard. Sound waves cannot be produced without an appropriate medium, such as the air particles composing the atmosphere.

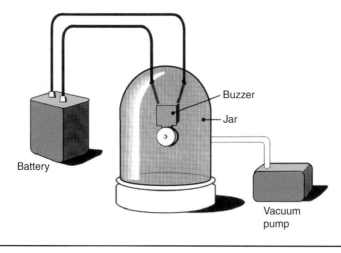

particles composing the atmosphere are normally moving in a random fashion. These random continual movements of air particles make up what is known as *brownian motion*. These random movements, however, can be ignored for the most part in our discussion of sound waves. It is sufficient to assume that each particle has an average initial or resting position.

When an object surrounded by air particles vibrates, the air particles adjacent to that object also vibrate. Thus, when a sufficient force is applied to the air particles by the moving object, the air particles will be moved or displaced in the direction of the applied force. Once the applied force is removed, a property of the air medium, known as its *elasticity*, returns the displaced particle to its resting state. The initial application of force sets up a chain of events in the surrounding air particles. This is depicted in Figure 2.1. The air particles immediately adjacent to the moving object (labeled A in Fig. 2.1) are displaced in the direction of the applied force. They then collide with more remote air particles once they have been displaced. This collision displaces the more remote particles in the direction of the applied force. The elasticity of the air returns the air particles to their resting position. As the more remote particles are colliding with air particles still farther away from the vibrating object, force

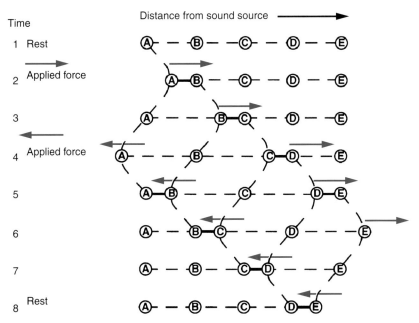

FIGURE 2.1 The movement of air particles (A through E) in response to an applied force at $t = 2$ and $t = 4$. The *arrows* indicate the direction of the applied force and the direction of particle displacement. Notice that each of the particles goes through a simple back-and-forth displacement. The wave propagates through the air, so that back-and-forth vibration of particle A eventually results in a similar back-and-forth vibration of particle E.

is applied to displace the object in the opposite direction. The void left by the former position of the object is filled by the adjacent air particles. This displaces the adjacent particle in the opposite direction. Note that the vibration of air particles passes on from one particle to another through this sequential series of collisions followed by a return to resting position. Thus, the displacement pattern produced by the object travels through the air particles via this chain of collisions.

Although we could measure this vibration in particles that are a considerable distance from the source of vibration, such as the particle labeled E in Figure 2.1, each particle in the chain of collisions has only moved a very small distance and then returned to its initial position. The air particles thus form the medium through which the vibration is carried. If the air particles adjacent to the vibrating object could actually be labeled, as is done in Figure 2.1, then it would be apparent that the vibration of air particles measured away from the vibrating object at point E would not involve the particles next to the object, labeled A. Rather, the particle labeled A remains adjacent to the object at all times and simply transmits or carries the displacement from resting position to the next air particle (B). In turn, B collides with C; C collides with D; D collides with E; and so on. A sound wave, therefore, is the movement or propagation of a disturbance (the vibration) through a medium, such as air, without permanent displacement of the particles.

Propagation of a disturbance through a medium can be demonstrated easily with the help of some friends. Six to eight persons should stand in a line, with the last person facing a wall and the others lined up behind that person. Each individual should be separated by slightly less than arm's length. Each person represents an air particle in the medium. Each individual should now place both hands firmly on the shoulders of the person immediately in front of him or her. This represents the coupling of one particle to another in the medium. Another individual should now apply some force to the medium by pushing forward on the shoulders of the first person in the chain. Note that the force applied at one end of the human chain produces a disturbance or wave that travels through the chain from one person to the next until the last person is pushed forward against the wall. The people in the chain remained in place, but the disturbance was propagated from one end of the medium to the other.

Vibration consists of movement or displacement in more than one direction. Perhaps the most fundamental form of vibration is simple harmonic motion. Simple harmonic motion is illustrated by the pendulum in Figure 2.2. Note that the pendulum swings back and forth with the maximum displacement of A. The direction of displacement is indicated by the sign (+ or −) preceding the magnitude of displacement. Thus, +A represents the maximum displacement of the pendulum to the left; 0 represents the resting position; and −A represents the

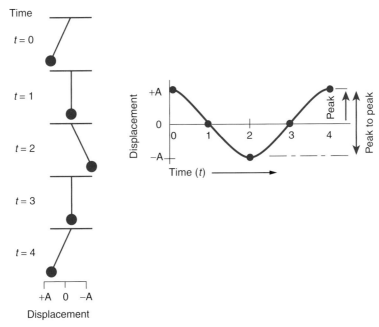

FIGURE 2.2 *Left:* Illustration of the movement of a pendulum at five instants in time, *t* = 0 through *t* = 4. *Right:* Notice that the simple back-and-forth vibration of the pendulum results in a sinusoidal waveform when displacement is plotted as a function of time.

maximum displacement to the right. An object that vibrates in this manner in air will establish a similar back-and-forth vibration pattern in the adjacent air particles; the surrounding air particles will also undergo simple harmonic motion.

The five illustrations of the pendulum on the left side of Figure 2.2 show the position or the displacement of the pendulum at five different instants in time (*t* = 0, 1, 2, 3, and 4). The plot in the right-hand portion of Figure 2.2 depicts the displacement as a function of time (*t*). Notice, for example, that, at *t* = 0, the pendulum is displaced maximally to the left, resulting in a data point (dot) at +A for *t* = 0 on the graph in the right-hand portion of Figure 2.2. Similarly, at the next instant in time, *t* = 1, the pendulum returns to the resting position, or 0 displacement. This point is also plotted as a dot in the right-hand portion of Figure 2.2. The solid line connects the displacement values produced at each moment in time. If *y* represents the displacement, then this *solid line* can be represented mathematically by the equation $y(t) = A \sin (2\pi ft + \varphi)$. The details regarding this equation are not of concern here. The term *t* in this equation refers to various instants in time. Note that displacement and time are related to one another in this equation via the sine function. As a result, simple harmonic motion is often also referred to as sinusoidal motion or **waveform**, "sine wave" for short.

Another common physical system that is used to represent simple harmonic or sinusoidal motion is a simple mass attached to an elastic spring. Such a system can be oriented horizontally or vertically. An example of a horizontally oriented mass-spring system is shown in Figure 2.3. The top panel shows the mass-spring system at rest. Next, at $t = 0$, force is applied to displace the mass to the right and to stretch the spring. When this applied force is removed, the elasticity of the spring pulls the mass toward the original resting position ($t = 1$). The inertial force associated with the moving mass, however, propels the mass beyond the resting position until it is displaced to the left of the original resting position ($t = 2$). This results in a compression of the spring. When the elastic restoring force of the spring exceeds the inertial force associated with the moving object, the motion of the object is halted and begins in the opposite direction ($t = 3$). As the moving mass reaches the original resting position, inertial forces again propel it past the resting position until it has once again been fully displaced to the right ($t = 4$). Notice that the displacement of the mass and the stretching of the spring at $t = 4$ are identical to those seen at $t = 0$. One complete cycle of back-and-forth displacement has been completed. The sinusoidal equation used previously to describe the back-and-forth motion of the pendulum can also be applied to this simple mass-spring system.

The mass-spring system, however, is often easier to relate to air particles in a medium than a pendulum system. For instance, one can think of the mass in Figure 2.3 as an air particle, with the spring representing the particle's connection to adjacent air particles. In this sense, the movement of air particles described previously in Figure 2.1 can be thought of as a series of simple mass-spring systems like the one shown in Figure 2.3.

All vibration, including sinusoidal vibration, can be described in terms of its *amplitude* (A), *frequency* (f), and *phase* (φ). This is true for both the pendulum and the mass-spring system. The primary ways of expressing the amplitude or magnitude of displacement are as follows: (a) peak amplitude, (b) peak-to-peak amplitude, and (c) root-mean-square (RMS) amplitude. RMS amplitude is an indicator of the average amplitude and facilitates comparisons of the amplitudes of different types of sound waves. The peak and peak-to-peak amplitudes are shown in the right-hand portion of Figure 2.2. Peak amplitude is the magnitude of the displacement from the resting state to the maximum amplitude. Peak-to-peak amplitude is the difference between the maximum displacement in one direction and the maximum displacement in the other direction. The amplitude of the sound can be considered to be roughly analogous to the perceptual attribute of loudness, although other characteristics of sound, including its duration, can impact loudness. In general, all else being equal between two sounds, a sound of higher amplitude is perceived as being louder than a sound of lower amplitude.

A cube (mass) attached to a spring which is attached to a wall at its other end. The mass is sliding back and forth across a surface (like a table top).

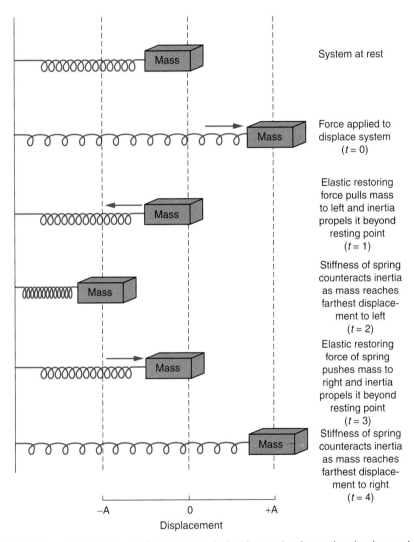

System at rest

Force applied to displace system
($t = 0$)

Elastic restoring force pulls mass to left and inertia propels it beyond resting point
($t = 1$)

Stiffness of spring counteracts inertia as mass reaches farthest displacement to left
($t = 2$)

Elastic restoring force of spring pushes mass to right and inertia propels it beyond resting point
($t = 3$)

Stiffness of spring counteracts inertia as mass reaches farthest displacement to right
($t = 4$)

−A   0   +A

Displacement

FIGURE 2.3 A simple mass-spring system in horizontal orientation is shown here to illustrate various stages of simple harmonic motion. The horizontal movement of the mass is depicted at five instants in time, $t = 0$ through $t = 4$. Notice that the simple back-and-forth vibration of this mass-spring system would result in a sinusoidal waveform of displacement as a function of time, just like the pendulum in Figure 2.2.

The period of the vibration is the time it takes for the pendulum to move from any given point and return to the same point. This describes one complete cycle of the pendulum's movement. Notice in Figure 2.2, for example, that, at $t = 4$, the pendulum has returned to the same position it occupied at $t = 0$.

The period in this case would be the difference in time between $t = 0$ and $t = 4$. For the mass-spring system in Figure 2.3, the time taken to progress from the system's state at $t = 0$ and to return to that state at $t = 4$ is the period or time required for one full cycle of displacement. If each interval in Figure 2.2 represented one-tenth of a second (0.1 s), the period would be 0.4 s. Hence, the period may be defined as the time it takes to complete one cycle of the vibration (seconds per cycle).

The frequency of vibration is the number of cycles of vibration completed in 1 second and is measured in cycles per second. Examination of the dimensions of period (seconds per cycle) and frequency (cycles per second) reflects a reciprocal relationship between these two characteristics of sinusoidal vibrations. This relationship can be expressed mathematically as $T = 1/f$ or $f = 1/T$, where T = period and f = frequency. Although the dimensions for frequency are cycles per second, a unit of measure defined as 1 cycle/s has been given the name hertz (Hz). Thus, a sinusoidal vibration that completed one full cycle of vibration in 0.04 s (i.e., $T = 0.04$ s) would have a frequency of 25 Hz ($f = 1/T = 1$ cycle/0.04 s). Although other factors contribute to the perceived pitch of sound, sound frequency can be thought to be roughly analogous to this perceptual attribute of sound. In general, sounds with higher frequencies have higher pitches, and those with lower frequencies have lower perceived pitches.

Finally, the phase (φ) of the vibration can be used to describe the starting position of the pendulum or mass (starting phase) or the phase relationship between two vibrating pendulums or masses. Two sinusoidal vibrations could be created that were identical in amplitude and frequency, but different in phase, if one vibration started with the pendulum or mass in the extreme positive position (to the left) while the other began at the extreme negative displacement (to the right). In this case, the two pendulums or masses would be moving in opposite directions. This is called a 180-degree phase relationship. The two pendulums or masses could have the same amplitude of vibration (extent of back-and-forth movement) and move back and forth at the same rate (same frequency), yet still have different patterns of vibration if they failed to have identical starting phases.

Figure 2.4 contrasts the various features used to describe sinusoidal vibration. In Figure 2.4A, the two displacement patterns shown have identical frequencies and starting phases, but the amplitude of vibration is approximately three times larger for wave X. The peak amplitude of the vibration pattern labeled X is A, whereas that of pattern Y is $0.3A$. In Figure 2.4B, on the other hand, amplitude and starting phase are equal, but the frequency of vibration for wave Y is twice as high as that for wave X. Notice, for example, that, at the instant in time labeled T in Figure 2.4B, vibration pattern X has completed one full cycle of vibration, whereas pattern Y has completed two cycles at that same

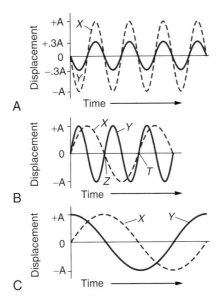

FIGURE 2.4 Sinusoidal waveforms differing only in amplitude (*A*), frequency (*B*), or starting phase (*C*).

instant. Interestingly, although these two functions start in phase (both beginning at $t = 0$ with 0 displacement), their phase relationship is very complex at other instants in time. At the point labeled *Z* in Figure 2.4B, for example, the phase relationship is 180 degrees. Thus, at the moment in time labeled *Z*, both function *X* and function *Y* are at 0 displacement, but one is moving in a positive direction and the other in a negative direction. Figure 2.4C illustrates two functions of identical amplitude and frequency that differ only in their starting phase. To fully describe sinusoidal vibration, all three parameters—amplitude, frequency, and starting phase—must be specified.

In the initial discussion of the vibration of air particles, a situation was described in which force was applied to an object, which resulted in the object itself displacing adjacent air particles. When the force was removed, the object and the air particles returned to their resting positions. This was a case of forced vibration. Before describing the features of forced vibration in more detail, its counterpart, free vibration, deserves brief mention. In free vibration, as in the case of the pendulum or the mass-spring system described above, once the vibration is started by applying force, the vibration continues without additional force being required to sustain it. For free vibration, the form of the vibration is always sinusoidal, and the frequency of oscillation for a particular object is always the same. This frequency is known as the object's natural or resonant frequency (Vignette 2.2). The amplitude, moreover, can be no larger than the initial displacement. If there is no resistance to oppose the sinusoidal

VIGNETTE 2.2 • EXPERIMENT

Conceptual Illustrations of Mass, Elasticity, and Resonance

#2

You will be conducting a small experiment that requires the following materials: a yardstick (or meter stick), tape, four wooden blocks, and heavy-duty rubber bands.

Place two of the wooden blocks so that the ends of the blocks are flush with the end of the yardstick, one block on each side of the yardstick, and secure tightly with rubber bands. Hold or clamp about 6 inches of the other end of the yardstick firmly to the top of a table. Apply a downward force to the far end of the yardstick (the end with wooden blocks) to bend it down approximately one foot. (Don't push down too hard, or the blocks may fly off of the yardstick when released.) Now release the far end of the yardstick, and count the number of complete up-and-down vibrations of the far end over a 10-s period. Repeat the measurements three times, and record the number of complete cycles of vibration during each 10-s period. This is experiment A.

Now add the other two wooden blocks to the end of the yardstick (two blocks on each side of the yardstick). Repeat the same procedure as above, and record the number of complete cycles three separate times. This is experiment B. If the number of complete cycles of vibration in each experiment is divided by 10 (for the 10-s measurement interval), the frequency (f) will be determined (in cycles per second). How has the system's natural or resonant frequency of vibration changed from experiment A to experiment B? By adding more blocks in experiment B, the mass of the system was increased. How was the system's natural or resonant frequency changed by increasing the mass of the system?

Now hold 18 inches of yardstick firmly against the table and repeat experiment B (four wooden blocks). This is experiment C. This increases the stiffness of the system. How has the resonant frequency been affected by increasing the stiffness?

The resonant frequency of an object or a medium, such as an enclosed cavity of air, is determined largely by the mass and stiffness of the object or medium. Generally, stiffness opposes low-frequency vibrations, whereas mass opposes high-frequency vibrations. In the figure for this vignette, the *solid lines* show the opposition to vibration caused by mass and stiffness. The point at which these two functions cross indicates the resonant frequency of the system. The opposition to vibration caused by either mass or stiffness is the lowest at this frequency. The vibration amplitude is greatest at the resonant frequency because the opposition to vibration is at its minimum value. The *dashed line* shows the effects of increasing the mass of the system. Note that the resonant frequency (the crossover point of the *dashed line* and the *solid line* representing the stiffness) has been shifted to a lower frequency. The frequency of vibration in experiment B (more mass) should have been lower than that of experiment A. Similarly, if stiffness is increased, then the resonant frequency increases. The frequency in experiment C should have been greater than that in experiment B.

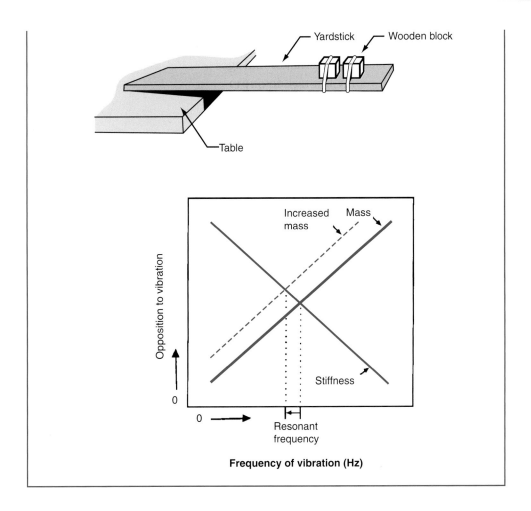

oscillation, then it will continue indefinitely. In the real world, however, this situation is never achieved. Friction opposes the vibration, which leads it to gradually decay in amplitude over time. To illustrate this, imagine that the mass depicted in the mass-spring system in Figure 2.3 is a smooth wooden cube that is sliding back and forth on a smooth glass surface. If the smooth glass surface is now replaced with a sheet of coarse sandpaper, then there will be greater friction created to oppose the back-and-forth movement of the block. The increased friction associated with the sandpaper surface will result in a quicker decay of the back-and-forth movement of the block in comparison with the original glass surface that offered much less resistance to the motion of the mass.

As illustrated in Vignette 2.2, objects with a specific mass and elasticity or stiffness will have a resonant frequency at which they prefer to vibrate. In speech communication, the vocal folds or vocal cords in the larynx represent a common example of this type of resonance in speech communication (Fig. 2.5). When air is forced through the vocal folds by the lungs, this causes them to

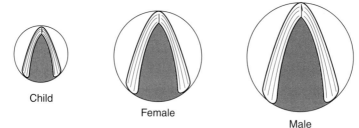

Child

Female

Male

FIGURE 2.5 The vocal folds of a typical child, adult woman, and adult man are illustrated here. Each is shown with the vocal folds open (*blue* air-filled space between them) and approximately the size of common U.S. coins (dime, nickel, and quarter, respectively). Assuming the stiffness or elasticity of each set of vocal folds is the same, one of the primary changes in the vocal folds from children to women to men is an increase in mass. As noted in Vignette 2.2, such an increase in mass will result in a decrease in resonant frequency. Thus, on average, men have lower voice fundamental frequencies than women, and women have lower fundamental frequencies than children. This largely, but not exclusively, determines the perceived pitch of the talker's voice.

vibrate at their natural frequency, which is determined by their mass and stiffness. As noted in Vignette 2.2, a system with higher mass, all else being equal between systems, will have a lower resonant frequency. The vocal folds of men, on average, have more mass than those of women, who, in turn, have vocal cords with more mass, on average, than those of children. As a result, the vocal cords typically have a lower resonant frequency in men than in women and in women than in children. It is this natural resonant frequency of the vocal folds, referred to as the fundamental frequency of the voice, that largely determines the pitch quality of voice. This is one of the primary reasons that the pitch of men's voices sounds lower than that of women's voices, which, in turn, sounds lower than that of children's voices.

This resonance involving mass and elasticity, however, is not the only type of resonance of interest in speech communication. Another type of resonance in acoustics that is of interest in speech communication is wavelength resonance. For our purposes, we will consider wavelength resonances as frequencies that are given preferential passage through air-filled tubes. Figure 2.6 illustrates a tube open at one end and closed at the other. If vibrations of various frequencies and equal amplitudes are applied to the closed end of the tube, certain frequencies will pass through this tube better than others. The frequency that passes through this tube the best is the resonant frequency of that tube. The length of the tube is the primary determiner of the wavelength resonance for such tubes. In general, the shorter the length of the tube is, the higher the resonant frequency. A common example of this in music is the overall higher pitch produced by a piccolo compared to the overall lower pitch of the trombone.

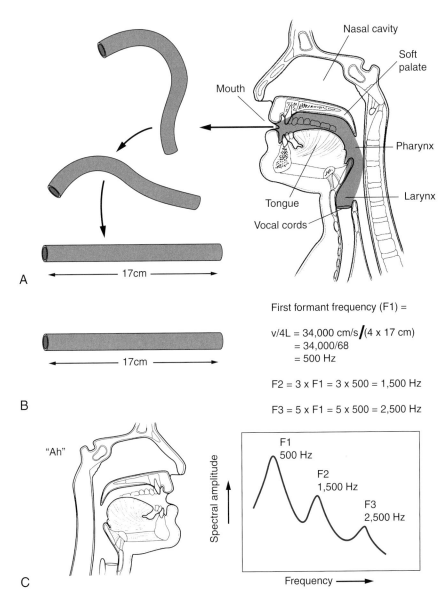

First formant frequency (F1) =

v/4L = 34,000 cm/s /(4 × 17 cm)
    = 34,000/68
    = 500 Hz

F2 = 3 × F1 = 3 × 500 = 1,500 Hz

F3 = 5 × F1 = 5 × 500 = 2,500 Hz

FIGURE 2.6 Illustration of the modeling of the human vocal tract in an average male as a 17-cm tube open at one end (lips) and closed at the other (vocal cords). *A:* Relation of 17-cm tube to actual vocal tract. *B:* Calculation of quarter-wavelength resonant frequencies associated with the first three formant frequencies of the 17-cm vocal tract. *C:* Illustration of the acoustical measurement of the formant frequencies for the average male vocal tract when producing a vowel that results in a fairly uniform vocal tract (tube) diameter throughout. This is the speech situation that is closest to the 17-cm uniform diameter tube assumed when making the calculations, and the measurements agree with the calculations.

In addition, for a given musical instrument, such as the trombone, the length of the tube can be changed by the musician such that shorter tubes have higher resonant frequencies and give rise to higher pitches than longer tubes.

Figure 2.6 illustrates how the "tube closed at one end" applies to the generation of speech sounds. Basically, the air-filled spaces from the vocal cords (closed end) to the lips (open end) can be modeled as an air-filled tube closed at one end and open at the other. When the column of air in the tube is vibrated by the vocal cords at the closed end, certain frequencies are passed through this tube better than others. This column of air between the vocal cords and lips is typically referred to as the vocal tract; the average length in adult males is 17 cm. For a tube of this length, the resonant frequency is 500 Hz, with additional secondary resonances at 1,500 and 2,500 Hz. These resonant frequencies of the vocal tract are very close to those that have been recorded for men when producing the vowel /U/ (as in "hood"). This vowel is produced with close to a uniform diameter of the vocal tract from the vocal cords to the lips and is the English vowel that is closest to the "tube closed at one end" model. Other vowels may be generated by a given talker by changing the shape or length of the vocal tract in various ways such that the resonant frequencies are changed. Additional details are beyond the scope of this text. Note, however, that children will have shorter vocal tracts, on average, than women; women, in turn, will have shorter vocal tracts, on average, than men. Thus, for a given speech sound, such as the vowel /U/, this difference in vocal tract length will also contribute to the speech of children being higher in pitch than that of women and the speech of women being higher in pitch than that of men, on average.

In summary, there are two primary types of resonance that impact the speech signal forming the link between the talker and the listener. One resonance involves the mass and stiffness of the vocal cords and is the primary determiner of the pitch quality of the speaker's voice. The other resonance is a wavelength resonance involving the length and shape of the vocal tract. These resonances provide important clues as to the identity of the specific speech sound uttered by the talker and have a secondary influence on the overall pitch of the talker's voice. Together, both types of resonances shape the sound generated by the speaker and ultimately impact the sound perceived by the listener. We will return to these speech acoustics concepts shortly, but first we must continue our discussion of general acoustics.

Now that some general features of vibration, including resonance, have been reviewed, let us return to the discussion of sound generation and propagation. Consider the following situation. The force applied to an object surrounded by air particles is sinusoidal, resulting in a sinusoidal back-and-forth displacement of the surrounding air particles. The object displaces adjacent air particles in one direction, causing a temporary buildup or increase in density of the air particles. As the object returns to the resting position because of its associated elastic restoring forces, the momentum associated with the mass of the object forces it past the resting state to its point of maximum displacement in the opposite direction. The immediately adjacent air particles attempt to fill the void left by the object, resulting in a less dense packing of air particles in this space. In doing so, the air particles surrounding the vibrating object undergo alternating periods of condensation and rarefaction. Therefore, the density of air particles is alternately increased and decreased relative to conditions at rest (no vibration). The increased concentration (density) of air particles results in an increase in air pressure according to a well-known law of physics, the ideal gas law. Thus, as the vibration propagates through the air medium, a volume of atmosphere goes through alternating periods of increased and decreased air particle density and, consequently, of high and low pressure. Waves of pressure fluctuations are created and travel through the medium.

Although the pressure variations associated with sound are small compared to normal atmospheric pressure for the air surrounding us, it is these small fluctuations in pressure that are important. The pressure fluctuations can be described using the same features discussed previously to describe changes in displacement over time. A sinusoidal driving force applied to an object vibrates the object and produces sinusoidal variations in pressure. These cyclic fluctuations in pressure can be described in terms of their amplitude, frequency, and phase. Pressure is the parameter most often used to describe sound waves because most measuring devices, such as microphones, respond to changes in sound pressure, and the ear, beginning at the eardrum, responds to changes in pressure.

The unit of sound pressure is *Pascal* (Pa). Recall that the term *hertz,* rather than *cycles per second,* is used to describe the frequency of a sound. The use of the term *hertz* for frequency and the term *pascal* for sound pressure reflects the contemporary practice of naming units of measure after notable scientists (Vignette 2.3).

Unfortunately for the student, this practice often obscures the dimensions of the quantity. Pressure, however, is force per unit area and has frequently been described in units of either newtons (N) per meter squared or dynes (d) per centimeter squared. Vignette 2.4 explains why there are two different types of units for force, dynes versus newtons, as well as the use of various prefixes in the metric system to modify these or other physical units.

Although sound pressure is the preferred quantity for depicting the amplitude of a sound wave, another commonly used quantity is acoustic intensity. *Acoustic intensity* and *sound power* are used synonymously in this book. It is possible to derive the acoustic intensity corresponding to a given sound pressure. For our purposes, however, it will suffice that acoustic intensity (I) is directly proportional to sound pressure (p) squared: $I \equiv p^2$.

VIGNETTE 2.3 • HISTORICAL NOTE

Units of Sound Named After Famous Scientists

Hertz (*A*)

The unit of frequency, the hertz (Hz), is named in honor of Heinrich Rudolph Hertz, a German physicist born in 1857 in Hamburg. Much of his career was devoted to the theoretical study of electromagnetic waves. This theoretical work led eventually to the development of radio, an area in which frequency is very important. Hertz died in 1894.

Pascal (*B*)

The unit of sound pressure, pascal (Pa), is named in honor of Blaise Pascal (1623–1662). Pascal was a French scientist and philosopher. He is well known for his contributions to both fields. As a scientist, he was both a physicist and a mathematician. In 1648, Pascal proved empirically that the mercury column in a barometer is affected by atmospheric pressure and not a vacuum, as was previously believed. Thus, his name is linked in history with research concerning the measurement of atmospheric pressure.

Newton (*C*)

The newton (N), the unit of force, is named in honor of the well-known English mathematician, physicist, and astronomer Sir Isaac Newton (1642–1727), who spent much of his career studying various aspects of force. Of his many discoveries and theories, perhaps the two best known are his investigations of gravitational forces and his three laws of motion.

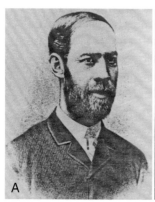
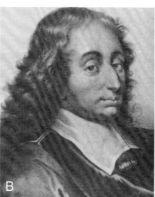
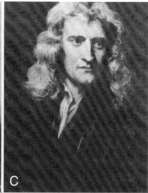

A   B   C

VIGNETTE 2.4 • FURTHER DISCUSSION

Review of Units of Measure and Metric Prefixes

As mentioned in the text, one may encounter a variety of physical units for various physical quantities. For sound pressure, for example, units of N/m^2 or $dynes/cm^2$ may both be found in various sources. Although both of these units of pressure in this example are metric, one expresses area in meters, and the other expresses area in centimeters. There are two basic measurement systems encountered in physics, the MKS system and the CGS system. The names for these two systems are derived from the units of measure within each system for the three primary physical quantities of length (meters in the MKS system and centimeters in the CGS system), mass (kilograms in the MKS system and grams in the CGS system), and time (seconds in both systems). The MKS system has been adopted as the standard international system for units of measure, so N/m^2 represents the preferred physical description of sound pressure. As noted previously, however, these physically meaningful units of force per unit area have been supplanted by units of pascals (Pa).

In the metric system, the use of standard prefixes is commonplace. It is important, for a variety of auditory processes and measures, to have a good grasp on many typically used prefixes. The table below provides a listing of many such prefixes.

Prefixes for Fractions of a Unit			Prefixes for Multiple Units		
10^{-9}	nano (n)	0.000000001	10^9	giga (G)	1,000,000,000
10^{-6}	micro (μ)	0.000001	10^6	mega (M)	1,000,000
10^{-3}	milli (m)	0.001	10^3	kilo (k)	1,000
10^{-2}	centi (c)	0.01	10^2	hecto (h)	100
10^{-1}	deci (d)	0.1	10^1	deka (da)	10

Let us suppose that a vibrating object completes two cycles of vibration when the appropriate driving force is applied. As the first condensation of air particles (or local high-pressure area) in the first cycle is created, it propagates through the medium and travels away from the source. During the second cycle of vibration, a new high-pressure area is created. By the time a second high-pressure area is completed, however, the first has traveled still farther from its point of origin. The *distance* between these two successive condensations or high-pressure areas is called the *wavelength* of the sound wave. (Recall that the *time* between successive condensations is the *period*.) If the frequency of vibration is high, the time interval between successive high-pressure areas (the period) is short, and the separation between successive high-pressure areas is small. Given a short period, the first high-pressure area is unable to travel far from the source before the second high-pressure area arises. Thus, the wavelength—the separation in distance between successive high-pressure areas—is small. The wavelength (l), frequency (f), and speed of sound (c) are related in the following manner: $l = c/f$. Wavelength varies inversely with frequency: the higher the frequency, the shorter the wavelength.

To clarify the concept of wavelength and its inverse relationship to frequency, consider once again the human chain that represented adjacent air particles. Suppose that, once a force was applied to the shoulders of the first person, it took 10 s for the disturbance (the push) to travel all the way to the end of the human chain. Let us also say that the chain had a length of 10 m. If a force was applied to the shoulders of the first person every 10 s, the frequency of vibration would be 0.1 Hz ($f = 1/T = 1/10$ s). Moreover, 10 s after the first push, the second push would be applied. Because we have stated that 10 s would be required for the disturbance to travel to the last person in the chain, when the second push is applied, the last person in the chain (10 m away) would also be pushing forward (on the wall). Thus, there would be a separation of 10 m between adjacent peaks of the disturbance or forward pushes. The wavelength (l) would be 10 m. If we double the frequency of the applied force to a value of 0.2 Hz, then the period is 5 s ($T = 1/f = 1/0.2 = 5$ s). Every 5 s, a new force will be applied to the shoulders of the first person in the chain. Because it takes 10 s for the disturbance to travel through the entire 10-m chain, after 5 s, the first disturbance will only be 5 m away as the second push is applied to the shoulders of the first person. Thus, the wavelength, or the separation between adjacent "pushes" in the medium, is 5 m. Notice that when the frequency of the applied force was doubled from 0.1 to 0.2 Hz, the wavelength was halved from 10 m to 5 m. Frequency and wavelength are inversely related. Vignette 2.5 illustrates the concepts of a wave's period and wavelength.

Another feature of sound waves that is obvious to almost anyone with normal hearing is that the sound pressure decreases in amplitude as the distance it travels increases. It would be fruitless, for example, to attempt to hail a taxicab a half block away with a soft whisper even on a quiet street. Because the amplitude of sound decays with increasing distance, it would probably require high vocal effort to generate enough sound amplitude at the source to be audible to the cab driver a half block away. One would have to yell "Taxi!" rather than whisper it.

Under special measurement conditions, in which sound waves are not reflected from surrounding surfaces and the sound source is a special source, known as a *point source*, the decrease in sound pressure with distance is well defined. Specifically, as the distance from the sound source is doubled, the sound pressure is halved. Similarly, because of the relationship between sound pressure and acoustic intensity described previously ($I \equiv p^2$), the same doubling of distance would reduce the acoustic intensity to one-quarter (or $[1/2]^2$) the initial value. This well-defined dependence of sound pressure and sound intensity on distance is known as the *inverse square law*.

So far, we have considered some of the characteristics or features of a single sound wave originating from one source. Moreover, we have assumed that the sound wave was propagating through a special environment in which the wave is not reflected from surrounding surfaces. This type of environment, one without reflected sound waves, is known as a *free field*. A diffuse field is the complement of a free field. In a diffuse field, sound is reflected from many surfaces. The inverse square law that was just described holds true only for free-field conditions. In fact, in a diffuse field, sound pressure is distributed equally throughout the measurement area, so that no matter how far we go from the sound source

VIGNETTE 2.5 • CONCEPTUAL DEMO

Illustration of the Period and Wavelength of a Wave

The figure below illustrates a giant wave pool, large enough to create waves for surfing. Waves in a wave pool are generated by displacing a wall at one end of the pool in a sinusoidal back-and-forth motion. The wave, once generated by the wall's displacement, travels through the water filling the wave pool. In the two *top* panels, the wall is moved back and forth at a higher frequency than in the two *lower* panels. In the *left*-hand panels, the surfers are sitting on their surf boards waiting to catch the crest of a wave. As they wait, they bob up and down in the water. When surfer A bobs up, we press a stopwatch and stop it when that same surfer bobs up again. This corresponds to the period of this wave. Which wave do you think has a shorter period? Since the wave in the top left panel has more waves or cycles per second (higher frequency), it has a shorter period, or fewer seconds per cycle (or wave).

In the *right*-hand panels, the three surfers each caught the crest of a successive wave and are riding it toward the far end of the wave pool. If we measured the distance between successive crests in the waves or, in this case, the distance between surfers riding those crests, we would find it to be a shorter distance in the *top right* panel than in the *lower left* panel. This separation of wave crests over distance corresponds to the wavelength for this wave. The higher the frequency, the closer the spacing of the wave crests over distance or the shorter the wavelength.

This analogy illustrates that the period can be considered to be the time separation of successive peaks of the sinusoidal waveform in seconds, whereas the wavelength is the length separation of successive peaks of the wave in meters. In both cases, the period and the wavelength are inversely related to the frequency of vibration. High frequencies yield short periods and short wavelengths, whereas low frequencies result in long periods and long wavelengths.

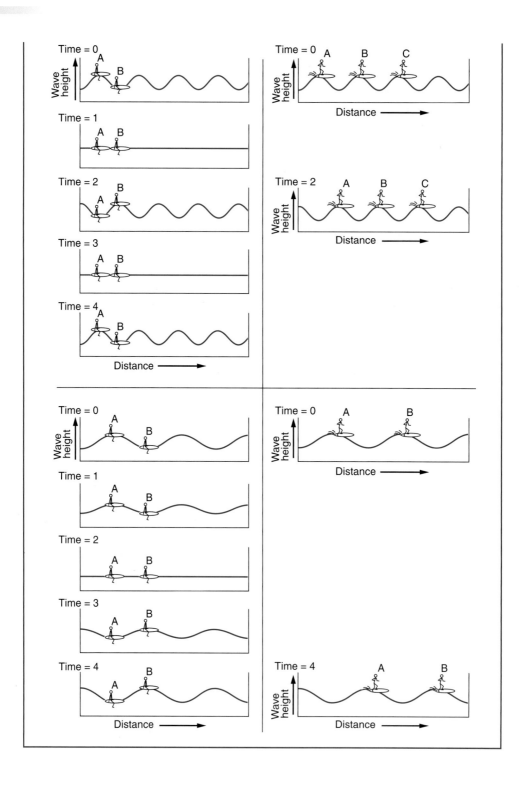

or where we are in the measurement area, the sound pressure is the same. Typical classrooms are environments that lie somewhere between a free field and a diffuse field, probably closer to the latter in most cases. The term *sound field* is sometimes used to describe a region containing sound waves. Free fields and diffuse fields, then, are special classes of sound fields.

Interference results when multiple sound waves encounter one another. Here, we will consider only the simplest case of interaction: *two* sound waves. The two sound waves may be two independent waves arising from separate sources (e.g., two loudspeakers or two people talking) or the original wave (usually called the incident sound wave) and its reflection off a wall, ceiling, floor, or other surface. The interference that results when two sound waves encounter one another may be either constructive or destructive. In constructive interference, the two sound waves combine to yield a sound wave that is greater in amplitude than either wave alone. This is illustrated in the left-hand portion of Figure 2.7. In the case shown here, in which the waves are of equal amplitude, the maximum possible constructive interference would be a doubling of amplitude. Negative interference occurs whenever the amplitude of the sound wave resulting from the interaction is less than the amplitude of either wave alone. The extreme case of negative interference results in the complete cancellation of the sound waves, as illustrated in the right-hand portion of Figure 2.7.

In addition to the interference that results when two sound waves interact, other interference effects result when a sound wave encounters an object or structure of some kind. When a sound wave encounters an object, the outcome of this encounter is determined in large part by the dimensions and composition of the object and the wavelength of the sound. When the dimensions of the object are large relative to the wavelength of the sound wave, a sound shadow is produced. This is analogous to the more familiar light shadow, in which an object in the path of light casts a shadow behind it. In the case of a sound shadow, the object creates an area without sound, or a dead area, immediately behind it, but not all objects cast sound shadows for all sound waves. The creation of a sound shadow depends on the dimensions of the object and the wavelength of the sound. For example, a cube having the dimensions 1 m × 1 m × 1 m will not cast a shadow for sound waves having a wavelength that is much larger than 1 m. Recall that wavelength and frequency vary inversely. In this example, a sound wave having a wavelength of 1 m has a frequency of 330 Hz ($f = c/l$; $c = 330$ m/s; $l = 1$ m/cycle). Thus, the object in this example would cast a sound shadow for frequencies greater than 330 Hz ($l < $ m) (Vignette 2.6).

Finally, consider what happens when a sound wave encounters a barrier of some type. First, let us discuss the case in which a hole is present in the barrier. In this case, as was the case for the sound shadow, the results depend on the wavelength (and therefore frequency) of the incident sound wave and the

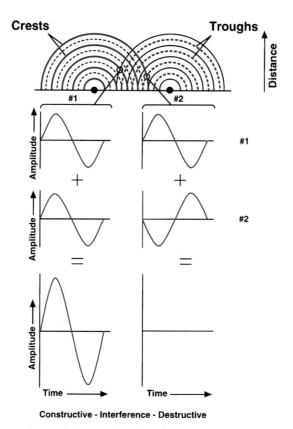

FIGURE 2.7 Constructive and destructive interference of two sound waves (#1 and #2). The origin of each wave is represented by the *black circles* in the *upper* portion of the figure. The graph at the *lower left* illustrates the combination of waves #1 and #2 when the crests coincide. The two waves are in phase at this point, and the resulting sound wave is greater than either wave alone. This is constructive interference. The graph at the lower right illustrates the combination of the crest of wave #1 and the trough of wave #2. The two waves are 180 degrees out of phase, resulting in complete cancellation of the two waves. This is destructive interference. (Adapted from Durrant JD, Lovrinic JH. *Bases of Hearing Science*. 2nd ed. Baltimore, MD: Williams & Wilkins; 1984:41.)

dimensions of the hole. For wavelengths much greater than the dimensions of the hole, the sound wave becomes diffracted. Diffraction is a change in direction of the sound wave. Thus, under these conditions, the direction of the incident sound wave can be altered.

Next, consider what happens if the sound wave encounters a barrier that contains no holes. In this case, varying degrees of sound transmission, absorption, or reflection can occur. The proportion of the sound wave's energy reflected by the barrier and the proportion transmitted through the barrier depend on the similarity of the barrier's and the medium's impedance. Impedance may

VIGNETTE 2.6 • FURTHER DISCUSSION

Sound Shadow Created by the Head

Sound shadow occurs whenever the dimensions of the object encountered by the sound wave are larger than the wavelength of the sound. Wavelength is inversely related to frequency, such that low frequencies have long wavelengths and high frequencies have short wavelengths. Consider the three frequencies 100, 1,000, and 10,000 Hz. The corresponding wavelengths, calculated as described in the text, are 3.3, 0.33, and 0.033 m, respectively.

The human head can be grossly approximated by a sphere (or a cube for blockheads) with a diameter of approximately 0.23 m (roughly 9 inches). Therefore, when the head (preferably accompanied by the body) is placed in a sound field, it is capable of producing a sound shadow for wavelengths shorter than 0.23 m. Using the three frequencies from the preceding paragraph, the average human head would create a sound shadow for 10,000 Hz, would possibly produce one at 1,000 Hz, and definitely would not produce one at 100 Hz, where the wavelength is several times greater than the diameter of the head.

The figure for this vignette illustrates how this so-called head shadow effect can be measured. In panel (A), two microphones spaced approximately 9 inches apart are positioned in a free field (a sound field without any reflections) with a loudspeaker to the *right* of the microphones at a distance of a few meters. The loudspeaker presents a pure tone of 100 Hz, and its sound level is measured at both microphones. This is repeated for pure tones of 1,000 and 10,000 Hz. All three pure tones are presented at equal levels. Because the left microphone is farther from the sound source than the right microphone, the sound level is a little lower at the left microphone, consistent with the inverse square law described in the text. The difference for these closely spaced microphones is small enough, however, that we can ignore it here and pretend that the sound levels are identical at both the left and right microphones.

Part (B) of this figure shows a head with a diameter of approximately 9 inches (0.23 m) between the two microphones. When we repeat the measurements at 100, 1,000, and 10,000 Hz, there is little change in sound level from panel (A) for 100 Hz and only a slight decrease in level at the left microphone for 1,000 Hz. At 10,000 Hz, however, the sound pressure has been reduced at the left microphone to a value that is only one-tenth of what it was in panel (A). In terms of sound level in decibels (described later in the text of this chapter), the sound level has been decreased at the left microphone by approximately 20 dB with the head present for the 10,000-Hz signal. The head is blocking the 10,000-Hz sound wave from reaching the left microphone. The 10,000-Hz sound would be perceived as being much louder at the ear nearest to the loudspeaker and softer at the ear farthest from the sound source.

This difference in sound level at the two ears that results from head shadow is a very strong cue for the location of a sound in the horizontal plane. The sound is generally assumed to come from the side that has the higher sound level. Given the dimensions of the human head and the wavelength of sound in air for various frequencies, the sound level difference between the two ears helps locate sounds with frequencies above 1,000 Hz. Below 1,000 Hz, the size of the head does not create a sound shadow, or difference in sound level, at the two ears. Cues other than the sound-level difference between the two ears are needed to locate low-frequency sounds (discussed in Chapter 3).

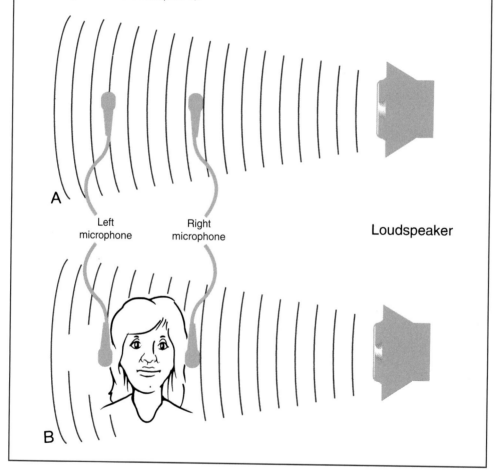

be thought of very generally as opposition to the flow of energy, in this case the advancement of the sound wave through the barrier. If the barrier and the medium have the same impedance, 100% of the energy of the sound wave will be transmitted through the barrier. If the difference in impedances, often referred to as the impedance mismatch, is large, most of the incident sound wave will be reflected, and little will be transmitted across the barrier (Vignette 2.7).

VIGNETTE 2.7 • CONCEPTUAL DEMO

Discussion of Impedance Mismatch between Air and Water

Consider the following situation. You and a friend are out on a boat in the ocean, scuba diving. Your friend is already underwater, and you want to talk to him. He's only a few feet below the surface, yet despite your yelling, he does not respond. Why not? The sound waves carrying your voice are traveling through an air medium. When the sound waves encounter the surface of the water, a change in impedance is encountered. The impedance of ocean water is a few thousand times greater than that of air. As a consequence, only approximately 0.1% of the sound energy will be transmitted beneath the surface of the water to your friend.

Approximately 99.9% of the airborne sound wave is reflected off the surface. Thus, the impedance mismatch between the air and ocean water results in almost all of the airborne sound energy being reflected away from the surface.

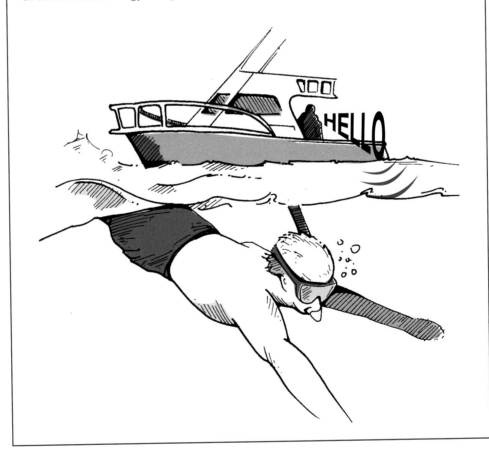

Aside from being reflected or transmitted, a portion of the sound wave may also be absorbed by the barrier. In the absorption of sound energy, the acoustic energy of the impinging sound wave is changed to heat. The materials out of which the barrier is constructed determine its ability to absorb sound.

More on the Concepts of Impedance, Admittance, and Resonance

In our discussion of the vibration and displacement of objects—whether the object was a pendulum, a mass-spring system, or an air particle—mass, elasticity, and resistance (friction) have been identified repeatedly as critical factors affecting the vibration. The mass-spring system described in Figure 2.3 probably best illustrated the interplay between mass, elasticity, and resistance in the back-and-forth sinusoidal vibration of a mass. This was also illustrated in Vignette 2.2, in which a simple vibrating system is constructed from a yardstick and a cup of marbles.

Systems having mass, elasticity, and resistance can be forced to vibrate in response to applied forces of various frequencies. The frequency at which the system vibrates maximally for equal applied force is the resonant frequency of the system. The resonant frequency and the amplitude of vibration at that frequency are both determined by the impedance of the system. Impedance is the net opposition to vibration resulting from the mass, elasticity, and resistance of the system. Admittance is the reciprocal of impedance: it indicates how easily energy is admitted through a system rather than impeded by it.

Inertia is a force of opposition associated with an object having mass and one that opposes acceleration of the object (speeding up or slowing down its movement). Elastic restoring forces are associated with a system's elasticity, and they oppose the displacement of the object. When a spring is stretched, for example, its elastic restoring force opposes that displacement and attempts to restore it to its original (resting) position. Finally, friction is a form of resistance that opposes the velocity or speed at which an object is moving. The faster an object is moving, the greater the opposition to that movement as a result of friction. Frictional forces usually oppose the movement of an object by converting the kinetic energy associated with the moving object to heat. Rubbing the palms of your hands together, for example, will be opposed by frictional forces and will generate heat. The faster you rub them together, the greater the opposition caused by friction and the greater the heat generated. Again, the net sum of the inertial, elastic, and frictional forces of opposition to motion is impedance. The higher the impedance, the greater the opposition to movement or vibration of the object, and the less the object moves or vibrates.

As noted in Vignette 2.2, the opposition to vibration associated with a system's mass increases with increase in frequency, whereas the opposition associated with a system's elasticity or stiffness decreases with increases in frequency. The opposition associated with a system's mass is referred to as mass reactance (Xm), whereas that caused by a system's elasticity is referred to as elastic reactance (Xe). Frictional forces, referred to as resistance (R), do not vary with frequency; they are frequency independent. For a system with mass M, the mass reactance can be calculated from the following equation: $Xm = 2\pi fM$. For a given mass, the forces of opposition associated with that mass increase with increase in frequency, f. In addition, the greater the mass of an object, the greater the opposition to movement or vibration. For a system with elasticity E, the elastic reactance associated with that system can be calculated from this equation: $Xe = 1/(2\pi fE)$. For a given E, the opposition caused by elasticity decreases as frequency (f) increases. In addition, as elasticity increases (and stiffness decreases), the opposition caused by elasticity decreases.

Impedance, the combination of Xm, Xe, and R, is usually symbolized as Z. Impedance is a complex vector quantity, as are Xm, Xe, and R. This simply means that it is a quantity with both magnitude and direction. Wind velocity is an everyday example of a vector quantity, a quantity in which both magnitude and direction are important. For example, a weather report might cite the wind at 25 miles per hour (mph) out of the southwest, rather than simply indicating its magnitude only (25 mph). Although impedance and its constituents are vector quantities with both magnitude and direction, we will focus here on the magnitude only. The magnitude of the impedance, Z, is calculated as follows: $Z = [R^2 + (Xm - Xe)^2]^{0.5}$. That is, the size of the impedance, Z, is equal to the square root of the sum of the resistance (R) squared and the net reactance (Xm – Xe) squared. Increases in R, Xm, or Xe result in increases in the magnitude or size of the impedance. The greater the impedance or net opposition to vibration, the lesser the amount of vibration or movement.

There exists some frequency, known as the resonant frequency, for which the impedance is at a minimum. Recall that Xm varies directly with frequency, whereas Xe varies inversely with frequency. As frequency increases upward from 0 Hz, Xm is increasing and Xe is decreasing. (The resistance, R, does not vary with frequency and remains constant.) At some frequency, Xe will equal Xm. At this frequency, the net reactance (Xm – Xe) will equal 0. According to the equation for impedance (Z), impedance will then be equal to the square root of R^2. In other words, at the resonant frequency, the opposing forces associated with the system's mass and elasticity cancel each other, and all that remains to oppose the vibration is the resistance. At resonance, $Z = R$. This is the smallest amount of opposition to vibration possible, so the system will vibrate maximally at this frequency. At frequencies other than the resonant frequency, Xm will not cancel Xe, and the impedance will be greater than that at resonance.

At resonance, how much and how long the object or system vibrates will be determined solely by R.

The reciprocal of impedance (Z) is admittance (Y). Just as impedance represented the net sum of resistance and reactance (X), admittance represents the net sum of conductance (G) and susceptance (B). Just as with reactance, a susceptance term is associated with the system's mass (Bm) and another associated with the system's elasticity (Be). Similarly, the formula for the calculation of admittance is as follows: $Y = [G^2 + (Bm - Be)^2]^{0.5}$. In general, as impedance increases, admittance decreases and vice versa. So at the resonant frequency, Z is minimum and Y is maximum. Admittance and impedance are alternative but equivalent ways of describing the flow of energy through a system. Impedance summarizes the overall opposition to vibration, whereas admittance reflects the ease with which the system is set into vibration. It's akin to having the option to describe a 12-oz glass filled with 6 oz of water as being either half full or half empty. Either description is accurate.

Although admittance-based and impedance-based descriptions of a system are equally appropriate, clinical measurement of the impedance or admittance of the middle ear system (see Chapter 7) has evolved from an initial favoring of impedance terminology to more recent consensus for admittance measures and terminology. The choice is not because one is more accurate or better than the other; it has to do with the ease with which one can be measured validly with the equipment available in the clinic.

Finally, the impedance and admittance concepts described here are for mechanical systems, although these concepts have been applied to numerous types of systems, including electrical and purely acoustical systems. Although the details change from one type of system to another, the concepts remain the same. Table 2.1 illustrates some of the parallels among mechanical, acoustical, and electrical impedance.

TABLE

2.1

Terms for Equivalent Components of Impedance (Z) for Mechanical, Electrical, and Acoustical Systems

Mechanical	Electrical	Acoustical
Mass reactance (Xm)	Inductive reactance (Xi)	Inertance (Xm)
Elastic reactance (Xe)	Capacitive reactance (Xc)	Elastic reactance (Xe)
Resistance (R)	Resistance (R)	Resistance (R)
Impedance (Zm)	Impedance (Ze)	Impedance (Za)
$Zm = [R^2 + (Xm - Xe)^2]^{0.5}$	$Ze = [R^2 + (Xi - Xc)^2]^{0.5}$	$Za = [R^2 + (Xm - Xe)^2]^{0.5}$

ANOTHER WAY TO LOOK AT SOUND WAVES: THE FREQUENCY DOMAIN

Many of the important features of a sound wave—such as its amplitude, frequency, and phase—can be summarized in either of two common formats. One format, the waveform, describes the acoustic signal in terms of amplitude variations as a function of time. The sinusoidal waveform described previously for simple harmonic motion is an example of a waveform or time-domain representation of an acoustic signal. The term "time domain" simply reflects the fact that variations in time are shown along the x-axis in a plot of the waveform. For every waveform, there is an associated representation of that signal in the frequency domain, called the amplitude and phase spectrum. Here, "frequency domain" simply means that frequency is shown along the x-axis in this representation of sound. Figure 2.8A illustrates the amplitude and phase spectrum for a simple sinusoidal waveform. Note that the x-axis of the spectrum is frequency, whereas the y-axis is either amplitude or phase. The amplitude scale

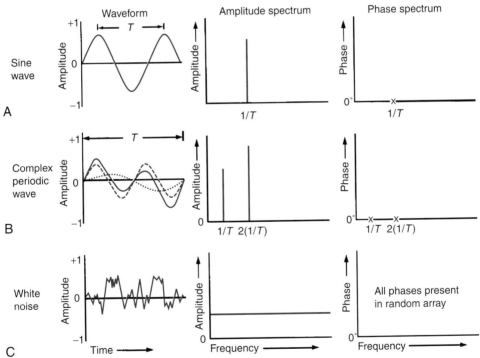

FIGURE 2.8 Illustration of the waveforms and corresponding amplitude and phase spectra for a continuous sine wave (A), a complex periodic wave (B), and white noise (C). All waveforms are assumed to be continuous, with only a brief snapshot of the waveform depicted here. In (B), the *solid line* is complex waveform; *dashed* and *dotted lines* are the two sine waves making up the complex sound.

can be peak-to-peak amplitude, peak amplitude, or RMS amplitude, as noted previously. The phase spectrum, in this case, illustrates the starting phase of the acoustic signal. There can only be one possible waveform associated with the amplitude and phase spectrum shown in the right-hand side of Figure 2.8A. Similarly, there is only one set of amplitude and phase spectra associated with the waveform in the left-hand side of Figure 2.8A. Thus, both the time-domain and frequency-domain representation of the acoustic stimulus uniquely summarize its features. Furthermore, knowing one, we can derive the other. For every waveform, there is only one amplitude spectrum and phase spectrum associated with it. For every amplitude and phase spectrum, there is only one possible waveform. Vignette 2.8 uses an analogy to reinforce the notion that the waveform and the spectrum are just two different ways of looking at any given sound. On some occasions, it is the frequency content of a sound that we wish to focus on, and the frequency domain provides an immediate indication of the frequencies comprising a sound, as well as their relative amplitudes and phases. On other occasions, it is the variations in amplitude over time that are of primary interest, and examining sound in the time domain is most appropriate.

4 tones

Simple sinusoidal sounds are more the exception than the rule in everyday encounters with sound. Although sine waves have all of their amplitude at one and only one frequency, most everyday sounds have amplitude at more than one frequency. Fortunately, well over a century ago, a mathematician named Fourier determined that all complex periodic sounds consisted of a sum of simple sinusoids. A periodic sound is one in which the waveform repeats itself every T seconds. In the left-hand portion of Figure 2.8B, a complex periodic waveform is illustrated by the solid line. The dashed and dotted waveforms illustrate the two sinusoidal signals that, when added together, yield the complex sound. The spectrum of the complex sound can be represented by the sum of the spectra of both sinusoidal components, as illustrated in the right-hand portion of Figure 2.8B. Complex periodic sounds, such as that shown in Figure 2.8B, have a special type of amplitude spectrum known as line spectra. The amplitude spectrum consists of a series of discrete vertical lines located at various frequencies and having specified amplitudes. Each line represents a separate sinusoidal component of the complex sound. The component having the lowest frequency is called the *fundamental frequency*. The fundamental frequency corresponds to $1/T$, where T is the period of the complex sound. Additional components, located at frequencies corresponding to integer multiples of the fundamental frequency, are referred to as *harmonics* of the fundamental. If the fundamental frequency is 200 Hz, for example, then the second and third harmonics of 200 Hz are 400 Hz (2×200 Hz) and 600 Hz (3×200 Hz), respectively. The first harmonic corresponds to the fundamental frequency. Additionally, the term *octave* means a doubling of frequency. Continuing the same example, 400 Hz

4 tones added

VIGNETTE 2.8 • CONCEPTUAL DEMO

Time-Domain and Frequency-Domain Representations of Sound: An Analogy Using Maps

As noted in the text, sound can be represented completely and equivalently in two different fashions: the time domain, or waveform, and the frequency domain, or spectrum. It is important to realize that these displays of sound just offer two different "pictures" of the same sound. By analogy, consider the piece of the Earth known as the state of Indiana in the United States. As shown in this figure, there are many ways one could display the features of this piece of property. The map on the *left* (A) is a road map for Indiana. The map in the *middle* (B) depicts the average annual rainfall in the state, and the one on the *right* (C) illustrates the relative elevation of various portions of the land within the state. Each map serves a specific purpose and function, but all three represent information about *the same* piece of the Earth, Indiana. If the reader wanted to know the best route to take from Indianapolis, Indiana to Fort Wayne, Indiana, for example, the road map would be the map of choice. The road map, however, conveys no information about annual rainfall or topography. If this information is of interest to the reader, then the other maps would need to be consulted. This is similar to the choices available for the analysis and display of sound. If the moment-to-moment variations in the amplitude of a sound are of interest, the waveform is the most appropriate representation. Likewise, if the frequency content of the sound is of interest, then the amplitude and phase spectra would be the most appropriate displays. In either case, the sound would be the same, but the "picture" of that sound could be displayed in either the time-domain or frequency-domain format.

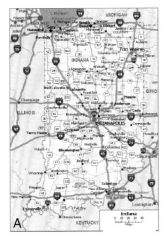
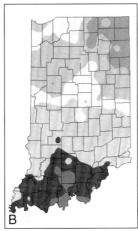
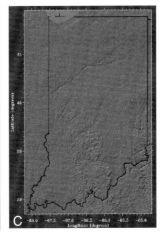

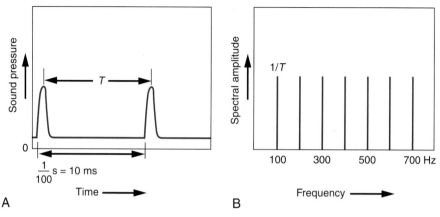

FIGURE 2.9 The waveform (*A*) and amplitude spectrum (*B*) of a series of glottal pulses measured (hypothetically) just above the vocal cords during voicing. Every time the vocal cords burst open from the air pressure generated by the lungs, the sound pressure increases rapidly and then decreases rapidly when the vocal cords close, as illustrated by the waveform in (*A*). The pulse repeats itself every 0.01 s. The corresponding amplitude spectrum (*B*) shows a series of vertical lines, beginning with the fundamental frequency [$1/T$ = 1/(0.01 s/cycle) = 100 Hz] and including all harmonics (integer multiples) of the fundamental frequency (200, 300, 400 Hz,…) at equal amplitude. It is this complex periodic sound generated by the vocal cords for voiced speech sounds, such as vowels, that is subsequently shaped by the resonances of the vocal tract. The fundamental frequency, in this case, 100 Hz, is the primary determiner of the pitch of the talker's voice.

would be 1 octave above the fundamental frequency (200 Hz), whereas 800 Hz would be 2 octaves (another doubling) above the fundamental frequency.

Figure 2.9 shows the waveform (left) and spectrum (right) for a hypothetical sound wave recorded by a microphone positioned just above the vocal cords. Notice that the waveform is essentially periodic (referred to as *quasi-periodic*, because there are typically minor cycle-to-cycle variations), but more complex than a simple sine wave. The period of this waveform (*T*) is 10 ms or 0.01 s. This informs us that the lowest frequency in this sound, the fundamental frequency, is 100 Hz (1/0.01 s), and this is most likely the voice of a man. However, what other frequencies are in the waveform in the left-hand portion of Figure 2.9? It is not easy to tell by looking at it. The corresponding representation of this sound in the frequency domain, however (shown in the right-hand panel of Fig. 2.9), immediately reveals the frequencies that are in this sound and their relative amplitudes. Note that each frequency in this periodic sound is represented by a vertical line with the horizontal location on the *x*-axis indicating its frequency, and the vertical height of each line represents the amplitude at that frequency. For simplicity, we have omitted the display of phase information at each frequency (i.e., the phase spectrum), but it should be remembered that, without this information, it would not be possible to go back and forth between the time-domain and frequency-domain versions of the sound. Also note that individual lines are positioned at the harmonics of the fundamental frequency. This particular sound has energy at all of the harmonics above the fundamental frequency (100, 200, 300, 400 Hz,...), but this is not always the case for complex waveforms. The key point illustrated in Figure 2.9 is that, although the waveform (left panel) and amplitude spectrum (right panel) provide equivalent depictions of sound, if the frequency content is the sound characteristic of interest, the amplitude spectrum provides an immediate illustration of this characteristic.

Figure 2.10 shows some additional waveforms and amplitude spectra for periodic vowel sounds. The left-hand panels depict various speech waveforms for individual vowels, and the right-hand panels show the corresponding amplitude spectra for a brief sample of the vowel sound at one instant in time. In the top two pairs of panels (A and B), notice that the period (T) of the waveform is longer in the top panel and shorter in the middle panel. As a result, the talker's voice is considerably higher in pitch for the middle panel than the top panel. This is also illustrated by the vertical lines in the corresponding amplitude spectra on the right. Notice that the first (lowest frequency) vertical component is lower in the top panel than in the middle panel. The fundamental frequency is 100 Hz for the top panel and 300 Hz for the middle panel. This also results in the other vertical lines in the amplitude spectrum at higher harmonics being more widely spaced in the middle panel than in the top panel. Notice, however, that the resonant peaks or the formant frequencies (F1 to F3) for this speech sound are identical. These formant frequencies correspond to those in the vowel /a/. Thus, based on the pattern of formant peaks in the amplitude spectra on the right, it is apparent that the same speech sound, /a/, is being spoken by two different voices or talkers, most likely a male adult (fundamental frequency = 100 Hz) and a young child (fundamental frequency = 300 Hz).

The bottom pair of panels in Figure 2.10 depicts the waveform and corresponding amplitude spectrum for another sample of speech. How do these compare to the pairs in the middle and top panels of Figure 2.10? Regarding the waveforms on the left, the period (T) is the same as that in the top panel. Therefore, the fundamental frequency and pitch of the voice are the same in the top and bottom panels. This is also revealed in the narrow spacing of the vertical lines in the amplitude spectrum on the right. Note, however, that the pattern of formant frequencies and amplitudes (F1 to F3) differs between the top and bottom amplitude spectra. The bottom panel represents the vowel /U/ (as in "hood") spoken by the same talker producing the vowel /a/ ("ah") in the top panel of this figure. Thus, the fundamental frequency ($1/T$) is a primary cue for the pitch of the talker's voice, and the formant frequencies

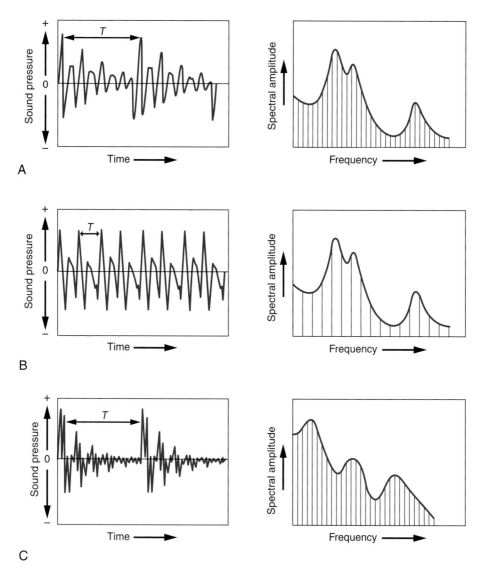

FIGURE 2.10 Illustrations of the differences between fundamental frequency and formant frequency. *The left-*hand panels show the waveforms for various speech sounds, and the *right-*hand panels illustrate the corresponding amplitude spectra at one moment in time. (Adapted from Denes PB, Pinson EN. *The Speech Chain.* **New York: WH Freeman; 1993.)**

(F1 to F3) are primary cues for the identity of the vowel that has been spoken. When the shape of the vocal tract is changed to produce different vowels by the talker, the corresponding change in the location and amplitude of the formant frequencies provides acoustic cues to the listener regarding the vowel's identity.

Vowel sounds are periodic, but many acoustic signals in our environment are not periodic. Noise is probably the most common example. Noise is said to be an aperiodic signal, because it fails to repeat itself at regular intervals. Rather, the waveform for noise shows amplitude varying randomly over time. This is illustrated in the left-hand portion of Figure 2.8C. The case shown here is an example of a special type of noise called *white noise*. White noise is characterized by an average amplitude spectrum that has uniform amplitude across frequency; in other words, there is equal sound energy at all frequencies. (White noise derives its name from white light—light that is composed of all wavelengths of light at equal amplitudes.) This is depicted in the right-hand portion of Figure 2.8C. Note that the amplitude spectrum no longer consists of a series of lines. Rather, a continuous function is drawn that reflects equal amplitude at all frequencies. Aperiodic waveforms, such as noise, have continuous amplitude spectra, not discrete line spectra.

White noise

Speech sounds are also often comprised of noises. For example, the "f" and "sh" sounds in the word *fish* are basically noises that are generated by passing air from the lungs through constrictions in the vocal tract. For the "f" sound, the constriction is made at the end of the vocal tract by placing the upper front teeth in contact with the lower lip, whereas the constriction for the "sh" sound is made by arching the tongue, so that it is in close proximity to the roof of the mouth. Again, the details of speech production are beyond the scope of this text. Suffice it to say that some speech sounds in English are basically aperiodic noises generated by forcing air from the lungs through constrictions in various locations along the vocal tract. In this case, the vocal cords are not required to vibrate to generate the speech sound, as was true when discussing the production of vowel sounds like "ah." It is also possible for some speech sounds, such as the "v" sound in the word *vat*, that both the vocal cords are vibrated, and turbulence is generated as the vibrated air passes through a constriction in the vocal tract.

As previously indicated, it is possible to represent an acoustic signal in both the frequency domain and the time domain. So far in our discussion of waveforms and spectra, we have assumed that the acoustic signals are continuous (≥1 s). Often, however, this is not the case. As a general rule, the shorter the duration of the signal, the broader the amplitude spectrum. Thus, a 1,000-Hz pure tone that is turned on and then turned off 0.1 s later will have sound energy at several frequencies other than 1,000 Hz. Approximately 90% of the sound energy will fall between 990 and 1,010 Hz. If the duration of the pure tone is decreased further to 0.01 s, then 90% of the sound energy will be distributed from 900 through 1,100 Hz. Hence, as the duration decreases, the spread of sound energy to other frequencies increases. The limit to the decrease in duration is an infinitely short pulse or click-like sound. For this hypothetical sound, energy would spread equally to all frequencies.

Such short-duration sounds, or transients, are increasingly common in clinical audiology, typically consisting of either brief bursts of a pure tone or clicks. As noted, as the duration of a sound decreases, its amplitude spectrum becomes broader. Because of the increasingly common use of transient acoustic signals in audiology, this tradeoff in the time and frequency domains is examined in more detail here.

Figure 2.11A illustrates the waveform and amplitude spectrum for a continuous pure tone with a peak amplitude of A, starting phase of $0°$, and a

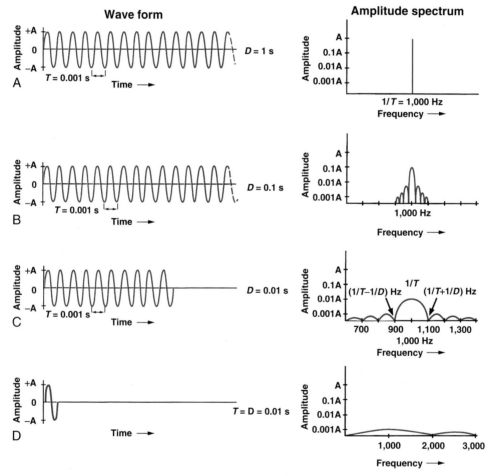

FIGURE 2.11 Trading relation between representations of an acoustic stimulus in the time and frequency domains. The *left* column shows the waveforms for a 1,000-Hz pure tone of various durations; the *right* column depicts the corresponding amplitude spectra. Duration of the 1,000-Hz tone is infinite (continuous) in (*A*), 0.1 s in (*B*), 0.01 s in (*C*), and 0.001 s in (*D*). As the duration decreases from *A* to *D*, the amplitude spectrum becomes flatter and broader.

frequency of 1,000 Hz. In principle, a continuous signal is one that is infinitely long. For practical purposes, however, acoustic signals having a duration, D, of 1 s or longer will be considered continuous. The 1,000-Hz waveform in this panel has a period, T, of 0.001 s, or 1 ms. The amplitude spectrum–plotting peak amplitude as a function of frequency therefore consists of a line with amplitude A at 1,000 Hz ($f = 1/T$).

In Figure 2.11B, the 1,000-Hz pure tone has been abruptly turned on and off for a total duration, D, of 0.1 s, or 100 ms. It is no longer considered a continuous periodic sound. Rather, it is a transient sound, one that occurs only once and for a duration of less than 1 s. Because it is an aperiodic transient sound, its corresponding amplitude spectrum no longer consists of lines, but is a continuous function of frequency. The spectrum of this 100-ms, 1,000-Hz tone burst has several key features, as shown in the right-hand portion of Figure 2.11B. First, the spectrum is broader than it was for the continuous 1,000-Hz pure tone shown in the top panel (Fig. 2.11A). Acoustic energy is present at frequencies other than 1,000 Hz for the tone burst, whereas this was not the case for the continuous pure tone. Second, although the peak in the amplitude spectrum is still at 1,000 Hz, the amplitude at that frequency has been decreased. In fact, the amplitude is now equal to the peak amplitude of the waveform (A) multiplied by the duration of the signal (D) in seconds (0.1), or 0.1 A. Reduction in the energy present at 1,000 Hz, however, is accompanied by a broader distribution of that energy across other frequencies, as noted earlier. Finally, the amplitude spectrum has several points at which the amplitude is 0, and these zero-amplitude regions occur at regular intervals above and below 1,000 Hz.

These points of zero amplitude are called nodes in the amplitude spectrum. They occur at frequencies above and below the pure-tone frequency and can be determined according to the following formula: n (1/D) and $-n$ (1/D), where n is 1, 2, 3, and so on. In the example shown in Figure 2.11B, D = 0.1 s; therefore, 1/D = 10 Hz. The nodes or points of zero amplitude occur at 1,000 + 10 Hz, 1,000 – 10 Hz, 1,000 + 20 Hz, 1,000 – 20 Hz, 1,000 + 30 Hz, 1,000 – 30 Hz, and so on, as shown in Figure 2.11B. The frequency region between the first positive node (1,010 Hz in Fig. 2.11B) and the first negative node (990 Hz) is referred to as the main lobe of the amplitude spectrum. The adjacent regions between successive nodes are referred to as side lobes. When the pure tone is instantly turned on and off, as in these examples, 90% of the signal energy is contained in the main lobe; the remaining 10% is contained in the side lobes. As we've progressed from a continuous pure tone in Figure 2.11A to one lasting only 0.1 s in Figure 2.11B, the amplitude spectrum has started to broaden such that we've progressed from 100% of the acoustic energy at 1,000 Hz to 90% spread from 990 to 1,010 Hz.

In Figure 2.11C, the duration of the 1,000-Hz pure tone has been decreased still further (D = 0.01 s, or 10 ms). The main lobe of the amplitude spectrum now stretches from 900 to 1,100 Hz, because 1/D is now 1/(0.01), or 100 Hz. Thus, the first positive node occurs at 1,000 – 100 Hz, and the first negative node occurs at 1,000 – 100 Hz. In addition, the peak amplitude at 1,000 Hz has been reduced still further to 0.01 A ($D \times A$), and 90% of the signal energy in the main lobe of the amplitude spectrum for this brief tone burst is now spread over a range of 200 Hz.

If the duration of the 1,000-Hz pure tone is shortened by another factor of 10, as in Figure 2.11D, the corresponding amplitude spectrum continues to flatten and broaden. In this case, the duration of the pure tone is 0.001 s, or 1 ms, which corresponds to a single cycle of the 1,000-Hz pure tone. Now, the main lobe containing 90% of the signal energy spans from 0 to 2,000 Hz, a signal that is very brief or compact in the time domain (short waveform) but very broad or spread out in the frequency domain (broad amplitude spectrum). Just the opposite was true for the continuous pure tone described in the top panel of this figure (Fig. 2.11A). For the continuous pure tone, the signal was widely spread in the time domain (a continuous waveform of ≥1 s) but very compact in the frequency domain (all of the amplitude at just one frequency).

This broadening of the spectrum with decrease in signal duration is apparent perceptually as well. As the listener is presented with each of the pure tones in Figure 2.11 in succession, the perception begins with that of a clear tonal sensation and progressively sounds more and more like a click. In fact, the amplitude spectrum for an ideal click (one that is infinitely short) is flat throughout the entire spectrum. The spectrum of the shortest duration tone burst (Fig. 2.11D) is beginning to look more like that associated with a click than that associated with the continuous pure tone (Fig. 2.11A).

In summary, the amplitude spectrum of a pure tone varies with its duration such that the shorter the tone, the broader the spectrum. In general, the amplitude spectrum for pure tones less than 1 s in duration having a period of T seconds, a peak amplitude of A, and turned on and off abruptly for a duration of D seconds will have a peak amplitude at 1/T Hz of $A \times D$ and a main lobe containing 90% of the signal's energy between the frequencies 1/T – 1/D and 1/T + 1/D Hz. In Figure 2.11, T was 0.001 s, which resulted in all the spectra being centered at 1,000 Hz (1/T), but these general formulas allow this same analysis to be applied to pure tones of any frequency.

In addition to these effects of duration, sound energy can spread to other frequencies by turning the sound on and off abruptly (instantaneously) as in this example. Adding a gradual onset and offset to the tone, known as the sound's rise and fall time, can reduce the spread of energy to other frequencies. If a short transient sound is desired for a particular clinical application, however, adding a brief rise and fall time will reduce but not eliminate the spread of energy to other frequencies. So in general, even with appropriate rise and fall times for a transient sound, the shorter the sound, the broader the spread of energy to other frequencies.

Sometimes, having snapshots of the waveform and spectrum of a sound is just not enough to truly represent the important features of the sound. The acoustic speech signal, for example, is a very complex and rapidly changing stimulus. The most complete picture of the speech signal is provided by looking at amplitude variations in both the frequency domain and time domain simultaneously. When this form of acoustic analysis is applied to speech stimuli, it is referred to as a *speech spectrogram*. Figure 2.12 (top) provides an

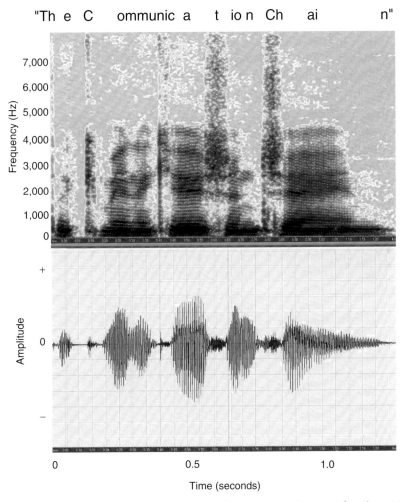

FIGURE 2.12 A speech spectrogram (*top*) and waveform (*bottom*) for the utterance, "the communication chain," illustrating the complex acoustic code sent from the talker to the listener. The spacing of the phase at the top corresponds to the approximate locations of those speech sounds in the spectrogram and waveform.

illustration of a speech spectrogram for the phrase "the communication chain." For speech spectrograms, the *y*-axis is sound frequency, with lower frequencies at the bottom and higher frequencies at the top, and the *x*-axis is time. To represent the important third dimension in this analysis of speech sounds, amplitude, gradients of color or of gray are used to reflect the amplitude at a particular frequency and moment in time. Figure 2.12 shows a grayscale version of the speech spectrogram with shades of gray representing variations in amplitude. On this scale, black is the highest amplitude and white is the lowest amplitude. Hundred-fold variations in amplitude can often be depicted using grayscale, with an even wider range of amplitudes represented when color is used. Through detailed acoustical analyses of speech-sound patterns, such as those in Figure 2.12, and corresponding experiments on the perception of these sounds, researchers have identified many of the cues needed to recognize speech sounds produced by the speaker. In fact, under good listening conditions and a constrained set of communication contexts, computer algorithms have been developed that will accurately identify 90% of the speech spoken clearly into a microphone. Interesting research is also being conducted on the use of complex acoustic codes for communication among animals; some of the tools used to analyze human speech, such as the spectrogram, have also been applied in this area (Vignette 2.9).

VIGNETTE 2.9 • CONCEPTUAL DEMO

Acoustic Codes for Communication

Humans use complex acoustic information or codes to communicate. As noted in the text, these codes can be analyzed in terms of the sound's waveform, spectrum, or a combination of both—the spectrogram. Are humans the only animals to use acoustic information to communicate? No. Many species use sound to communicate warnings for perceived threats such as approaching predators, intentions such as aggression or submission, or location such as when locating a suitable mate for reproduction.

Some animals appear to make use of even more complex acoustic codes and for more elaborate forms of communication. The acoustic productions of the bottlenose dolphin, for example, have been studied extensively. One interesting sound generated by the bottlenose dolphin is referred to as a "signature whistle." This sound is believed to be unique to each dolphin's social group and, perhaps, to each individual dolphin; similar to the identifiers used by humans in communication ("I'm Larry Humes from Bloomington, Indiana.")

The figure below shows examples of three signature whistles recorded from three bottlenose dolphins. The *top* panel of each pair shows the waveform for the signature whistle, whereas the *bottom* panel of each pair displays the corresponding sound spectrogram. Clearly, each waveform and spectrogram reveals a complex acoustic code and one that is unique for each of the three animals. By manipulating these signature whistles with a computer, researchers were able to basically change the voice (fundamental frequency) while leaving the shape of the sound spectrogram unchanged. This is roughly equivalent to having different talkers speak the same vowel sounds (Fig. 2.6) or words. Dolphins were able to recognize the signature whistles produced by different "voices" as well as the originals. Thus, bottlenose dolphins appear to be able to use complex acoustic signals as labels or identifiers of specific individuals, whether the identifier is produced by that animal or another animal; just as humans can understand the sound sequence that corresponds to "Larry Humes from Bloomington, Indiana," whether spoken by Larry Humes or someone else referring to him.

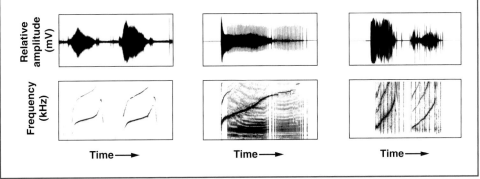

SOUND MEASUREMENT

As mentioned previously, the amplitude of a sound wave is typically expressed as sound pressure (p) in pascal units (Pa). Recall that one of the major reasons for this was that most measuring devices are pressure detectors. Devices such as microphones are sensitive to variations in air pressure and convert these pressure variations to variations in electrical voltage. In more general terms, the microphone can be referred to as an *acousticoelectrical transducer*. A transducer is any device that changes energy from one form to another. In this case, the conversion is from acoustical to electrical energy. (Usually, however, microphones are referred to as electroacoustical, rather than acousticoelectrical, transducers.)

Although the overall amplitude of sound waves is best expressed in terms of RMS pressure, the use of the actual physical units to describe the level of sound is cumbersome. In humans, the ratio of the highest tolerable sound pressure to the sound pressure that can just be heard exceeds 10,000,000:1. Moreover, the units dictate that one would be dealing frequently with numbers much smaller than 1. The lowest sound pressure that can just be heard by an average young adult with normal hearing, for instance, is approximately 0.00002 Pa (2×10^{-5} Pa) or 20 μPa (micropascals).

Rather than deal with this cumbersome system based on the physical units of pressure, scientists devised a scale known as the decibel scale. The decibel scale quantifies the sound level by taking the logarithm (base 10) of the ratio of two sound pressures and multiplying it by 20. The following formula is used to calculate the sound level in decibels from the ratio of two sound pressures (p_1 and p_2): $20 \log_{10} (p_1/p_2)$. Let's use the range of sound pressures from maximum tolerable (200,000,000 μPa) to just audible (20 μPa) to see how this range would be represented in decibels. To do this, we begin by substituting 200,000,000/20 for p_1/p_2, which reduces to a ratio of 10,000,000/1. The $\log_{10}$ of 10,000,000 (or 10^7) is 7. When the number 7 is multiplied by 20, the result is 140 dB. This represents the maximum tolerable sound level. Now, for the just-audible sound pressure of 20 μPa, the ratio of p_1/p_2 is 20/20, or 1. The log of 1 is 0, and 20×0 is 0. Thus, the just-audible sound pressure is represented by a sound level of 0 dB. We have taken a scale represented by a range of physical sound pressures of 200,000,000:20 and compressed it to a much more manageable range of 140 to 0 dB. The greatest sound pressure that can be tolerated is 140 dB larger than the softest sound pressure that can be heard. Note that this statement does not indicate what either of those sound pressures is in pascal units, which is because a ratio of two sound pressures has been used in the calculation of decibels, and ratios are dimensionless quantities (e.g., 0.2 Pa/0.2 Pa = 1; *not* 1 Pa). Thus, we are calculating the decibel increase of one sound relative to another. Sometimes all we are interested in is a relative change in sound pressure. Recall from the discussion of the inverse square law, for example, that as the distance was doubled from the sound source, the sound pressure was decreased to half its original value. The corresponding change in decibels associated with this halving of sound pressure can be calculated by using a ratio of 0.5/1. The $\log_{10}$ of 0.5 is −0.301, which, when multiplied by 20, yields a change in sound pressure of approximately −6 dB. We can restate the inverse square law by indicating that, as the distance from the sound source is doubled, the sound pressure level (SPL) decreases by 6 dB. Again, this does not indicate what the values are for the two sound pressures involved in this change. The sound pressure may begin at 10 Pa and be halved to 5 Pa or may start at 10,000 Pa and decrease to 5,000 Pa. Either of these cases corresponds to a halving of the initial sound pressure, which corresponds to a 6-dB decrease in sound level.

Often, an indication of the SPL, which provides an absolute rather than a relative indication of the sound level, is needed. To accomplish this, all sound pressures relative to the same reference sound pressure must be evaluated. Thus, the denominator of the decibel equation becomes a fixed value called

VIGNETTE 2.10 • FURTHER DISCUSSION

Decibel Values of Common Sounds

SOUND LEVEL	COMMON SOUND AT THIS dB LEVEL	
0 dB SPL	Softest sound level heard by average human listener	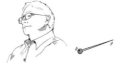
20 dB SPL	Leaves rustling in a breeze	
40 dB SPL	Whispered speech measured 1m away	Pssst
60 dB SPL	Average, conversational speech measured 1m away	Hello
80 dB SPL	Loud, shouting voice measured 1m away	HEY YOU! 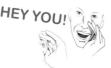
100 dB SPL	City subway, nearby thunder	
120 dB SPL	Typical level at a rock concert for audience	
140 dB SPL	Jet engine at takeoff	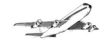

the *reference sound pressure*. The reference sound pressure for a scale known as the SPL scale is 2×10^{-5} Pa, or 20 µPa. As noted above, this corresponds to the softest sound pressure that can be heard by humans under ideal conditions. Calculation of the SPL for a specific sound pressure (p_1) can be accomplished by solving the following equation: SPL in dB = 20 log $[p_1/(2 \times 10^{-5}$ Pa$)]$. Perhaps, the simplest case to consider is the lowest sound pressure that can just be heard: 2×10^{-5} Pa. If $p_1 = 2 \times 10^{-5}$ Pa, then the ratio formed by the two sound pressures is $(2 \times 10^{-5}$ Pa$)/(2 \times 10^{-5}$ Pa$)$, or 1. The log of 1 is 0, which, when multiplied by 20, yields a sound level of 0 dB SPL. Consequently, 0 dB SPL does not mean absence of sound. Rather, it simply corresponds to a sound with a sound pressure of 2×10^{-5} Pa. Sound pressures lower than this value will yield negative dB SPL values, whereas sound pressures greater than this yield positive values.

Let us consider another example: A sound pressure of 1 Pa corresponds to how many decibels SPL? This can be restated by asking the reader to solve the following equation: SPL in dB = 20 log $[1.0$ Pa$/(2 \times 10^{-5}$ Pa$)]$. We begin by first reducing $1.0/(2 \times 10^{-5})$ to 5×10^4. The log of 5×10^4 is approximately 4.7, which, when multiplied by 20, yields an SPL of 94 dB. Thus, a sound pressure of 1 Pa yields an SPL of 94 dB SPL. This sound level is within the range of typical noise levels encountered in many factories and would be perceived to be quite loud.

Fortunately, laborious calculations are not required every time measurements of SPL are required. Rather, simple devices have been constructed to measure the level of various acoustic signals in decibels SPL. These devices, known as sound level meters, use a microphone to change the sound pressure variations to electrical voltage variations. The RMS amplitude of these voltage variations is then determined within the electronic circuitry of the meter, and an indicator (e.g., needle, pointer, or digital display) responds accordingly. In the case of 1 Pa RMS sound pressure input to the microphone, for example, the meter would either point to or display a value of 94 dB SPL (Vignette 2.10).

SUMMARY

The fundamentals of acoustics were reviewed in this chapter. Understanding the basics of sound is critical because sound waves form the primary link between the sender and receiver in the communication chain. We began the review of basic acoustics with simple harmonic motion or sinusoidal vibration, the simplest of all periodic sounds. The effects of varying the amplitude, frequency, and starting phase of the sinusoidal waveform were examined. The relation between the representations of sound in the time domain, the waveform, and sound in the frequency domain, the amplitude and phase spectra, were then reviewed. Resonance was also discussed. Special emphasis was placed on the complex acoustic code representing human speech. Finally, the measurement of sound levels in decibels was reviewed.

CHAPTER REVIEW QUESTIONS

1. Draw the waveform and amplitude spectrum for a sine wave or pure tone that has a peak amplitude of 10, a frequency of 1,000 Hz, and a starting phase of 0 degrees. Label all axes. What is the period for this sine wave?
2. Draw the waveform and amplitude spectrum for a sine wave that has half the amplitude and twice the frequency of the sine wave in Question 1 (starting phase remains at 0 degrees). Label all axes. What is the period of this sine wave?
3. Draw the waveform and amplitude spectrum for a sine wave that has half the amplitude and twice the frequency of the sine wave in Question 2 (starting phase remains at 0 degrees). Label all axes. What is the period of this sine wave?
4. Compare your answers to Questions 1 to 3. What happened to the period of the sine wave as the frequency was doubled (increased by 1 octave)? Why?
5. Assume that the amplitude axis for Questions 1 to 3 is in units of sound pressure (pascals). How would the sound level in dB SPL change as one progressed from Question 1 to Question 2 and from Question 2 to Question 3?

REFERENCES AND SUGGESTED READINGS

Beranek LL. *Acoustics*. New York, NY: McGraw-Hill; 1954.

Berlin CI. *Programmed Instruction on the Decibel*. New Orleans, LA: Kresge Hearing Research Laboratory of the South, Louisiana State University School of Medicine; 1970.

Cudahy E. *Introduction to Instrumentation in Speech and Hearing*. Baltimore, MD: Williams & Wilkins; 1988.

Denes PB, Pinson EN. *The Speech Chain*. New York, NY: WH Freeman; 1993.

Durrant JD, Lovrinic JH. *Bases of Hearing Science*. 3rd ed. Baltimore, MD: Williams & Wilkins; 1995.

Janik VM, Sayigh LS, Wells, RS. Signature whistle shape conveys identity information to bottlenose dolphins. *PNAS* 2006;103(21):8293–8297.

Small AM. *Elements of Hearing Science: A Programmed Text*. New York, NY: John Wiley & Sons; 1978.

Speaks C. *Introduction to Sound: Acoustics for the Hearing and Speech Sciences*. 3rd ed. San Diego, CA: Singular Publishing Group; 1999.

Yost WA. *Fundamentals of Hearing: An Introduction*. 4th ed. New York, NY: Academic Press; 2000.

3

Structure and Function of the Auditory System

Chapter Objectives

- To be able to identify basic anatomical landmarks of the outer ear, middle ear, inner ear, and auditory portions of the central nervous system;

- To understand the primary functions of the outer ear, middle ear, inner ear, and auditory portions of the central nervous system;

- To gain insight into how the primary functions of each portion of the auditory system are supported by underlying anatomy and physiology; and

- To understand some basic perceptual aspects of sound such as hearing threshold, loudness, pitch, and masking.

Key Terms and Definitions

- **Auditory periphery:** The outer ear, middle ear, and inner ear, ending at the nerve fibers exiting the inner ear.

- **Auditory central nervous system:** The ascending and descending auditory pathways in the brainstem and cortex.

- **Tonotopic organization:** The systematic mapping of sound frequency to the place of maximum stimulation within the auditory system that begins in the cochlea and is preserved through the auditory cortex.

- **Transducer:** A device or system that converts one form of energy to another. The cochlea can be considered a mechanoelectrical transducer, because it converts mechanical vibrations to electrical energy to stimulate the afferent nerve fibers leading to the brainstem.

Recall that the primary purpose of the communication chain is to support the transfer of thoughts, ideas, or emotions between two people, the sender and the receiver. Thus far, we have seen that the sender can translate the thought to be communicated into a code of sound sequences representing meaningful words and sentences in the language shared by these two individuals. How is this acoustic code converted into information that can be understood by the mind of the receiver or listener? The mind of the receiver makes use of neural electrical signals generated by the central nervous system. Thus, one of the primary functions of the auditory system is to convert the acoustic energy produced by the talker—human speech sounds—into neural energy that can be deciphered by the brain of the listener. This process is the central topic of this chapter.

This chapter is divided into three main sections. The first two deal with the anatomy, physiology, and functional significance of the peripheral and central sections of the auditory system. The peripheral portion of the auditory system is defined here as the structures from the outer ear through the auditory nerve. The auditory portions of the central nervous system begin at the cochlear nucleus and end at the auditory centers of the cortex. The third section of this chapter details some fundamental aspects of the perception of sound.

PERIPHERAL AUDITORY SYSTEM

Figure 3.1 shows a cross section of the peripheral portion of the auditory system. This portion of the auditory system is usually further subdivided into the outer ear, middle ear, and inner ear.

Outer Ear

The outer ear consists of two primary components: the pinna and the ear canal. The pinna, the most visible portion of the ear, extends laterally from the side of the head. It is composed of cartilage and skin. The ear canal is the long, narrow canal leading to the eardrum. The entrance to this canal is called the external auditory meatus. The deep bowl-like portion of the pinna adjacent to the external auditory meatus is known as the concha.

Figure 3.2 is a detailed drawing of the right pinna of a normal adult. This cartilaginous structure has several noteworthy anatomic landmarks. First, the bowl-shaped depression in the middle is the concha, which terminates at its medial end at the entrance to the ear canal (the external auditory meatus). Along the anterior inferior (front lower) portion of the concha are two cartilaginous protuberances known as the tragus and antitragus, which are separated, as shown in the figure, by the intertragal notch. The posterior and superior

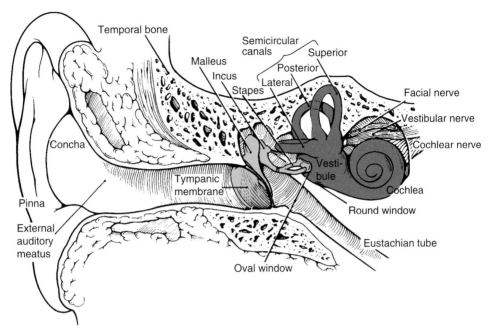

FIGURE 3.1 A cross section of the peripheral portion of the auditory system revealing some of the anatomic details of the outer, middle, and inner ear. (Adapted from Kessel RG, Kardon RH. *Tissues and Organs: A Text-Atlas of Scanning Electron Microscopy*. San Francisco, CA: Freeman; 1979.)

(rear and upper) borders of the concha are formed by a cartilaginous ridge known as the antihelix, which is closely paralleled along the posterior edge of the pinna by the helix. The helix and antihelix diverge in the superior portion of the pinna and then converge as they progress anteriorly and inferiorly. The slight depression formed between the helix and antihelix in the anterior superior portion of the pinna is the triangular fossa.

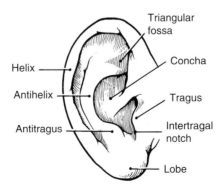

FIGURE 3.2 Detailed drawing of the right pinna showing various anatomic landmarks.

Medial to the external auditory meatus is the ear canal. The lateral two-thirds of the ear canal are cartilaginous, with the medial third composed of bone (osseous portion). An epithelium (skin) covering over the cartilaginous and osseous portions of the ear canal is contiguous with the tympanic membrane, or eardrum. That is, the lateralmost portion of the tympanic membrane is a layer of epithelium that is a part of the skin lining the ear canal.

The outer ear serves a variety of functions. First, the long (2.5 cm), narrow (5 to 7 mm) canal makes the more delicate middle and inner ear relatively inaccessible to foreign bodies. The outer third of the canal, moreover, is composed of skin and cartilage lined with glands and hairs. These glands, known as ceruminous glands, secrete a substance that potential intruders, such as insects, find terribly noxious. So, both the long, narrow, tortuous path of the canal and the secretions of these glands serve to protect the remaining portions of the peripheral auditory system.

Second, the various air-filled cavities composing the outer ear, the two most prominent being the concha and the ear canal, have a natural or resonant frequency to which they respond best. This is true of all air-filled cavities. For an adult, the resonant frequency of the ear canal is approximately 2,500 Hz, whereas that of the concha is roughly 5,000 Hz. The resonance of each of these cavities is such that each structure increases the sound pressure at its resonant frequency by approximately 10 to 12 dB. This gain or increase in sound pressure provided by the outer ear can best be illustrated by considering the following hypothetical experiment.

Let us begin the experiment by using two tiny microphones. One microphone will be placed just outside (lateral to) the concha, and the other will be positioned very carefully inside the ear canal to rest alongside the eardrum. Now if we present a series of sinusoidal sound waves, or pure tones, of different frequencies, which all measure the 70-dB sound pressure level (SPL), at the microphone just outside the concha, and if we read the SPLs measured with the other microphone near the eardrum, we will obtain results like those shown by the *solid line* in Figure 3.3. At frequencies less than approximately 1,400 Hz, the microphone near the eardrum measures sound levels of approximately 73-dB SPL. This is only 3 dB higher than the sound level just outside the outer ear. Consequently, the outer ear exerts little effect on the intensity of low-frequency sound. The intensity of the sound measured at the eardrum increases to levels considerably above 70-dB SPL, however, as the frequency of the sound increases. The maximum sound level at the eardrum is reached at approximately 2,500 Hz, which corresponds to a value of approximately 87-dB SPL. Thus, when a sound wave having a frequency of 2,500 Hz enters the outer ear, its sound pressure is increased by 17 dB by the time it strikes the eardrum. The function drawn with a *solid line* in Figure 3.3 illustrates the role that the entire

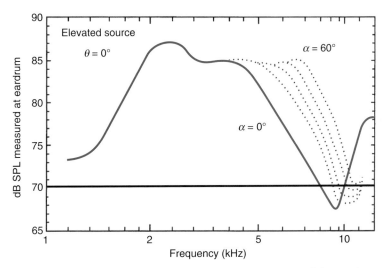

FIGURE 3.3 The response of the head, outer ear, and ear canal for various angles of elevation (a) of the sound source. Zero degree corresponds to a sound source at eye level and straight ahead (0-degree azimuth, 0-degree elevation), whereas 60 degrees represents a source straight ahead but at a higher elevation. If the listener's head and outer ear had no influence on the sound level measured at the eardrum, a flat line at 70-dB SPL would result. This figure illustrates the amplification of high-frequency sound by the outer ear and the way this amplification pattern changes with elevation of the sound source. (Adapted from Shaw EAG. The external ear. In: Keidel WD, Neff WD, eds. *Handbook of Sensory Physiology*. Vol 1. New York, NY: Springer Verlag; 1974:463.)

outer ear serves as a resonator or amplifier of high-frequency sounds. Experiments similar to this one can be conducted to isolate the contribution of various cavities to the resonance of the total outer ear system. Again, the results of such experiments suggest that the two primary structures contributing to the resonance of the outer ear are the concha and the ear canal.

The resonance of the outer ear, which is represented by the *solid line* in Figure 3.3, was obtained with a sound source directly in front of the subject at eye level. If the sound source is elevated by various amounts, a different resonance curve is obtained. Specifically, the notch or dip in the solid function at 10 kHz in Figure 3.3 moves to a higher frequency, and the peak of the resonant curve broadens to encompass a wider range of frequencies as the elevation of the sound source rises. This is illustrated in Figure 3.3 by the *dotted lines*. Each dotted line represents a different angle of elevation. An elevation of 0 degree corresponds to eye level, whereas a 90-degree elevation would position the sound source directly overhead. The response of the outer ear changes as the elevation of the sound source changes. This results from the angle at which the incident sound wave strikes the various cavities of the outer ear.

The result is that a code for sound elevation is provided by the outer ear. This code is the amplitude spectrum of the sound, especially above 3,000 Hz, which strikes the eardrum. Thus, the outer ear plays an important role in the perception of the elevation of a sound source.

Finally, the outer ear assists in another aspect of the localization of a sound source. The orientation of the pinnae is such that the pinnae collect sound more efficiently from sources in front of the listener than from sources behind the listener. The attenuation of sound waves originating from behind the listener assists in the front/back localization of sound. This is true especially for high-frequency sounds (i.e., sounds with short wavelengths).

In summary, the outer ear serves four primary functions. First, it protects the more delicate middle and inner ears from foreign bodies. Second, it boosts or amplifies high-frequency sounds. Third, it provides the primary cue for the determination of the elevation of a sound's source. Fourth, it assists in distinguishing sounds that arise from in front of the listener from those that arise from behind the listener.

Middle Ear

The tympanic membrane forms the anatomic boundary between the outer and middle ears. The tympanic membrane itself is a multilayered structure. Approximately 85% of the surface area of the tympanic membrane is composed of three types of layers: a lateral epithelial layer, a medial membranous layer that is contiguous with the lining of the middle ear cavity, and a fibrous layer sandwiched in between the epithelial and membranous layers. The fibrous layer actually contains two sets of fibers: one that is oriented like a series of concentric circles (as in a bull's-eye target) and another that is oriented in a radial fashion (like spokes on a bicycle wheel with the bull's eye as the hub of the wheel). These fibrous layers give the tympanic membrane considerable strength while maintaining elasticity.

For a small portion of the tympanic membrane, an area in the superior anterior portion that represents approximately 15% of the total eardrum surface area, the two sets of fibers between the epithelial and membranous layers of the eardrum are missing. This portion of the eardrum is known as the *pars flaccida* (*pars*, part, and *flaccida*, flaccid or loose). The portion of the tympanic membrane that contains all three types of layers and constitutes the majority (85%) of the eardrum is the *pars tensa*.

As previously mentioned, the most medial layer of the eardrum is a membranous layer that is contiguous with the membranous lining of the middle ear cavity. The middle ear consists of a small (2 cm³) air-filled cavity lined with a mucous membrane. It forms the link between the air-filled outer ear and the fluid-filled inner ear (Fig. 3.1). This link is accomplished mechanically via three tiny bones, the ossicles. The lateralmost ossicle is the malleus. The malleus is in contact with the eardrum, or tympanic membrane. At the other end of the outer ear-inner ear link is the smallest, medialmost ossicle, the stapes. The broad base of the stapes, known as the footplate, rests in a membranous covering of the fluid-filled inner ear referred to as the oval window. The middle ossicle in the link, sandwiched between the malleus and stapes, is the incus. The ossicles are suspended loosely within the middle ear by ligaments, known as the axial ligaments, extending from the anterior and posterior walls of the cavity. There are other connections between the surrounding walls of the middle ear cavity and the ossicles. Two connections are formed by the small middle ear muscles, known as the tensor tympani and the stapedius. The tensor tympani originates from the anterior (front) wall of the cavity and attaches to a region of the malleus called the neck, whereas the stapedius has its origin in the posterior (back) wall of the tympanic cavity and inserts near the neck of the stapes.

We have mentioned that the middle ear cavity is air-filled. The air filling the cavity is supplied via a tube that connects the middle ear to the upper part of the throat, or the nasopharynx. This tube, known as the auditory tube or the eustachian tube, has one opening along the bottom of the anterior wall of the middle ear cavity. The tube is normally closed but can be readily opened by yawning or swallowing. In adults, the eustachian tube assumes a slight downward orientation. This facilitates drainage of fluids from the middle ear cavity into the nasopharynx. Thus, the eustachian tube serves two primary purposes. First, it supplies air to the middle ear cavity and thereby enables equalization of the air pressure on both sides of the eardrum. This is desirable for efficient vibration of the eardrum. Second, the eustachian tube allows fluids that accumulate in the middle ear to drain into the nasopharynx.

Although the bones and muscles within the middle ear are key structural components, the middle ear cavity itself has several additional noteworthy anatomic landmarks. To review these landmarks and orient you to their location within this tiny cavity, imagine that we've surgically removed the three ossicles while leaving everything else intact and that you've been struck by a shrink ray that has reduced you in size, so that you can stand on the floor of the middle ear cavity after being inserted through a tiny surgical slit in the right eardrum ("Honey, I've shrunk the reader!"). As shown in Figure 3.4, you would find yourself standing on a mucus-covered membranous lining not unlike that which lines the inside of your nose and throat. A bulge running through the floor underneath your feet represents the tunnel, or fossa, for the jugular vein, one of the main blood vessels carrying blood to the brain.

As you gazed straight ahead, you would notice a small opening in the lower portion of the front wall and some ligaments and a tendon dangling loosely

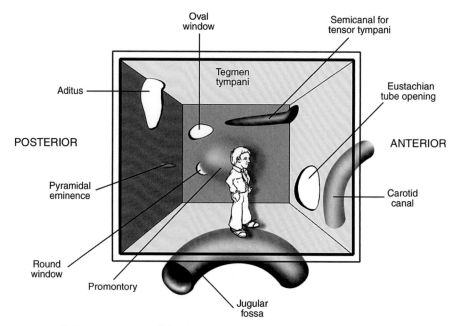

FIGURE 3.4 "Shrunken reader" in the center of the right middle ear with the ossicles removed.

from the upper right portion of the wall. The opening is the entrance, or orifice, for the eustachian tube; the ligaments are those previously attached to the anterior process of the malleus, the lateralmost of the three middle ear ossicles; and the tendon is protruding from a bony structure that houses one of the two middle ear muscles, the tensor tympani. This muscle would normally be connected via the tendon to the neck of the malleus.

As you looked above you, you would notice a partial ceiling that appears to be constructed of bone, although covered, like all of the cavity surfaces, with a mucous membrane. This is the tegmen tympany. The unfinished portion of the ceiling, or hole in the ceiling above you, is the aditus. It opens up into an "attic" known as the epitympanic recess, which leads to a series of air-filled caverns that penetrate the surrounding bone of the skull. The air-filled caverns and pockets are the mastoid air cells.

Directing your gaze to the rear or posterior wall, you would observe two primary landmarks. One is the pyramidal eminence, a bony pyramid-shaped structure in the medial superior portion of this wall. It houses the other muscle of the middle ear, the stapedius, which connects via tendon to the stapes. The other landmark, on the lateral superior portion of the wall, is the posterior portion of the axial ligaments that attaches to the incus. The axial ligaments, one attaching to the malleus from the anterior wall and the other attaching to the incus from the posterior wall, hold the ossicles in place and help to form the primary axis of rotation for the ossicular chain when it is vibrated by a sound wave striking the eardrum.

Now, as you returned to your original position facing the anterior wall, to your right along the lateral wall of the middle ear cavity you would observe the membranous layer of the eardrum; to your left, along the medial wall, you would find the oval window and round window. (Remember, you are in the *right* middle ear cavity, not the left.) A bulge running most of the way across the medial wall would also be apparent. This bulge is the promontory. It is formed by the large basal turn of the adjacent cochlea, the hearing portion of the inner ear.

These are some of the highlights of the many anatomic landmarks found in this tiny middle ear cavity. There are certainly others, such as various nerve fibers and blood vessels, but the effects of the shrink ray are starting to wear off, and we don't want to leave you trapped in here! ("Phew! Honey, it's okay. I've unshrunk the reader!")

What is the purpose of the elaborate link between the air-filled outer ear and the fluid-filled inner ear formed by the three ossicles? Recall from the example in Chapter 2 in which two people attempted to communicate, one underwater and one above the water, that the barrier formed by the interface between the media of air and sea water resulted in a "loss" of approximately 99.9% of the sound energy. That is, 99.9% of the energy in the impinging sound wave was reflected away, and only 0.1% was transmitted into the water. This loss amounts to a decrease in sound energy of approximately 30 dB. If the middle ear did not exist and the membranous entrance of the fluid-filled inner ear (oval window) replaced the eardrum, sound waves carried in air would impinge directly on the fluid-filled inner ear. This barrier is analogous to the air-to-water interface described in Chapter 2. Consequently, if such an arrangement existed, there would be a considerable loss of sound energy.

The middle ear compensates for this loss of sound energy when going from air to a fluid medium through two primary mechanisms. The first of these, the areal ratio (ratio of the areas) of the tympanic membrane to the footplate of the stapes, accounts for the largest portion of the compensation. The effective area of the tympanic membrane (i.e., the area involved directly in the mechanical link between the outer ear and inner ear) is approximately 55 mm^2. The corresponding area of the stapes footplate is 3.2 mm^2. Pressure (p) may be defined in terms of force (F) per unit area (A) ($p = F/A$). If the force applied at the eardrum is the same as that reaching the stapes footplate, the pressure at the smaller footplate must be greater than that at the larger eardrum. As an analogy, consider water being forced through a hose. If the area of the opening at the far end of the hose is the same as that of the faucet to which it is connected, the water will exit the hose under the same water pressure as it would at the faucet. If a nozzle is attached to the far end of the hose and it is adjusted to decrease the size of the opening at that end of the hose, the water pressure at that end will be increased in proportion to the degree of constriction produced by the nozzle. The smaller the opening, the greater the water pressure at the nozzle (and the farther the water will be ejected from the nozzle). Applying the same force that exists at the faucet to push the water through a smaller opening created by the nozzle has increased the water pressure at the nozzle. Another analogy explaining the pressure gain associated with areal ratios is one that explains why carpentry nails have a broad head and sharp, narrow point (Vignette 3.1).

For the middle ear, given application of equal force at the tympanic membrane and the stapes footplate ($F_1 = F_2$), the pressure at the smaller footplate ($F_1/3.2$) is greater than that at the larger tympanic membrane ($F_2/55$). The ratio of these two areas is 55/3.2, or 17. Consequently, the pressure at the oval window is 17 times that at the tympanic membrane for a given driving force simply because of their difference in area. An increase in sound pressure by a factor of 17 corresponds to an increase of 24.6 dB. Thus, of approximately 30 dB that would be lost if the air-filled outer ear were linked directly to the fluid-filled inner ear, almost 25 dB is recovered solely because of the areal ratio of the eardrum to the stapes footplate.

The other primary mechanism that might contribute to compensation for the existing impedance mismatch has to do with a complex lever system presumed to exist within the ossicles. The lever is created by the difference in length between the malleus and a portion of the incus known as the long process. This lever factor recovers only approximately 2 dB of the loss caused by the impedance mismatch. The assumptions underlying the operation of this lever mechanism, moreover, are not firmly established.

The middle ear system, therefore, compensates for much of the loss of sound energy that would result if the airborne sound waves impinged directly on the fluid-filled inner ear. The middle ear compensates for approximately 25 to 27 dB of the estimated 30-dB impedance mismatch. The ability of the middle ear system to amplify or boost the sound pressure depends on signal frequency. Specifically, little pressure amplification occurs for frequencies below 100 Hz or above 2,000 to 2,500 Hz. Recall, however, that the outer ear amplified sound energy by 20 dB for frequencies from 2,000 to 5,000 Hz. Thus, taken together, the portion of the auditory system peripheral to the stapes footplate increases sound pressure by 20 to 25 dB in a range of approximately 100 to 5,000 Hz. This range of frequencies happens to correspond to the range of frequencies in human speech that are most important for communication.

Another less obvious function of the middle ear also involves the outer ear–inner ear link formed by the ossicles. Because of the presence of this mechanical link, the preferred pathway for sound vibrations striking the eardrum will be

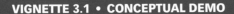

VIGNETTE 3.1 • CONCEPTUAL DEMO

An Analogy for Pressure Amplification

The common carpentry nail illustrates the pressure amplification that occurs when the same force is applied over a smaller versus larger surface area. As shown, the head of the nail has more surface area than the point. When force is applied to the head of the nail with a hammer, that force is channeled through to the point. However, because the area of the point is approximately one-tenth the area at the head of the nail, the pressure applied at the point is 10 times greater. (Pressure is equal to force per unit of area: pressure = force/area.) The increased pressure at the point of the nail helps it to penetrate the material (e.g., wood) into which it is being driven. Of course, other practical factors affect the design of the common carpentry nail (e.g., the broader head also makes it easier to strike and to remove), but the pressure amplification is one of the key elements in the design. Also, it supplies a nice analogy to the pressure amplification achieved by the areal ratio of the tympanic membrane and stapes footplate in the middle ear.

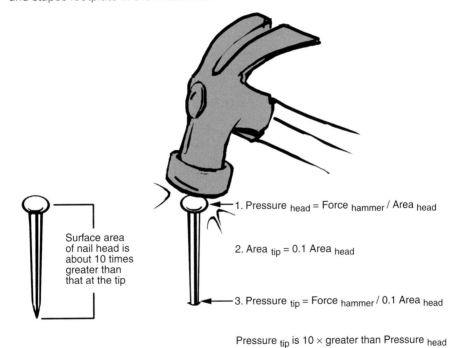

Surface area of nail head is about 10 times greater than that at the tip

1. Pressure $_{head}$ = Force $_{hammer}$ / Area $_{head}$

2. Area $_{tip}$ = 0.1 Area $_{head}$

3. Pressure $_{tip}$ = Force $_{hammer}$ / 0.1 Area $_{head}$

Pressure $_{tip}$ is 10 × greater than Pressure $_{head}$

along the chain formed by the three ossicles. Sound energy, therefore, will be routed directly to the oval window. Another membranous window of the inner ear also lies along the inner or medial wall of the middle ear cavity. This structure is known as the round window (Fig. 3.1). For the inner ear to be stimulated appropriately by the vibrations of the sound waves, the oval window and round window must not be displaced in the same direction simultaneously. This situation would arise frequently, however, if the sound wave impinged directly on the medial wall of the middle ear cavity where both the oval window and the round window are located. Thus, routing the vibrations of the eardrum directly to the oval window via the ossicles ensures appropriate stimulation of the inner ear.

Finally, we mentioned previously that two tiny muscles within the middle ear make contact with the ossicular chain. These muscles can be made to contract in a variety of situations. Some individuals can contract these muscles voluntarily. For most individuals, however, the contraction is an involuntary reflex arising either from loud acoustic stimuli or from nonacoustic stimuli (such as a puff of air applied to the eyes or scratching the skin on the face just in front of the external auditory meatus) or accompanying voluntary movements of the oral musculature, as in chewing, swallowing, or yawning. For acoustic activation, sound levels must generally exceed 85-dB SPL to elicit a reflexive contraction of the middle ear muscles.

The result of middle ear muscle contraction is to compress or stiffen the ossicular chain and essentially to pull the ossicular chain away from the two structures it links, the outer ear and inner ear. This results in an attenuation or decrease of sound pressure reaching the inner ear. The attenuation, amounting to 15 to 20 dB, depends on frequency. Recall from Chapter 2 that increases in a system's stiffness have the greatest effect on low-frequency vibrations. Consequently, the attenuation produced by the middle ear muscles contracting and increasing the stiffness of the ossicles exists only for frequencies below 2,000 Hz. The attenuation measured for acoustically elicited contractions, moreover, appears to apply only to stimuli of high intensities. Low-level signals, such as those near threshold, are not attenuated when middle ear muscle contraction is elicited, but high-level signals (~80-dB SPL) may be attenuated by as much as 15 to 20 dB. The middle ear reflex is known as a consensual reflex, meaning that when either ear is appropriately stimulated, the muscles contract in both ears.

Inner Ear

The inner ear is a complex structure that resides deep within a very dense portion of the skull known as the petrous portion of the temporal bone. Because of the complexity of this structure, it is often referred to as a labyrinth. The inner ear

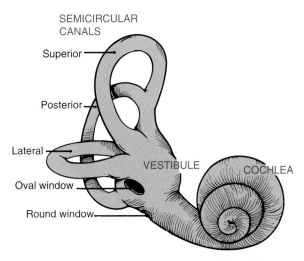

SEMICIRCULAR
CANALS

Superior

Posterior

Lateral

VESTIBULE   COCHLEA

Oval window

Round window

FIGURE 3.5 The osseous labyrinth and its landmarks. (Adapted from Durrant JD, Lovrinic JH. *Bases of Hearing Science*. 2nd ed. Baltimore, MD: Williams & Wilkins; 1984:98.)

consists of a bony outer casing, the osseous labyrinth. Within this bony structure is the membranous labyrinth. The osseous labyrinth, as shown in Figure 3.5, can be divided into three major sections: the *semicircular canals* (*superior, lateral*, and *posterior*), the *vestibule*, and the *cochlea*. The first two sections house the sensory organs for the vestibular system. The vestibular system assists in maintaining balance and posture. The focus here, however, is on the remaining portion of the osseous inner ear, the cochlea. It is the cochlea that contains the sensory organ for hearing. The coiled, snail-shaped cochlea has approximately $2^3/_4$ turns in human beings. The largest turn is called the basal turn, and the smallest turn, at the top of the cochlea, is referred to as the apical turn. Two additional anatomic landmarks of the inner ear depicted in Figure 3.5 are the *oval window* and the *round window*. Recall that the footplate of the stapes, the medialmost bone of the three ossicles in the middle ear, is attached to the oval window.

The cochlea is cut in cross section from top (apex) to bottom (base) in Figure 3.6. The winding channel running throughout the bony snail-shaped structure is further subdivided into three compartments. The compartment sandwiched between the other two is a cross section of the membranous labyrinth that runs throughout the osseous labyrinth. All three compartments are filled with fluid. The middle compartment, known as the *scala media*, is filled with a fluid called endolymph. The two adjacent compartments, the *scala vestibuli* and *scala tympani*, contain a different fluid called perilymph. At the apex of the cochlea is a small hole called the *helicotrema* that connects the two compartments filled with perilymph, the scala tympani and scala vestibuli. The oval window forms an interface between the ossicular chain of the middle ear and the fluid-filled scala

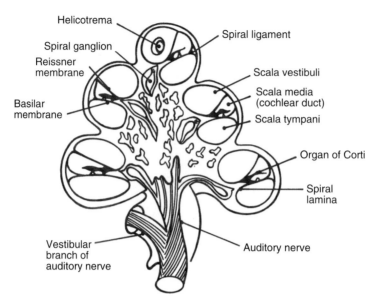

FIGURE 3.6 Modiolar cross section of the cochlea illustrating the scalae through each of the turns. (Adapted from Zemlin WR. *Speech and Hearing Science: Anatomy and Physiology*. 2nd ed. Englewood Cliffs, NJ: Prentice-Hall; 1988:464.)

vestibuli of the inner ear. When the oval window vibrates as a consequence of vibration of the ossicular chain, a wave is established within the scala vestibuli. Because the fluid-filled compartments are essentially sealed within the osseous labyrinth, the inward displacement of the cochlear fluids at the oval window must be matched by an outward displacement elsewhere. This is accomplished via the round window, which communicates directly with the scala tympani. When the oval window is pushed inward by the stapes, the round window is pushed outward by the increased pressure in the inner ear fluid.

When the stapes footplate rocks back and forth in the oval window, it generates a wave within the cochlear fluids. This wave displaces the scala media in a wave-like manner. This displacement pattern is usually simplified by considering the motion of just one of the partitions forming the scala media, the *basilar membrane*. The motion depicted for the basilar membrane also occurs for the opposite partition of the scala media, *Reissner membrane* (Fig. 3.6). Although we will be depicting the displacement pattern of the basilar membrane, the reader should bear in mind that the entire fluid-filled scala media is undergoing similar displacement.

Figure 3.7 illustrates the displacement pattern of the basilar membrane at four successive points in time. When this displacement pattern is visualized directly, the wave established along the basilar membrane is seen to travel from the base to the apex. The displacement pattern increases gradually in

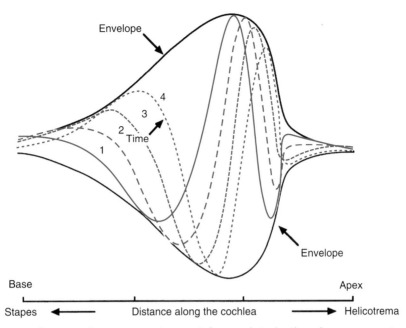

FIGURE 3.7 The traveling wave pattern at four points in time in response to a mid-frequency sound. The *thin solid black lines* connect the maximum and minimum displacements at each location along the cochlea and for each point in time. These lines represent the envelope of the displacement patterns. (Adapted from von Bekesy G. *Experiments in Hearing.* New York, NY: McGraw-Hill; 1960:462.)

amplitude as it progresses from the base toward the apex until it reaches a point of maximum displacement. At that point, the amplitude of displacement decreases abruptly. The *thin solid black line* connecting the amplitude peaks at various locations for these four points in time describes the displacement envelope. The envelope pattern is symmetrical in that the same pattern superimposed on the positive peaks can be flipped upside down and used to describe the negative peaks. As a result, only the positive, or upper, half of the envelope describing maximum displacement is usually displayed.

Figure 3.8 displays the envelopes of the displacement pattern of the basilar membrane that have been observed for different stimulus frequencies. As the frequency of the stimulus increases, the peak of the displacement pattern moves in a basal direction closer to the stapes footplate. At low frequencies, virtually the entire membrane undergoes some degree of displacement. As stimulus frequency increases, a more restricted region of the basilar membrane undergoes displacement. Thus, the cochlea is performing a crude frequency analysis of the incoming sound. In general, for all but the very low frequencies (50 Hz), the place of maximum displacement within the cochlea is associated with the frequency of an acoustic stimulus. The frequency of the acoustic stimulus striking

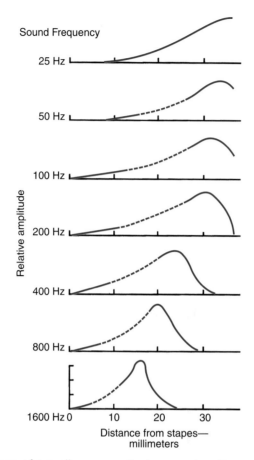

FIGURE 3.8 Envelopes of traveling wave displacement patterns for various stimulus frequencies. Low frequencies (*top*) produce a maximum displacement of the basilar membrane in the apex (farthest distance from the stapes), whereas higher frequencies (*bottom*) produce maximum displacement in the basal portion of the cochlea (nearer to the stapes). (Adapted from von Bekesy G. *Experiments in Hearing.* New York, NY: McGraw-Hill; 1960:448.)

the eardrum and displacing the stapes footplate will be analyzed or distinguished from sounds of different frequency by the location of the displacement pattern along the basilar membrane.

Because the pressure wave created within the cochlear fluids originates near the base of the cochlea at the oval window, one might think that this is the reason the traveling wave displacement pattern appears to move from the base to the apex. On the contrary, experiments with models of the inner ear have shown that the source of vibration (oval window) can be anywhere along the cochlea, including the apex, with no effect on the displacement pattern of the basilar membrane (Vignette 3.2). The primary physical feature of the inner ear responsible for the direction in which the traveling wave progresses is the stiffness gradient of the basilar membrane. The stiffness of the basilar membrane is greatest in the base and decreases from the base to the apex. As we saw in Chapter 2, stiffness offers greatest opposition to displacement for low-frequency vibrations. Thus, the greater stiffness of the basilar membrane in the basal portion of the cochlea opposes displacement when stimulated by low-frequency sound and forces the

---

VIGNETTE 3.2 • FURTHER DISCUSSION

Discussion of the Traveling-Wave Paradox

Regardless of where the vibration is introduced into the cochlea, the traveling wave always travels from base to apex. This phenomenon is known as the traveling-wave paradox. The early tests of hearing that were routinely performed decades ago with tuning forks made use of this phenomenon. A tuning fork was struck, and the vibrating tongs were placed next to the outer ear. The tester asked the listener to indicate when the tone produced by the vibrating tuning fork could no longer be heard. Immediately after the listener indicated that the sound was no longer audible, the base of the tuning fork was pressed against the mastoid process, the bony portion of the skull behind the ear. If the listener could hear the tone again, it was assumed that the hearing sensitivity of the inner ear alone was better than that of the entire peripheral portion of the auditory system as a whole (outer ear, middle ear, and inner ear).

When the base of the tuning fork was placed on the mastoid process, the skull vibrated. The cochlea is embedded firmly within the temporal bone of the skull, such that skull vibrations produce mechanical vibration of the inner ear. Even though the vibration is not introduced at the oval window by the vibrating stapes, the tone produced by the tuning fork placed against the skull is heard as though it were. The traveling wave within the inner ear behaves the same, regardless of where the mechanical vibration is introduced.

For normal listeners, the typical means of stimulating the inner ear is through the outer and middle ears. This is air conduction hearing. Sound can also be introduced by vibrating the skull at the mastoid process, forehead, or some other location. This is called bone conduction hearing. Whether the tone is introduced into the inner ear by bone conduction or air conduction, the traveling wave and the resulting sensation are the same.

Modern-day air conduction and bone conduction tests are described in more detail in Chapter 7. They are of great assistance in determining which portion of the peripheral auditory system is impaired in listeners with hearing loss.

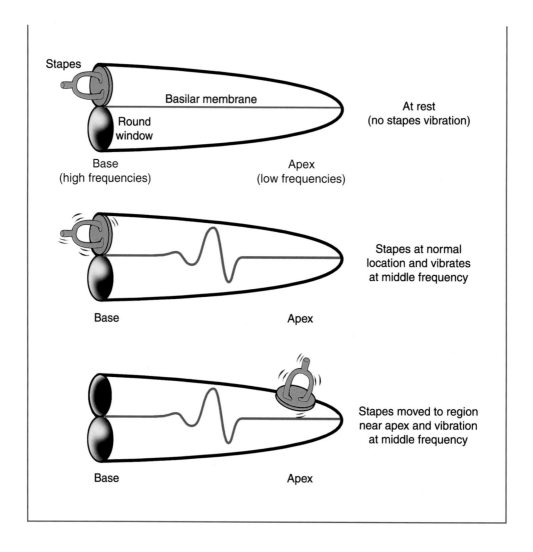

wave to travel further up the cochlea toward the apex to a region having less stiffness and less opposition to low-frequency vibration.

A more detailed picture of the structures within the scala media is provided in Figure 3.9 The sensory organ of hearing, the organ of Corti, is seen to rest on top of the basilar membrane. The organ of Corti contains several thousand sensory receptor cells called *hair cells*. Each hair cell has several tiny hairs, or cilia, protruding from the top of the cell. As shown in Figure 3.9, there are two types of hair cells in the organ of Corti. The inner hair cells make up a single row of receptors closest to the modiolus, or bony core, of the cochlea. The cilia of these cells are freestanding (i.e., they do not make contact with any other structures). Approximately 90% to 95% of the auditory nerve fibers that carry information to the brain make contact with the inner hair cells. The outer hair

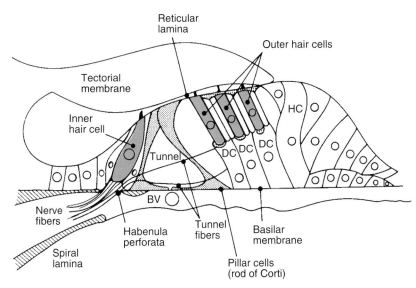

FIGURE 3.9 Detailed cross section of the organ of Corti. *BV*, basilar vessel; *DC*, Deiter cell; *HC*, Hensen cell. (Adapted from Pickles JO. *An Introduction to the Physiology of Hearing*. 2nd ed. London, UK: Academic; 1988:29.)

cells are much greater in number and are usually organized in three rows. The cilia of the outer hair cells are embedded within a gelatinous structure known as the *tectorial membrane*, draped over the top of the organ of Corti.

The organ of Corti is bordered by two membranes: the basilar membrane below and the tectorial membrane above. The modiolar or medial points of attachment for these two membranes are offset; the tectorial membrane is attached to a structure called the spiral limbus, which is nearer to the modiolus than the comparable point of attachment for the basilar membrane (a bony structure called the spiral lamina). Figure 3.10 illustrates one of the consequences of these staggered points of attachment. When the basilar membrane is displaced upward (toward the scala vestibuli), the cilia of the outer hair cells embedded in the tectorial membrane undergo a shearing force in a radial direction (a horizontal direction in the figure). Displacement downward develops a radial shearing force in the opposite direction. This shearing force is believed to be the trigger that initiates a series of electrical and chemical processes within the hair cells. This, in turn, leads to the activation of the auditory nerve fibers that are in contact with the base of the hair cell.

A critical element in the conversion of mechanical movements of the basilar membrane to electrical impulses in the auditory nerve is the transduction function served by the inner and outer hair cells in the organ of Corti. The shearing forces applied to the cilia on the tops of these hair cells in response to acoustic stimulation give rise to electrical potentials known generally as receptor

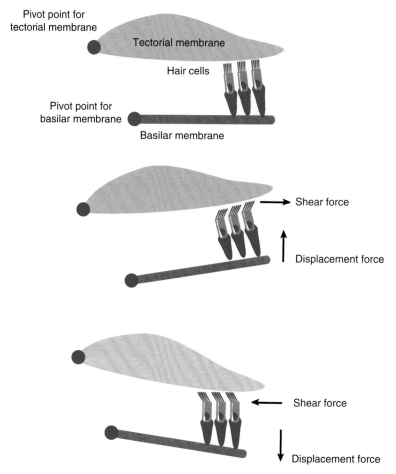

FIGURE 3.10 The mechanism responsible for generation of shearing forces on the cilia of the outer hair cells. Because the pivot points for the tectorial membrane and basilar membrane (*small black circles*) are offset horizontally, vertical displacement of the basilar membrane creates radial shearing forces across the cilia (i.e., a push or pull of the cilia in left to right in the drawings). (Adapted from Zemlin WR. *Speech and Hearing Science: Anatomy and Physiology.* 2nd ed. Englewood Cliffs, NJ: Prentice-Hall; 1998:484.)

potentials. Receptor potentials are common in sensory cells and are produced only in response to a stimulus, unlike resting potentials, which are present in cells at all times in the living organism. Two types of receptor potentials are found in the cochlea: the cochlear microphonic (CM) potential and the summating potential (SP). These potentials are generally referred to as gross electrical potentials in that they are measured with electrodes inserted in the cochlea (and sometimes can be recorded from the ear canal) and represent the collective response of hundreds or even thousands of hair cells. In addition, the CM is an alternating-current (ac) potential that varies in instantaneous amplitude over time (the waveform of the potential mimics that of the stimulating sound, the same way a microphone does). The SP is a steady-state direct-current (dc) potential that maintains a constant value in response to sound.

Scientists have been able to record electrical potentials generated by individual hair cells. Again, both resting potentials and receptor potentials have been recorded from individual hair cells. Receptor potentials of single hair cells, referred to as the ac and dc receptor potentials, are somewhat analogous to the grossly recorded CM and SPs, respectively. The exact role of the hair cells, their receptor potentials, and the interaction between the two types of hair cells (inner and outer) is unclear. It is clear, however, that damage to the hair cells and the elimination of the receptor potentials produced by the cells greatly diminish the cochlea's ability to perform a frequency analysis on incoming sounds and reduce the sensory response for sounds of low and moderate intensity.

One of the critical functions of the hair cells in the organ of Corti is the conversion (**transducer** function) of mechanical energy from the middle ear vibration to electrical energy that stimulates the connecting nerve fibers. As noted previously, this is a critical link in the communication chain in converting the acoustic signal from the sender to a neural electrical signal that can be deciphered by the brain of the receiver. The conversion takes place within the inner ear in the organ of Corti. Intact inner and outer hair cells are needed for this conversion to take place. As we will see later, many agents—such as noise, genetic disorders, or aging—can harm or destroy these hair cells and cause a breakdown in the communication chain. Although exciting research is underway that may alter this statement in the near future, at the moment, such loss of hair cells in the organ of Corti is irreversible.

Some research conducted since the mid-1980s has indicated that the receptor potentials generated by the hair cell trigger mechanical changes in the length of the bodies of the hair cells. When the cilia on the top of the hair cell are sheared in one direction, the receptor potential produced makes the cell body of the hair cell contract. Deflection of the cilia in the opposite direction changes the receptor potential, which causes the body of the hair cell to elongate or stretch. This expansion and contraction of the hair cells along the length of their cell bodies have been likened to similar events in muscle fibers. Although, actin, a protein found in muscle fibers that is critical to the fiber's ability to expand and contract, has also been found in hair cells, it is a different protein, prestin, that supports the contractile properties of the hair cells. The net effect of these mechanical changes in the length of the hair cell is to amplify, or boost, the displacement of the basilar membrane and to create a more vigorous electrical response to the stimulus. The ultimate effect of this elaborate micromechanical system is a much more precise analysis of frequency and a stronger mechanical and electrical response to sounds of low and moderate intensity.

Researchers frequently refer to this facilitatory effect of the hair cell movement as the cochlear amplifier because of its enhancement of low- and moderate-intensity sounds (Vignette 3.3).

To understand how changes in the length of the hair cell bodies in response to sound can enhance the basilar membrane's response, consider the following analogy. Imagine that you are bouncing up and down on a large trampoline. You adjust your bounce so that the trampoline is vibrated in an up-and-down motion with a vertical displacement of 1 foot in each direction. A partner is now positioned beneath the trampoline and is wearing a special helmet, the top of which is attached to the underside of the trampoline's surface at the location corresponding to your point of contact with the trampoline. When your partner squats, the trampoline is pulled down, and when he or she stands, it is returned to a horizontal position. By synchronizing your partner's active vertical movements (using the muscles in his or her legs to alternately squat and stand) with the "passive" vertical displacement of the trampoline produced by your bouncing, the height of your jump (and the displacement of the trampoline) can be increased or amplified considerably. The trampoline surface is like the basilar membrane, and your partner represents the contracting and expanding hair cell body sandwiched between the basilar membrane and the

---

VIGNETTE 3.3 • FURTHER DISCUSSION

The Cochlear Amplifier

The ability of the outer hair cells to contract and elongate in response to sound stimulation results in the amplification of the mechanical response of the inner ear (the basilar membrane) at low sound intensities. This has been determined through research involving a variety of techniques and approaches over the years. Some of these techniques involved either temporarily or permanently disabling the outer hair cells while leaving the rest of the inner ear intact. When this is done, the amplitude of vibration measured for the basilar membrane is less at low intensities but unchanged at high intensities. This also affects the frequency resolving, or filtering, power of the inner ear at low intensities. Both of these effects, on low-intensity displacement and low-intensity tuning or filtering, are illustrated in the nearby figure. These well-established physiologic effects have considerable significance for audiologists, since, as noted in subsequent chapters, many cases of sensorineural hearing loss involve primarily the loss of outer hair cells. As a consequence, based on research findings like those illustrated here, one would expect such individuals to have trouble hearing soft sounds but not loud sounds and in performing frequency analysis of low-intensity sounds.

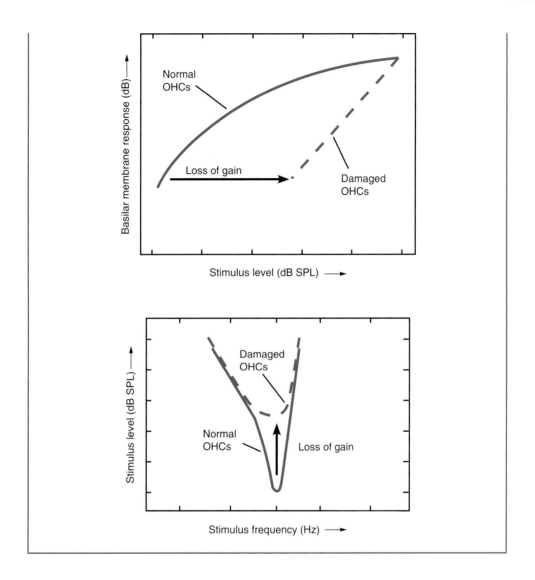

tectorial membrane. The electrical potentials that perfectly mimic the displacement pattern of the basilar membrane (and the waveform of the sound) keep the two partners synchronized to enhance the vertical displacement. Otherwise, without synchronization, your partner could be pushing upward while you were moving downward on the trampoline and effectively cancel the vertical displacement. Working together, however, the combined efforts of you and your partner produce more activity than you could accomplish by yourself.

If such an active cochlear amplifier exists, one would expect to be able to measure vibrations coming out of the inner ear when the hair cells have been pushing and pulling on the basilar membrane. Further, if they vibrate the basilar membrane, the oval window and stapes footplate should also vibrate, which should vibrate the rest of the middle ear ossicles and the eardrum, which in turn should produce a measurable sound in the ear canal. In fact, such sounds, known as otoacoustic emissions (OAEs) (*oto*, of the ear, and *acoustic*, sound), have been the focus of an incredible amount of research since their discovery in 1978. They have been measured by placing a tiny microphone deep inside the ear canal.

There are two broad classes of otoacoustic emissions, or OAEs: spontaneous and evoked. Evoked emissions require a stimulus of some sort to produce them, whereas spontaneous emissions simply occur, as the name implies, spontaneously (without a stimulus). Using the trampoline analogy, spontaneous emissions can be thought of as being produced by your partner's continued up-and-down movement, even when you are no longer on the trampoline. Spontaneous OAEs occur in at least 50% of the normal-hearing young adult population, are more prevalent in females, and are not of much clinical value at present. Evoked OAEs, however, have been demonstrated to be sensitive to damage to the hair cells in the cochlea and have become a key clinical tool for the detection and diagnosis of hearing loss (Vignette 3.4).

There are basically three types of evoked OAEs: (a) transient-evoked OAE (TEOAE), (b) distortion-product OAE (DPOAE), and (c) stimulus-frequency OAE (SFOAE). The SFOAEs are the most difficult to measure and have been studied the least. They are produced by presenting the ear with a pure tone and then examining the sound recorded in the ear canal. The frequency of the emission sound, however, is the same as that of the stimulus tone, and its level is much lower than that of the stimulus. This makes it difficult to measure and study.

TEOAEs were the first OAEs measured in humans. They are recorded by stimulating the ear with a brief click while recording the sound level in the ear canal with a tiny microphone. A click is a brief sound that has energy spread over a wide range of frequencies. Thus, a wide range of the basilar membrane can be stimulated in an instant. Because of the nature of the traveling wave mechanism in the cochlea, the basilar membrane initially responds to a click with maximum displacement in the high-frequency basal region. The peak displacement of the basilar membrane then travels toward the apex, where maximum displacement occurs in response to low-frequency sounds. Thus, even though the click stimulus instantly presents the ear with sounds of low, mid, and high frequency, it takes longer for the low-frequency sounds to travel to the apex and stimulate the basilar membrane. Assuming that it takes 3 ms for the peak displacement to travel from the basal to the apical portion of the basilar membrane, the low frequencies would maximally stimulate the basilar membrane at the appropriate place about 3 ms after the high frequencies present in the click. Further, the vibrations producing the emissions travel back out of the cochlea at the same rate, so that low-frequency sounds would come back out

VIGNETTE 3.4 • CLINICAL APPLICATIONS

Use of OAEs as a Screening Tool for Babies

The development of tools to measure OAEs clinically has led to many exciting applications. For the first time in the history of clinical audiology, a tool to measure the integrity of the sensory receptors in the generally inaccessible inner ear was available.

One of the clinical applications explored and refined during the 1990s was the use of OAEs as a screening tool for hearing loss in infants. Some of the advantages associated with the use of OAEs for this application included the ability to record these responses without requiring the active participation of the infant, the ability to assess each ear separately, and the capability of evaluating a fairly broad range of frequencies. In addition, normal OAE responses would be possible only with normal outer, middle, and inner ears. The focus in OAE-based screening is clearly on the auditory periphery. Problems localized to any of these sections of the auditory periphery, moreover, are most amenable to intervention, either medical (for the outer and middle ears) or audiologic (in the form of hearing aids or other prosthetic devices for those with inner ear problems; see Chapter 9).

In recent years, most states have adopted legislation to require that all infants be screened for hearing loss at birth (referred to as universal screening; see Chapter 8). Screening tools based on OAEs are among the most commonly used devices in universal newborn screening programs.

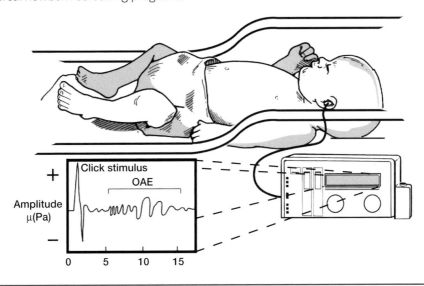

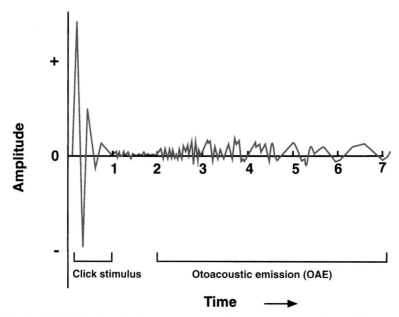

FIGURE 3.11 A TEOAE. The plot is a waveform showing as a function of time the sound levels recorded by a tiny microphone in the ear canal. The large initial portion of the waveform is a recording of the click stimulus presented in the ear canal by the earphone. The lower-level and later-appearing portion of the waveform is the echo coming back out into the ear canal from the inner ear.

of the cochlea and be measurable by a microphone in the ear canal about 6 ms after the high frequencies appeared.

Figure 3.11 illustrates a representative TEOAE from a normal-hearing young adult. The plot is essentially the acoustic waveform that is recorded in the ear canal by the tiny microphone. The first, large, abrupt portion of the waveform is the click stimulus presented by the earphone. After a brief period of silence, another waveform emerges: a low-level echo! In fact, TEOAEs have frequently been referred to as cochlear echoes. Careful scrutiny of the echo reveals that the first portion has shorter periods or higher frequencies than the later parts of the echo. This is entirely consistent with the scenario described earlier based on the delays introduced by the traveling wave along the basilar membrane.

TEOAEs are observed only in response to clicks of low and moderate sound level. Animal research has demonstrated that TEOAEs are sensitive to damage, even reversible injury, to the hair cells. If the measurements described in Figure 3.11 were repeated on an individual with hair cell damage in the high-frequency basal portion of the cochlea, the early parts of the echo would be missing, and only the later-emerging low-frequency emissions originating from the healthy apical region would be observed.

DPOAEs are also being used for clinical applications. Although DPOAEs can be generated in a variety of ways, the most commonly employed method makes use of two stimulus tones simultaneously introduced into the ear canal. The frequencies of these two pure tones are denoted f_1 and f_2, with f_2 being higher in frequency than f_1. Distortion is a characteristic of many systems, including mechanical systems, and can be measured in a variety of ways. One manifestation of distortion in a system is the emergence of tones in the response or output of the system that were not part of the sound stimulus presented to the system. These additional tones are referred to as distortion products. When two tones are presented to the auditory system, the most prominent distortion product that emerges is one that has a frequency corresponding to $2f_1 - f_2$. For reasons beyond the scope of this book, this distortion product is often referred to as the cubic difference tone, or CDT. The CDT is lower in frequency than the two input tones. For example, for $f_1 = 1,000$ Hz and $f_2 = 1,200$ Hz, the frequency of the CDT is 800 Hz ([2 × 1,000 Hz] – 1,200 Hz). Although other distortion products have been explored for measurement of DPOAEs, the CDT has been the most thoroughly studied and is the one receiving the most emphasis clinically. Hereafter, unless noted otherwise, the term DPOAE implies measurement of the CDT distortion product.

Because the DPOAE occurs at a frequency close to, but separate from, the input frequencies, it is possible to use sounds of longer duration to evoke the emission. The distortion product is separated from the input frequencies by a fast frequency analysis of the sound recorded in the ear canal. Unlike the TEOAE, the DPOAE can be measured over a wide range of sound levels from moderately low to very high. Although there is considerable uncertainty as to whether the same distortion processes are involved over this entire range of sound levels, it appears that the DPOAEs evoked by low-intensity stimuli are just as sensitive to hair cell damage in the cochlea as TEOAEs. They continue to be explored for a variety of clinical applications.

The two primary functions of the auditory portion of the inner ear can be summarized as follows. First, the inner ear performs a frequency analysis on incoming sounds so that different frequencies stimulate different regions of the inner ear. Second, mechanical vibration is amplified and converted into electrical energy by the hair cells. The hair cells are frequently referred to as mechano-electrical transducers. That is, they convert mechanical energy (vibration) into electrical energy (receptor potentials).

Auditory Nerve

The action potentials generated by auditory nerve fibers are called all-or-none potentials, because they do not vary in amplitude when activated. If the nerve fibers fire, they always fire to the same degree, reaching 100% amplitude.

The action potentials, moreover, are very short-lived events, typically requiring less than 1 to 2 ms to rise in amplitude to maximum potential and return to the resting state. For this reason, they are frequently referred to as spikes. They can be recorded by inserting a tiny microelectrode into a nerve fiber. When this is done, spikes can be observed even without the presentation of an acoustic stimulus, because the nerve fiber has spontaneous activity that consists of random firings of the nerve fiber. The lowest sound intensity that gives rise to a criterion percentage increase (e.g., 20% increase) in the rate at which the fiber is firing is called the threshold for that particular stimulus frequency. As stimulus intensity rises above threshold, the amplitude of the spikes does not change. They always fire at maximum response. The rate at which the nerve fiber responds, however, does increase with stimulus level. This is illustrated in Figure 3.12, in which an input-output function for a single auditory nerve fiber is displayed. The discharge rate, or *spike rate*, increases steadily with input level above the spontaneous rate until a maximum discharge rate is reached approximately 30 to 40 dB above threshold. Consequently, a single nerve fiber can code intensity via the discharge rate over only a limited range of intensities. Again, an increase in intensity is encoded by an increase in the firing rate (more spikes per second), not by an increase in the amplitude of the response.

Solid line c in Figure 3.13 depicts the frequency threshold curve (FTC) of a single auditory nerve fiber. Combinations of stimulus intensity and frequency lying within the *striped area* bordered by the FTC will cause the nerve fiber to increase its firing rate above the spontaneous rate. Combinations of frequency

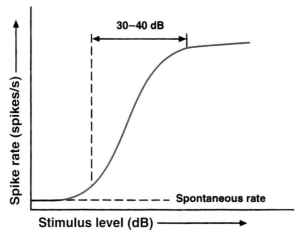

FIGURE 3.12 An input-output function for a single auditory nerve fiber. As stimulus intensity increases, the firing rate of the nerve fiber increases but only over a narrow range of 30 to 40 dB.

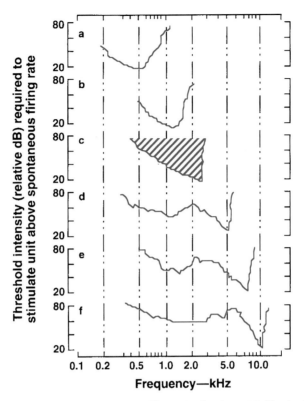

FIGURE 3.13 FTCs for six auditory nerve fibers (a–f). The FTC illustrates the intensity required at each frequency to produce a barely measurable response in the nerve fiber. The frequency requiring the lowest intensity for a response is known as the best frequency or characteristic frequency. The best frequency for each of the six nerve fibers increases from *top* (a) to the *bottom* (f). The area within each curve, illustrated in c by the striped region, represents the response area of the nerve fiber. Any combination of frequency and intensity represented in that area will yield a response from the nerve fiber.

and intensity lying outside this region fail to activate the nerve fiber. The *striped region*, therefore, is frequently referred to as the nerve fiber's response area (Vignette 3.5).

The FTC for the nerve fiber in Figure 3.13, area c, indicates that the nerve fiber responds best to a frequency of about 2,000 Hz; that is, 2,000 Hz is the frequency requiring the least amount of stimulus intensity to evoke a response from the nerve fiber. This frequency is often referred to as the best frequency or characteristic frequency of the nerve fiber. Some nerve fibers have a low characteristic frequency, and some have a high characteristic frequency. This is illustrated in the other areas of Figure 3.13. Fibers with high characteristic frequencies come from hair cells in the base of the cochlea, whereas those with

Illustration of Response Area and FTC of Nerve Fiber

The FTC of an auditory nerve fiber maps out the response area of the fiber. Combinations of stimulus frequency and intensity falling within the response area produce a response from the nerve fiber, whereas those lying outside this area fail to do so.

The figure illustrates how this area can be mapped out. A series of response histories from an auditory nerve are displayed. The vertical location of these response tracings from the nerve fiber corresponds to the level of the sound presented to the ear, as noted along the *y*-axis. The lowest tracing shows the spikes or action potentials (short vertical lines) recorded from this nerve fiber for a sound that had a level of 0-dB SPL as it increased gradually in frequency from 100 Hz (left-hand portion) to 10,000 Hz (right-hand portion). Only a few spikes occurred during the several seconds required to progress from a sound of 100 Hz to one of 10,000 Hz. This tracing essentially describes the spontaneous activity of the nerve fiber: the sound was not intense enough to produce a response in the nerve fiber.

Next, the sound stimulus is increased to 10-dB SPL (second tracing from bottom) and, again, gradually increased in frequency from 100 to 10,000 Hz. Now, there is an increase in the rate of firing (more vertical lines) near the frequency of 2,000 Hz. Thus, this particular nerve fiber appears to respond best (i.e., at the lowest sound intensity) at a frequency of 2,000 Hz. This frequency corresponds to this nerve fiber's best, or characteristic, frequency (BF or CF).

As the pure tone increases by another 10 dB to a level of 20-dB SPL, the nerve fiber reveals a broader range of frequencies to which it responds at a rate greater than its spontaneous firing rate. This range now extends from approximately 1,500 to 2,200 Hz. As the level of the tone continues to increase in 10-dB steps and sweeps the frequency from 100 to 10,000 Hz, the frequency range over which the nerve fiber responds continues to broaden. A line connecting the border between spontaneous activity and increased firing rate at each level to those at adjacent levels defines the response area. This border is essentially the FTC for the nerve fiber. The FTC is sometimes referred to as the tuning curve of the nerve fiber, because it indicates the frequency to which the nerve fiber is tuned (in this case, 2,000 Hz). The FTC indicates the response area of the fiber and its best frequency. With a best frequency of 2,000 Hz, this auditory nerve fiber originated from somewhere in the middle of the cochlea between the high-frequency basal portion and the low-frequency apex.

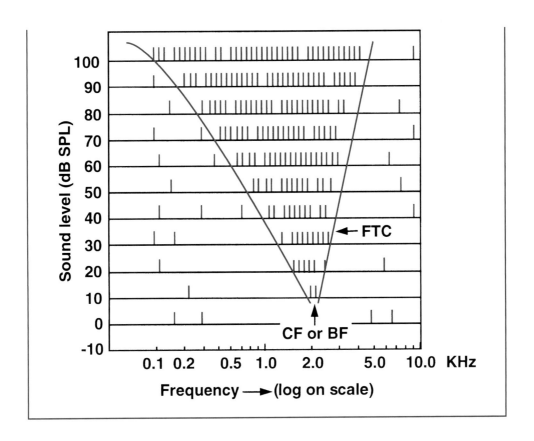

low characteristic frequencies supply the apex. As the nerve fibers exit through the bony core of the cochlea, or modiolus, on their way to the brainstem, they maintain an orderly arrangement. The bundle of nerve fibers composing the cochlear branch of the auditory nerve is organized, so that fibers with high characteristic frequencies are located around the perimeter, whereas fibers with low characteristic frequencies make up the core of the cochlear nerve. Thus, the auditory nerve is organized, as is the basilar membrane, so that each characteristic frequency corresponds to a place within the nerve bundle. This mapping of the frequency of the sound wave to place of maximum activity within an anatomic structure is referred to as **tonotopic organization**. It is a fundamental anatomic property of the auditory system from the cochlea through the auditory cortex.

Temporal or time domain information is also coded by fibers of the auditory nerve. Consider, for example, the discharge pattern that occurs within a nerve fiber when that stimulus is a sinusoid that lies within the response area of the nerve fiber. The pattern of spikes that occurs under such conditions is illustrated in Figure 3.14A. When the single nerve fiber discharges, it always does so at essentially the same location on the stimulus waveform. In Figure 3.14A,

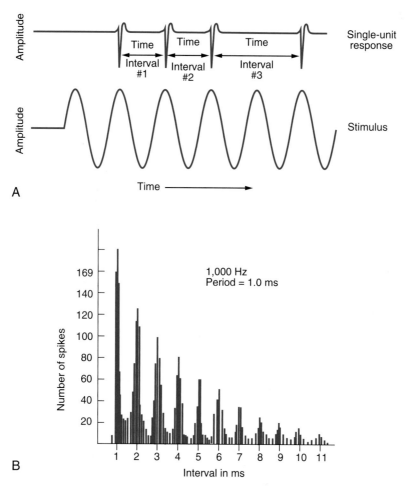

FIGURE 3.14 *A:* The synchronization of nerve fiber firings to the stimulus waveform. The nerve fiber always fires at the same point of the waveform, although it may not fire every cycle. The intervals between successive firings of the nerve fiber can be measured and stored for later analysis. *B:* A histogram of the interspike intervals measured in *A*. An interval of 1 ms was the most frequently occurring interval, having occurred approximately 180 times. This corresponds to the period of the waveform in *A*.

this happens to be the positive peak of the waveform. Notice also that it may not fire during every cycle of the stimulus waveform. Nonetheless, if one were to record the interval between successive spikes and examine the number of times each interval occurred, a histogram of the results would look like that shown in Figure 3.14B. This histogram, known simply as an interval histogram, indicates that the most frequent interspike interval corresponds to the period of the waveform. All other peaks in the histogram occur at integer multiples of the period. Thus, the nerve fiber is able to encode the period of the waveform. This holds true for nerve fibers with characteristic frequencies less than approximately 5,000 Hz. As discussed in Chapter 2, if we know the period of a sinusoidal waveform, we know its frequency ($f = 1/T$). Hence, the nerve fibers responding in the manner depicted in Figure 3.14 could code the frequency of the acoustic stimulus according to the timing of discharges. For frequencies up to 5,000 Hz, the neural firing is synchronized to the sound stimulus, as in Figure 3.14A. By combining synchronized firings for several nerve fibers, it is possible to encode the period of sounds up to 5,000 Hz in frequency.

The electrical activity of the auditory nerve can also be recorded from more remote locations. In this case, however, the action potentials are not being measured from single nerve fibers. Recorded electrical activity under these circumstances represents the composite response from a large number of nerve fibers. For this reason, this composite electrical response is referred to frequently as the whole-nerve action potential (WNAP). The WNAP can be recorded in human subjects from the ear canal or from the medial wall of the middle ear cavity by placing a needle electrode through the eardrum (with local anesthesia applied, of course!). Because the WNAP represents the summed activity of several nerve fibers, the more fibers can be made to fire simultaneously, the greater the amplitude of the response. For this reason, brief abrupt acoustic signals, such as clicks or short-duration pure tones, are used as stimuli. Recall, however, that the traveling wave begins in the base and travels toward the apex. It takes roughly 2 to 4 ms for the wave to travel the full length of the cochlea from the base to apex. Even for abrupt stimuli, such as clicks, the nerve fibers are not triggered simultaneously throughout the cochlea. Fibers associated with the basal high-frequency region respond synchronously to the stimulus presentation. Fibers originating farther up the cochlea will fire later (up to 2 to 4 ms later). Those firing in synchrony will provide the largest contribution to the WNAP. Consequently, the WNAP does not represent the activity of the entire nerve, but reflects primarily the response of the synchronous high-frequency fibers associated with the base of the cochlea.

The input-output function for the WNAP differs considerably from that described previously for single nerve fibers. For the WNAP, the response is measured in terms of its amplitude or latency, not its spike rate. The input-output function of the WNAP shows a steady increase in amplitude with increase in stimulus level. This is illustrated in Figure 3.15. Also shown is a plot of the latency of the response as a function of stimulus intensity. Latency refers to the interval between stimulus onset and the onset of the neural response. As stimulus intensity increases, the latency of the response decreases. Thus, as response amplitude increases with intensity, response latency decreases. The plot of response latency as a function of stimulus intensity is called a latency intensity function. The latency intensity function is of primary importance in clinical electrophysiologic assessment of auditory function.

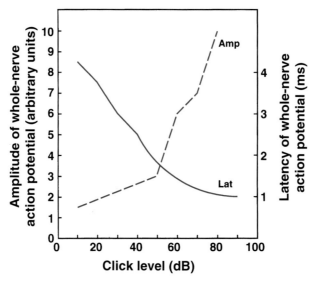

FIGURE 3.15 Amplitude intensity (*left* ordinate) and latency intensity (*right* ordinate) functions for the WNAP. As intensity increases, the amplitude (Amp) of the action potential increases, and the latency (Lat) of the response decreases.

AUDITORY CENTRAL NERVOUS SYSTEM

Once the action potentials have been generated in the cochlear branch of the auditory nerve, the electrical activity progresses up toward the cortex. This network of nerve fibers is frequently referred to as the **auditory central nervous system** (auditory CNS). The nerve fibers that carry information in the form of action potentials up the auditory CNS toward the cortex form part of the ascending or afferent pathways. Nerve impulses can also be sent toward the periphery from the cortex or brainstem centers. The fibers carrying such information compose the descending or efferent pathways.

Figure 3.16 is a simplified schematic diagram of the ascending auditory CNS. All nerve fibers from the cochlea terminate at the cochlear nucleus on the same side. From here, however, several possible paths are available. Most nerve fibers cross over, or decussate, at some point along the auditory CNS, so that the activity of the right ear is represented most strongly on the left side of the cortex and vice versa. The crossover, however, is not complete. From the superior olives through the cortex, activity from both ears is represented on each side. All ascending fibers terminate in the medial geniculate body before ascending to the cortex. Thus, all ascending fibers within the brainstem portion of the auditory CNS synapse at the cochlear nucleus and at the medial geniculate body, taking one of several paths between these two points, with many paths having additional intervening nerve fibers. Vignette 3.6 describes measurement of the auditory brainstem response (ABR) and its correlation with anatomic structure.

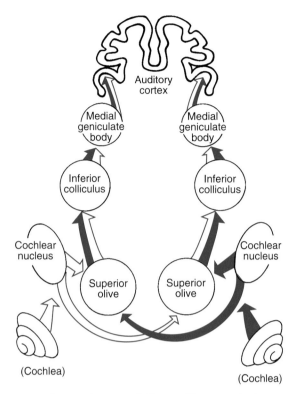

FIGURE 3.16 The ascending pathways of the auditory central nervous system. *White arrows*, input from the right ear; *blue arrows*, input from the left ear. (Adapted from Yost WA, Nielsen DW. *Fundamentals of Hearing: An Introduction*. 2nd ed. New York, NY: Holt Rinehart & Winston; 1985:98.)

VIGNETTE 3.6 • CLINICAL APPLICATIONS

Auditory Brainstem Response Measurements

It was mentioned earlier that the WNAP represented the summed response of many single nerve fibers firing synchronously in response to an abrupt acoustic signal. It was also mentioned that this potential could be recorded remotely from the ear canal. The left-hand portion of the drawing that accompanies this vignette shows a patient with electrodes pasted to the skin of the forehead, the top of the head (vertex), and the area behind the pinna (the mastoid prominence). The tracing in the right-hand portion of this illustration shows the electrical activity recorded from the patient. The acoustic stimulus is a brief click that produces synchronized responses from nerve fibers in the cochlea and the brainstem portion of the auditory CNS. The tracing represents the average of 2,000 stimuli presented at a moderate intensity at a rate of 11 clicks per second. Approximately 3 minutes is required to present all 2,000 stimuli and to obtain the average response shown here. The time scale for the *x*-axis of the tracing spans from 0 to 10 ms. This represents a 10-ms interval beginning with the onset of the click stimulus. The tracing shows several distinct bumps or waves, with the first appearing at approximately 1.5 ms after stimulus onset. This first wave, labeled *I*, is believed to be a remote recording of the WNAP from the closest portion of the auditory nerve.

Approximately 1 ms later, 2.5 ms after stimulus onset, wave *II* is observed. This wave is believed to be the response of the more distant portion of the auditory nerve. Another millisecond later, the electrical activity has traveled to the next center in the brainstem, the cochlear nucleus, and produces the response recorded as wave *III*. Wave *IV* represents the activity of the superior olivary complex. Wave *V* represents the response of the lateral lemniscus, a structure lying between the superior olives and the inferior colliculus. Waves *VI* and *VII* (the two unlabeled bumps after wave *V*) represent the response of the latter brainstem structure.

The response shown in the right-hand tracing is known as an ABR. It has proved very useful in a wide variety of clinical applications, from assessment of the functional integrity of the peripheral and brainstem portions of the ascending auditory CNS to assessment of hearing in infants or difficult-to-test patients.

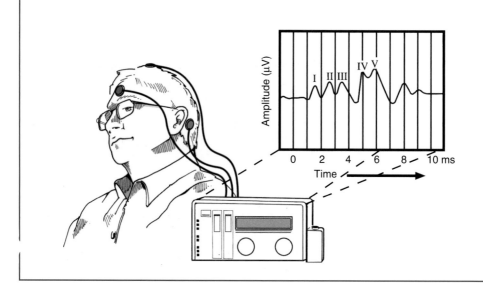

We have already reviewed the simple coding of information available in the responses of the auditory nerve fibers. The mapping of frequency to place within the cochlea, for example, was preserved in the responses of the nerve fibers in that fibers having high characteristic frequencies originated from the high-frequency base of the cochlea. The period of the waveform could also be coded for stimulus frequencies less than 5,000 Hz. In addition, the intensity of the stimulus was coded over a limited range (30 to 40 dB) by the discharge rate of the fiber. At the level of the cochlear nucleus, it is already apparent that the ascending auditory pathway begins processing information by converting this fairly simple code into more complex codes. The coding of timing information, for example, is much more complex in the cochlear nucleus. In addition, some nerve fibers within the cochlear nucleus have a much broader range of intensities (up to 100 dB) over which the discharge rate increases steadily with sound intensity. As one probes nerve fibers at various centers within the auditory CNS, a tremendous diversity of responses is evident.

Despite this increasing anatomic and physiologic complexity, one thing that appears to be preserved throughout the auditory CNS is tonotopic organization. At each brainstem center and within the auditory portions of the cortex, there is an orderly mapping of frequency to place. This can be demonstrated by measuring the characteristic frequency of nerve fibers encountered at various locations within a given brainstem center or within the cortex.

Another principle underlying the auditory CNS is redundancy. That is, information represented in the neural code from one ear has multiple representations at various locations within the auditory system. Every auditory nerve fiber, for example, splits into two fibers before entering the cochlear nucleus, with each branch supplying a different region of the cochlear nucleus. In addition, from the superior olives through the auditory areas of the cortex, information from both ears is represented at each location in the auditory CNS. This redundancy in the auditory CNS helps to protect the communication chain against breakdowns. A lesion, such as a tumor, on one side of the brainstem, for example, will not necessarily prevent information from both ears reaching the auditory portions of the cortex.

Our knowledge of the ascending pathway of the auditory CNS is far from complete. We know even less about the descending pathways. This is a result, in part, of the small number of efferent nerve fibers involved in this pathway. There are approximately 2 descending efferent fibers for every 100 ascending afferent nerve fibers. Essentially, the same brainstem centers are involved in the descending pathway as were involved in the ascending path, although an entirely separate set of nerve fibers is used. The last fiber in this descending pathway runs from the superior olivary complex to enter the cochlea on the same side or the cochlea on the opposite side. These fibers are referred to as either the crossed or the uncrossed olivocochlear bundles. Most (60% to 80%) of these fibers cross over from the superior olivary complex on one side to the cochlea on the other side and innervate the outer hair cells. The remaining fibers make up the uncrossed bundle and appear to innervate the inner hair cells.

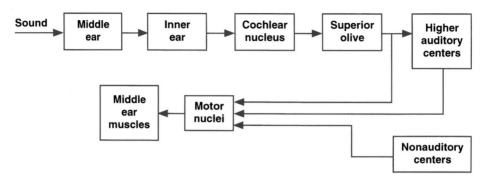

FIGURE 3.17 The reflex arc for the middle ear muscle reflex.

Not all descending fibers terminate at the cochlear nerve fibers. Descending fibers may modify incoming neurally coded sensory information at any of the centers along the auditory CNS. In addition, they may either facilitate or inhibit responses along the ascending auditory pathway. In other words, electrical stimulation of some descending fibers increases the discharges recorded from fibers at lower centers, whereas stimulation of other descending fibers results in decreased activity at lower centers. Thus, the descending efferent system regulates, modifies, and shapes the incoming sensory information.

Reflexive contractions of the middle ear muscles caused by the presentation of a sound stimulus may also be considered a regulating mechanism for the incoming sensory information. The reflex pathway is illustrated schematically in Figure 3.17. Incoming sensory information enters through the peripheral auditory system and ascends to the superior olive. If the sound is sufficiently intense, descending information is routed to motor nuclei that control the contraction of the middle ear muscles. This explains why the reflexive contraction of middle ear muscles caused by sound stimuli is a consensual phenomenon, as mentioned previously. Information from the cochlear nucleus goes to both superior olives, so that sound stimulation on one side yields middle ear muscle contraction on both sides.

CLINICAL AUDITORY ELECTROPHYSIOLOGY

In our discussion of auditory electrophysiology earlier in this chapter, we focused primarily on peripheral electrophysiology, mainly the cochlear receptor potentials and the action potentials from the auditory nerve. Much of the information reviewed was for receptor potentials from individual hair cells or action potentials from individual nerve fibers.

Although this is the most fundamental form of electrophysiologic information, clinical electrophysiology never makes use of electrical potentials from individual cells. Rather, clinical auditory electrophysiology involves the recording of gross electrical potentials representing the activity of hundreds or thousands of individual hair cells or nerve fibers. These tiny electrical potentials are usually recorded from remote locations on the surface of the head and require amplification and computer averaging of at least several hundred stimulus presentations to be visible.

To give you some perspective on the size and temporal sequence of many of the more common electric potentials used in audiology, consider the hypothetical electrical waveform in Figure 3.18. We have assumed that a special recording electrode has been placed in each ear canal and that a third electrode has been applied to the top of the scalp (vertex). The stimulus is a 2-ms burst of a 2,000-Hz pure tone, as shown in the top waveform. This stimulus is presented 1,000 times at 11 tone bursts per second, and the electrical potentials recorded have been averaged to produce the electrical waveform in the lower portion of the figure. The first electrical potentials to be recorded are the gross CM, which looks like a miniature version of the sound stimulus, and the SP, which appears as a vertical shifting of the CM away from the zero line. Next is the WNAP, which also corresponds to waves I and II of the ABR. The ABR consists of a series of five to seven bumps or waves in the electrical waveform that appear in the first 10 ms after the stimulus has been presented. Next, we have a larger and

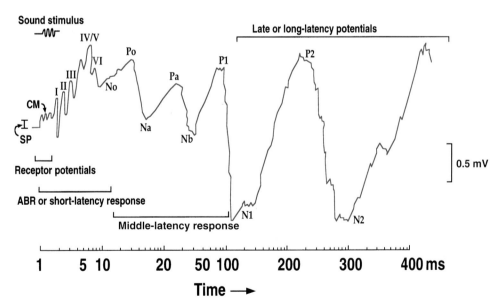

FIGURE 3.18 Hypothetical clinical electrophysiologic response recorded from the scalp of a human, showing the electrical responses from early responses of the auditory nerve through later responses from the higher centers of the auditory system (*bottom* portion) in response to a brief (2-ms) 2,000-Hz pure tone (*top* portion). *CM*, cochlear microphonic; *SP*, summating potential.

later electrical response known as the middle latency response (MLR), followed by a still larger and later potential referred to as the late evoked potential. The MLR is believed to originate from the upper portions of the auditory brainstem, and the late potential comes from the auditory cortex. Thus, the hypothetical electrical waveform shows the progression of electrical activity from the cochlea to the auditory cortex. This waveform is hypothetical in that the recording procedures and stimulus characteristics that are ideal for one type of electrical potential are often not the same ones used to record one of the other potentials. Nonetheless, it suffices to introduce the various electrical potentials that can be recorded easily from surface electrodes by the audiologist.

Of the electrical potentials available to the audiologist, the one that has received the most investigation and most frequent use clinically is the ABR. The ABR is of value because it is very robust and can be recorded reliably and easily, yet it is sensitive to dysfunction occurring from the **auditory periphery** to the upper brainstem portions of the auditory CNS. Thus, it is useful in assisting with detection of neurologic problems along a large portion of the auditory CNS; also, it can be used to estimate the hearing loss in a patient. Although a normal ABR waveform does not indicate normal auditory function (i.e., a problem could lie further up the auditory pathway), an abnormal or absent ABR waveform in response to acoustic stimulation does indicate significant hearing loss or neurologic dysfunction in approximately 95% of such cases. ABR has been used to screen the hearing of newborns and to estimate hearing thresholds in patients who are difficult to test. It is an extremely valuable clinical tool for the audiologist. Vignette 3.7 illustrates how the combined use of OAEs and the ABR led to the discovery of an intriguing disorder referred to as auditory neuropathy.

VIGNETTE 3.7 • CLINICAL APPLICATIONS

OAEs, ABR, and "Auditory Neuropathy"

Audiologists are keenly interested in applying emerging science and technology to obtain a better understanding of challenging cases encountered in the clinic. Although ABR has been used as a clinical tool since the 1970s, widespread clinical application of OAEs emerged only in the mid 1990s. In many diagnostic evaluations, both the ABR and OAEs were obtained from the same patients. After doing so with hundreds or thousands of cases, some clinicians began to notice a surprising pattern in some of these patients.

A robust ABR could not be measured, or wave latencies were prolonged considerably, despite the presence of perfectly normal OAEs! The presence of normal

OAEs, as noted previously, is an indication that the entire auditory periphery, from the outer ear to the outer hair cells within the inner ear, is normal. Yet, the ABR suggested that pathology was present in the auditory system at or below the brainstem. Most often, the abnormalities in ABR waveforms appeared first in the early waves of the response. Subsequent radiologic or surgical investigation of many of these individuals failed to detect the presence of significant brainstem or auditory nerve pathology, such as tumors. This pattern of results in the OAE and ABR measures is called auditory neuropathy and is believed to indicate a dysfunction of the inner hair cells or the first-order afferent fibers of the auditory nerve. It has been suggested that another common feature of such cases is difficulty understanding speech, especially in noisy conditions, which is greater than one would expect given the measured hearing loss. Although auditory neuropathy is believed to be a fairly rare clinical disorder, further research is being conducted to further validate its existence and to establish its prevalence. The case of auditory neuropathy, however, is just a relatively recent example of how audiologists attempt to capitalize on emerging hearing science to solve sometimes puzzling clinical problems, whether of a diagnostic or rehabilitative nature.

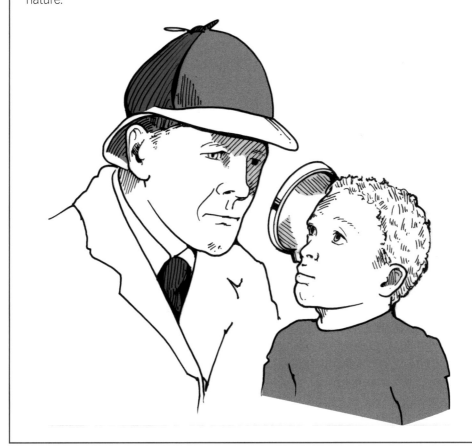

THE PERCEPTION OF SOUND

The basic structure and some key aspects of the physiologic function of the auditory system have been reviewed; the remainder of this chapter reviews some fundamental aspects of the perception of sound by humans. We have examined the acoustics involved in the generation and propagation of a sound wave and have reviewed its conversion into a complex neural code. This code of incoming sensory information can influence the behavior of a human subject, whether the sound is the loud whistle of an oncoming train or the cry of a hungry infant. The study of behavioral responses to acoustic stimulation is referred to as psychoacoustics.

Psychoacoustics

Psychoacoustics is the study of the relationship between the sound stimulus and the behavioral response it produces in the subject. We have already discussed how the important parameters of the acoustic stimulus can be measured. Much of psychoacoustics concerns itself with the more challenging task of appropriately measuring the listener's response. Two primary means have evolved through which the psychoacoustician measures responses from the listener. The first, known generally as the discrimination procedure, is used to assess the smallest difference that would allow a listener to discriminate between two stimulus conditions. The end result is an estimate of a threshold of a certain type. A tone of specified amplitude, frequency, and starting phase, for example, can be discriminated from the absence of such a signal. In this particular case, one is measuring the absolute threshold for hearing. That is, the absolute threshold is a statistical concept that represents the lowest SPL at which the tone can be heard a certain percentage of the time. This threshold is often referred to as a detection threshold, because one is determining the stimulus parameters required to detect the presence of a signal.

Discrimination procedures have also been used to measure difference thresholds. A difference threshold is a statistical concept that indicates the smallest change in a stimulus that can be detected by the listener. A standard sound that is fixed in intensity, frequency, starting phase, and duration is employed. A comparison stimulus that differs typically in one of these stimulus parameters is then presented. The difference threshold indicates how much the comparison stimulus must differ from the standard signal to permit detection of the difference by the listener a certain percentage of the time.

Many of the discrimination procedures used to measure absolute and difference thresholds were developed over a century ago. Three such procedures, referred to as the classic psychophysical methods, are (a) the method of limits, (b) the method of adjustment, and (c) the method of constant stimuli. Research conducted in more recent years has resulted in two important developments regarding the use of these procedures. First, it was recognized that thresholds measured with these procedures were not uncontaminated estimates of sensory function. Rather, thresholds measured with these procedures could be altered considerably by biasing the subject through various means, such as the use of different sets of instructions or different schedules of reinforcement for correct and incorrect responses. The threshold for the detection of a low-intensity pure tone, for example, can be changed by instructing the listener to be very certain that a tone was heard before responding accordingly or by encouraging the listener to guess when uncertain. The magnitude of sensation evoked within the sensory system during stimulus presentation should remain unchanged under these manipulations. Yet, the threshold was noticeably affected. Threshold as measured with any of these traditional psychophysical procedures is affected by factors other than the magnitude of sensation evoked by the signal. For the audiologist, however, the traditional psychophysical procedures have proven to be valid and reliable tools with which to measure various aspects of hearing in clinical settings as long as care is used in instructing the listeners and administering the procedures.

The second recent development that led to a modification of the classic psychophysical procedures was the creation of adaptive test procedures. The current procedure advocated for the measurement of absolute threshold of hearing (discussed in Chapter 7) uses an adaptive modification of the method of limits. Adaptive procedures increase the efficiency of the paradigm without sacrificing the accuracy or reliability of the procedure.

In addition to discrimination procedures, a second class of techniques has been developed to quantify a subject's responses to acoustic signals. These procedures, known generally as scaling techniques, attempt to measure sensation directly. In the study of hearing, they are used most frequently to measure the sensation of loudness, though they have also been used to quantify other sensations, such as pitch. The results from one of these procedures, magnitude estimation, are shown in Figure 3.19. In the magnitude estimation technique, subjects simply assign numbers to the perceived loudness of a series of stimuli. In the case shown in Figure 3.19, the stimuli differed only in intensity. The average results fall along a straight line when plotted on log-log coordinates. Both the x-axis and the y-axis in Figure 3.19 are logarithmic. Recall that the decibel scale, the x-axis in this figure, involved the logarithm of a pressure ratio: SPL in decibels = 20 log (p_1/p_2). Comparable results have been obtained for other sensations, such as brightness, vibration on the fingertip, and electric shock. In all cases, a straight line fits the average data very well when plotted on log-log coordinates. From these extensive data, a law was developed to relate the perceived magnitude of sensation (S) to the physical intensity of the stimulus (I) in the following manner: $S = kI^x$, where k is an arbitrary constant, and x is an

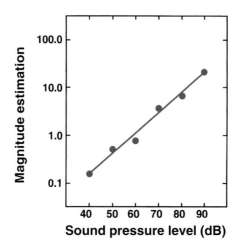

FIGURE 3.19 Hypothetical results from a magnitude estimation experiment in which the perceived loudness was measured for various sound levels. The results fall along a straight line when both axes are logarithmic (recall use of logarithms in the calculation of decibels).

exponent that varies with the sensation under investigation. This law is known as Stevens power law in honor of the scientist S. S. Stevens, who discovered and developed it. A convenient feature of a power function plotted on log-log coordinates is that the slope of the line fit to the data is the exponent, x.

Finally, a procedure that has been used extensively in psychoacoustics to measure auditory sensations via the subject's response is the matching procedure. The matching procedure is a cross between discrimination procedures and scaling procedures. The technique is similar to that of the method of adjustment (one of the classic psychophysical methods), but its goal is to quantify a subjective attribute of sound, such as loudness or pitch. The matching procedures enable the experimenter to determine a set of stimulus parameters that all yield the same subjective sensation. A pure tone fixed at 1,000 Hz and 70-dB SPL, for example, may be presented to one ear of a listener and a second pure tone of 8,000 Hz presented to the other ear in an alternating fashion. The subject controls the intensity of the 8,000-Hz tone until it is judged to be equal in loudness to the 1,000-Hz, 70-dB SPL reference tone. Data in the literature indicate that the 8,000-Hz tone would have to be set to 80- to 85-dB SPL to achieve a loudness match in the case presented above.

Hearing Threshold

Let us now examine how these procedures have been applied to the study of the perception of sound. The results obtained from the measurement of hearing thresholds at various frequencies are depicted in Figure 3.20. The SPL that

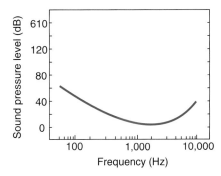

FIGURE 3.20 Average normal threshold SPL plotted as a function of frequency for binaural (two-ear) listening in a free field. (Adapted from Sivian LJ, White SD. Minimum audible pressure and minimum audible field. *J Acoust Soc Am* 1933;4:288–321.)

is just detectable varies with frequency, especially below 500 Hz and above 8,000 Hz. The slope of the function in the low frequencies is a result of the attenuation of lower frequencies by the middle ear. The frequency contour of the hearing threshold has a minimum in the 2,000- to 4,000-Hz range. This is attributable, in large part, to the amplification of signals in this frequency range by the outer ear, as discussed earlier in this chapter. The range of audibility of the normal-hearing human ear is described frequently as 20 to 20,000 Hz. Acoustic signals at frequencies above or below this range typically cannot be heard by the normal human ear.

Masking

The phenomenon of masking has also been studied in detail. Masking refers to the ability of one acoustic signal to obscure the presence of another acoustic signal so that it cannot be detected. A whisper might be audible, for example, in a quiet environment. In a noisy industrial environment, however, such a weak acoustic signal would be masked by the more intense factory noise.

The masking of pure tone signals by noise has been studied extensively. To consider the results, however, we must first examine some important acoustic characteristics of the masking noise. Briefly, two measures of intensity can be used to describe the level of a noise. These two measures are the total power (TP) and the noise power per unit (1-Hz) bandwidth, or spectral density (N_o). The TP in decibels SPL is the quantity measured by most measuring devices, such as sound level meters. The N_o of the noise in decibels is not measured directly with a sound level meter. Rather, it is calculated from the following equation: $10 \log_{10} N_o = 10 \log_{10} TP - 10 \log_{10} BW$, where BW is the bandwidth of the noise in hertz. The quantity $10 \log 10\ N_o$ is the spectrum level in units of decibels SPL per hertz and

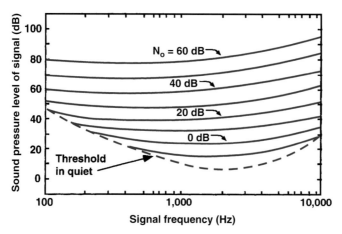

FIGURE 3.21 Threshold in quiet and masked threshold for various noise spectrum levels (N_o). Threshold was measured at several frequencies in the presence of a broadband noise. (Adapted from Hawkins JE Jr, Stevens SS. The masking of pure tones and of speech by white noise. *J Acoust Soc Am* 1950;22:6–13.)

represents the average noise power in a 1-Hz band. For broadband noises, the spectrum level determines the masking produced at various frequencies.

Figure 3.21 illustrates data obtained from one of the early studies of masking produced by broadband noise. These data have been replicated several times since. The lowest curve in this figure depicts the threshold in a quiet environment; all other curves represent masked thresholds obtained for various levels of the noise masker. These levels are expressed as the spectrum level of the masker. The lowest noise levels are not effective maskers at low frequencies. That is, hearing thresholds measured for low-frequency pure tones in the presence of a broadband noise having N_o = 0 dB SPL/Hz are the same as thresholds in quiet. At all frequencies, however, once the noise begins to produce some masking, a 10-dB increase in noise intensity produces a 10-dB increase in masked threshold for the pure tone. Once the noise level that just begins to produce masking has been determined, the desired amount of masking can be produced simply by increasing the noise level by a corresponding amount.

How might the masking produced by a noise be affected by decreasing the bandwidth of the noise? Figure 3.22 illustrates data obtained several decades ago from a now-classic masking experiment. The results of this experiment, referred to frequently as the band-narrowing experiment, have been replicated several times since. Masked threshold in decibels, SPL is plotted as a function of the bandwidth of the masker in hertz. Results for two different pure-tone frequencies are shown. The *open circles* represent data for a 1,000-Hz pure tone, and the *solid circles* depict data for a 4,000-Hz pure tone. When the band of masking noise was narrowed, the tone was kept in the center of the noise,

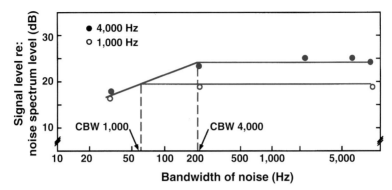

FIGURE 3.22 Results from a band-narrowing experiment. Data for two frequencies, 1,000 and 4,000 Hz, are shown. The critical bandwidths at each frequency are illustrated by *dashed vertical lines*. For bandwidths greater than the critical bandwidth (CBW), masking remained unchanged. (Data from Fletcher H. Auditory patterns. *Rev Mod Phys* 1940;12:47–65.)

and the spectrum level of the noise was held constant. For both frequencies, the masked threshold remains the same as the bandwidth decreases to a level called the critical bandwidth. Continued decreases in bandwidth beyond the critical bandwidth reduce the masking produced by the noise, as reflected in the decrease in masked threshold.

The critical bandwidth, first derived from the band-narrowing masking experiment, has proved to apply to a wide variety of psychoacoustic phenomena. For the audiologist, however, one of the most important implications drawn from the band-narrowing experiment is that noise having a bandwidth just exceeding the critical bandwidth is as effective a masker for a pure tone centered in the noise as a broadband noise of the same spectrum level. As Chapter 7 shows, the audiologist frequently must introduce masking into a patient's ear. A broadband masking noise can be uncomfortably loud to a patient. The loudness can be reduced by decreasing its bandwidth while maintaining the same spectrum level. A masking noise having a bandwidth only slightly greater than the critical bandwidth will be just as effective as broadband noise in terms of its masking but much less loud. The narrow band of noise is more appropriate for use as a masking sound when measuring hearing threshold for pure tones in patients because of its reduced loudness but equal masking capability.

Loudness

Loudness is another psychoacoustic phenomenon that has been studied extensively. The effects of signal bandwidth on loudness, alluded to in the discussion of masking, have been investigated in detail. Basically, as the bandwidth of the stimulus increases beyond the critical bandwidth, an increasing number of adjacent critical bands are stimulated, resulting in an increase in loudness. Thus, broadband signals are louder than narrow-band signals at the same spectrum level.

For pure tones, loudness also varies with frequency. This has been established using the matching procedure described previously. Figure 3.23 depicts so-called equal-loudness contours that have been derived with this technique. A given contour displays the SPL at various frequencies necessary to match the loudness of a 1,000-Hz pure tone at the level indicated by the contour. For example, on the curve labeled *20*, the function coincides with an SPL of 20-dB SPL at 1,000 Hz, whereas on the curve labeled *60*, the function corresponds to 60-dB SPL at 1,000 Hz. The contour labeled *60* indicates combinations of frequencies and intensities that were matched in loudness to a 60-dB SPL, 1,000-Hz pure tone. All combinations of stimulus intensity and frequency lying along that contour are said to have a loudness level of 60 phons (pronounced *phones*, as in *telephones*). Thus, a 125-Hz pure tone at 70-dB SPL (point labeled *A* in Fig. 3.23) and an 8,000-Hz tone at 58 dB SPL (point labeled *B*) are equivalent

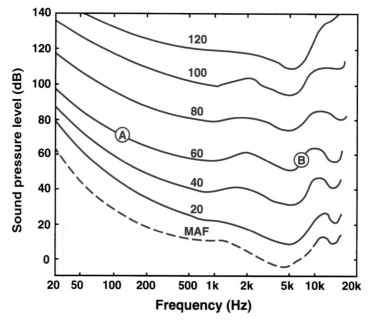

FIGURE 3.23 Equal-loudness contours. Each curve displays the combinations of frequency and intensity judged to be equal in loudness to a 1,000-Hz tone having SPL as indicated above each contour. Point A indicates that a 125-Hz tone at 75-dB SPL is as loud as a 1,000-Hz tone at 60 dB. (Frequency scale is logarithmic.) *MAF*, minimum audible field, or the threshold contour for free-field testing. (Adapted from Fletcher H, Munson WN. Loudness, its definition, measurement, and calculation. *J Acoust Soc Am* 1933;5:82–108.)

in loudness to a 60-dB SPL, 1,000-Hz pure tone. All three of those stimuli have a loudness level of 60 phons.

In Figure 3.23 stimulus intensity must be increased by 110 dB to go from a loudness level of 10 phons (threshold) to 120 phons at 1,000 Hz. At 100 Hz, only an 80-dB increase is required to span that same change in loudness. From this, we can conclude that loudness increases more rapidly at low frequencies than at intermediate frequencies. It took only an 80-dB increase in sound level to go from a sound that was just audible (10 phons) to one that was uncomfortably loud (120 phons) at 100 Hz, whereas an increase of 110 dB was needed to cover this same range of loudness at 1,000 Hz.

Another scale of loudness is the sone scale, derived by first defining the loudness of a 1,000-Hz, 40-dB SPL pure tone as 1 sone. Next, the listener is asked to set the intensity of a second comparison stimulus so that it produces a loudness sensation either one-half or twice that of the 1-sone standard stimulus. These intensities define the sound levels associated with 0.5 and 2 sones, respectively. This procedure is repeated, with the sound having a loudness of either 0.5 or 2 sones serving as the new standard signal. Figure 3.24 illustrates the relationship between the increase of loudness in sones and the increase in sound intensity. Consistent with Stevens law, described previously, we find that the loudness-growth function is a straight line, with the exception of intensities near threshold, when plotted on log-log coordinates. The slope of this line is 0.6, indicating that Stevens law for loudness is $L = k\, P^{0.6}$, where L is loudness, k is a constant, and P is sound pressure. Over the linear range of the function in Figure 3.24, a 10-dB increase in SPL yields a doubling of loudness.

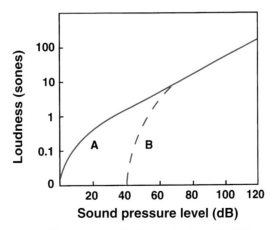

FIGURE 3.24 The growth of loudness with intensity in quiet (A) and in the presence of a background noise that produced 40 dB of masking (B). (Loudness scale is logarithmic.) Functions comparable to *B* are also obtained in listeners who have sensorineural hearing loss.

At 1,000 Hz, an increase in SPL from 40 to 50 dB SPL or from 80 to 90 dB SPL corresponds to a doubling of loudness.

The *dashed line* in Figure 3.24 illustrates a loudness growth function obtained at 1,000 Hz in the presence of a broadband-masking noise. The intersection of the x-axis by the *dashed line* at 40-dB SPL indicates that the threshold has been elevated 40 dB (from 0 to 40 dB SPL) because of the masking noise. As intensity increases slightly above threshold, comparison of the two functions indicates that the loudness of a 50-dB SPL tone is greater in the quiet condition (2 sones) than in the masked condition (0.2 sones). At higher intensities, however, the two functions merge, so that an 80-dB SPL tone has a loudness of 16 sones in both cases. Thus, in the masked condition, loudness grows very rapidly to catch up with the loudness perceived in the unmasked condition. This rapid growth of loudness is also a characteristic of ears that have sensorineural hearing loss, which affects the hair cells in the cochlea. The rapid growth of loudness in ears with sensorineural hearing loss is known as loudness recruitment. Its presence helps signify that the hearing loss is caused by pathology within the cochlea. As will be noted later, this represents a potential "break" in the communication chain with input to the higher centers distorted by a loss of hair cells in the cochlea. In this particular case of loss of outer hair cells only, the conventional hearing aid represents a reasonable approach to the repair of the communication chain. Unfortunately, loudness recruitment presents the audiologist with considerable difficulties in attempting to fit affected patients with amplification devices, such as hearing aids. Low-level sounds must be amplified a specified amount to make them audible to the listener with hearing loss. If high-level sounds are amplified by the same amount, however, they are uncomfortably loud, just as they would be in a normal ear.

Loudness is clearly one of the more salient perceptual features of a sound, and it has considerable clinical importance. Pitch is another very salient perceptual feature of sound, but it has less clinical relevance. Some basic aspects of pitch perception in normal listeners have been summarized in Vignette 3.8 as illustrated through the case of the missing fundamental.

Binaural Hearing

The final section of this chapter deals with the manner in which the information encoded by one ear interacts with that encoded by the other ear. The processing of sound by two ears is referred to as binaural hearing.

The localization of sound in space is largely a binaural phenomenon. A sound originating on the right side of a listener will arrive first at the right ear because it is closer to the sound source. A short time later, the sound will reach the more distant left ear. This produces an interaural (between-ear) difference

VIGNETTE 3.8 • FURTHER DISCUSSION

Pitch Perception and the Case of the Missing Fundamental

The pitch of a sound is often one of its most salient perceptual characteristics. Musicians and hearing scientists have been interested in how humans perceive pitch for centuries, but probably the greatest progress in our understanding of pitch perception occurred during the twentieth century.

In the late nineteenth century, probably the most widely accepted theory of pitch perception was based on a "place principle" akin to tonotopic organization, described in the discussion of basic auditory structure and function. Although many details of early place principle theories of pitch perception were incorrect, the basic premise that certain portions of the auditory system, especially the inner ear, were tuned to specific frequencies was correct. Basically, low-frequency pure tones produced a low pitch sensation and high-frequency pure tones produced a high pitch sensation because each frequency stimulated a different region or place within the inner ear.

In the late nineteenth and early twentieth centuries, however, several researchers in the Netherlands produced a low-frequency pitch using sounds that were composed of only higher frequencies. An example of the amplitude spectrum for one such sound is shown in the figure. This sound is composed of pure tones at frequencies of 800, 1,000, 1,200, and 1,400 Hz. Yet, the pitch of this sound was judged to be 200 Hz by listeners. A frequency of 200 Hz would correspond to the fundamental frequency of these sounds, with 800 Hz being the fourth harmonic of 200 Hz (i.e., 800 Hz = 4 × 200 Hz), 1,000 Hz being the fifth harmonic, 1,200 Hz being the sixth harmonic, and 1,400 Hz being the seventh harmonic of 200 Hz. For this reason, the pitch of such a series of pure tones is often referred to as the missing fundamental.

Now, the place theorists simply argued that the equipment or the ear (the middle ear was believed to be the culprit at the time) generated a distortion product that corresponded to the 200-Hz frequency, and the listener's pitch perception was dominated by this low-frequency distortion tone. Therefore, the fundamental frequency (200 Hz) wasn't really missing after all. In this way, the results were entirely consistent with the place theory. The complex of four pure tones from 800 to 1,400 Hz generated a distortion product at 200 Hz, and this 200-Hz distortion product stimulated the place associated with a 200-Hz pure tone yielding a corresponding pitch.

To counter this argument, the Dutch researchers conducted the following experiment. A low-frequency noise was introduced with enough acoustical energy below 400 Hz to mask low-frequency tones of moderate intensity (e.g., as demonstrated with a pure tone at 200 Hz). The four pure tones from 800 to 1,400 Hz were played in this background of low-frequency noise, and a pitch of 200 Hz was again perceived. Basically, the low-frequency masking noise rendered the low-frequency region of the inner ear unusable, and yet a low-frequency pitch was still perceived when the four tones from 800 to 1,400 Hz were presented. Clearly, the place theory could not account for these findings.

Recognizing the limitations of the place theory as a single explanation for the perception of pitch, hearing scientists began to focus on possible timing, or periodicity, cues in the four-tone complex. Today, although several details of pitch perception remain unexplained, most findings can be described by a duplex theory. This theory relies on exclusive use of place cues above approximately 5,000 Hz (synchronization of nerve fiber firing breaks down at frequencies above approximately 5,000 Hz, making periodicity cues unavailable). It also rests on exclusive use of timing cues for very low frequencies, below approximately 50 Hz, and a combination of periodicity and place cues for frequencies from 50 to 5,000 Hz.

Incidentally, there is a standardized scale of pitch sensation, the mel scale (no, not named after a famous scientist named Mel, but derived from *melody*). A pure tone of 1,000 Hz at 40-dB SPL is said to have a pitch of 1,000 mels (as well as a loudness of 1 sone and a loudness level of 40 phons). A sound with a pitch judged to be twice as high as this standard would have a pitch of 2,000 mels, whereas one with half the pitch of the standard sound would be assigned a pitch value of 500 mels. Often, however, pitch is measured by matching the frequency of a pure tone to the perceived pitch of the sound under evaluation.

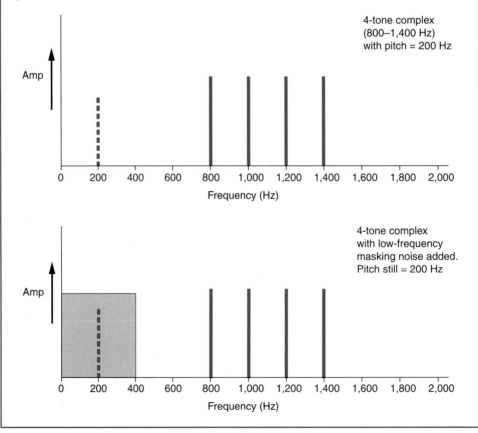

in the time of arrival of the sound at the two ears. The ear being stimulated first will signal the direction from which the sound arose. As might be expected, the magnitude of this interaural time difference will increase as the location of the sound source changes from straight ahead (called 0-degree azimuth) to straight out to the side (90-degree or 270-degree azimuth). As shown in Figure 3.25A, when the sound originates directly in front of the listener, the length of the path to both ears is the same, and there is no interaural difference in time of arrival of the sound. At the extreme right or left, however, the difference between the length of the path to the near ear and the length of the path to the far ear is

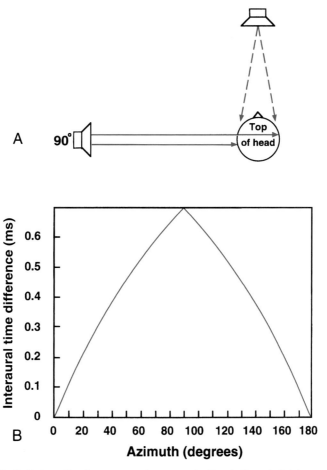

FIGURE 3.25 *A:* Path lengths from sound source to the left and right ears for 0-degree azimuth (*dashed lines*) and 90-degree azimuth (*solid lines*). *B:* The interaural time differences as a function of azimuth for the spherical head assumed in *A.* At 0 degree and 180 degrees, the sound arrives at the left and right ears simultaneously, resulting in no interaural time difference. The maximum interaural time difference occurs at 90 degrees.

greatest (and corresponds to the width of the head). This then will produce the maximum interaural time difference. Figure 3.25B illustrates the dependence of the interaural time difference on the azimuth of the sound source.

For frequencies below approximately 1,500 Hz, the interaural time difference could also be encoded meaningfully into an interaural phase difference. Figure 3.25B shows that a 60-degree azimuth results in an interaural time difference of approximately 0.5 ms. This occurs for all frequencies. For a pure tone that completes one cycle in 1 ms (frequency = 1,000 Hz), this means that the signal to the far ear would be starting 0.5 cycles after the signal to the near ear. The two signals therefore would have a 180-degree phase difference between the two ears. A pure tone of 500 Hz having a 2-ms period and originating from a 60-degree azimuth, however, would only be delayed one-fourth of the period (0.5 ms/2.0 ms), corresponding to a 90-degree interaural phase difference. Thus, although interaural time differences are the same for all frequencies, the interaural phase differences resulting from these time differences vary with frequency.

Interaural intensity differences are also produced when a sound originates from a location in space. These differences result from a sound shadow being cast by the head. Recall from Chapter 2 and Vignette 2.5 that when the wavelength of the sound is small relative to the dimensions of the object, a sound shadow is produced. The magnitude of the sound shadow created by the head increases with frequency above 500 Hz. It produces interaural intensity differences of 20 dB at 6,000 Hz for 90-degree or 270-degree azimuth. The intensity of a 6,000-Hz pure tone at the near ear is 20 dB greater than that measured at the far ear when the sound originates straight to the side of the listener (90-degree or 270-degree azimuth). At 500 Hz, the maximum interaural intensity difference is less than 4 dB. The interaural intensity difference decreases to 0 dB at all frequencies for 0-degree azimuth (sound source straight ahead).

Thus, there are two primary acoustic cues for the localization of sound in space (specifically, the horizontal plane): interaural time differences and interaural intensity differences. The duplex theory of sound localization in the horizontal plane (left to right) maintains that both cues may be used over a wide range of frequencies by the listener in identifying the location of a sound source but that interaural time differences predominate at low frequencies and interaural intensity differences predominate at high frequencies. In contemporary theories of sound localization, several additional monaural and binaural cues are included, but interaural time and intensity differences are considered the strongest cues.

Masking has also been explored in considerable detail in the binaural system. Experiments conducted in the late 1940s and the 1950s indicated that certain combinations of binaural signals and maskers could make the signal more detectable than others. Consider the following example. A noise masker and a pure-tone signal are presented equally and identically to both ears. The signal threshold, that is, the sound level of the signal required to make it barely heard in the presence of the noise, is determined. Then, the pure-tone signal is removed from one ear, and the signal becomes *easier* to detect! This release from masking, named the masking level difference (MLD), corresponds to the change in threshold between two test conditions. The initial or reference threshold is usually determined for identical maskers and signals delivered to both ears. This is referred to as a diotic condition. Diotic stimulus presentations are those that deliver identical stimuli to both ears. Sometimes the reference threshold involves a masker and signal delivered to only one ear. This is called a monotic or monaural condition. After establishing the masked threshold in one of these reference conditions, the signal threshold is measured again under any one of several dichotic conditions. A dichotic test condition is one in which different stimuli are presented to the two ears. In the example in which the signal was removed from one ear, the removal of the signal made that condition a dichotic one. That is, one ear received the masker and the pure-tone signal, while the other received only the masker. In general, a signal is more readily detected under dichotic masking conditions than under diotic or monaural masking conditions. For a given dichotic condition, the MLD is greatest at low frequencies (100 to 500 Hz), increases with the intensity of the masker, and is typically 12 to 15 dB under optimal stimulus conditions.

SUMMARY

In this chapter, we have seen how the acoustic information, serving as the link between the sender and the receiver in the communication chain, is encoded by the auditory system. Initially, the pressure fluctuations corresponding to the acoustic speech sounds are converted into mechanical vibrations of the middle ear and the organ of Corti. These mechanical vibrations are converted to electrical signals by the organ of Corti and ultimately lead to the generation of electrical signals in the auditory nerve. The sensory input representing the acoustic speech stimulus is now in the "electrical language" of the brain and is subject to further processing by the auditory centers of the brainstem and cortex. This neural auditory information in the auditory cortex is then processed, as needed, by other centers of the brain, such as various language-processing centers, to make sense of the incoming sensory information. Impairments in the auditory periphery or auditory portions of the central nervous system can result in "breaks" in the communication chain, with degraded neural information reaching the higher centers of the auditory system. The identification of such impairments is the focus of the Chapter 7.

CHAPTER REVIEW QUESTIONS

1. What are the primary functions of the outer ear?
2. What is the primary function of the middle ear, and what is the main anatomical feature that supports this function?
3. The eustachian tube serves two main functions. What are they?
4. Define tonotopic organization. Where does it originate? Based on this anatomical organization, if an individual lost all inner and outer hair cells in the base of the cochlea, what sound frequencies would this person have difficulty hearing?
5. What is meant by the "transducer function" of the cochlea?
6. Frequency can be encoded by the auditory periphery using a placed-based code or a timing-based code. Explain what this means.
7. What structures represent the beginning and ending of the auditory central nervous system?
8. Aside from the initial letter in their spelling, what is the difference between "afferent" and "efferent" nerve fibers?
9. In very general terms, loudness and pitch can be considered to be the perceptual correlates of what two physical aspects of sound waves?

REFERENCES AND SUGGESTED READINGS

Durrant JD, Lovrinic JH. *Bases of Hearing Science*. 2nd ed. Baltimore, MD: Lippincott Williams & Wilkins; 1995.

Geisler CD. *From Sound to Synapse*. New York, NY: Oxford University Press; 1998.

Gelfand SA. *Hearing: An Introduction to Psychological and Physiological Acoustics*. 3rd ed. New York, NY: Marcel Dekker; 1997.

Hall JW. *Handbook of Auditory Evoked Responses*. Needham, MA: Allyn & Bacon; 1992.

Kidd J. Psychoacoustics. In: Katz J, ed. *Handbook of Clinical Audiology*. 5th ed. Philadelphia, PA: Lippincott Williams & Wilkins; 2002.

Möller AR. *Auditory Physiology*. New York, NY: Academic Press; 1983.

Moore BCJ. *An Introduction to the Psychology of Hearing*. 4th ed. London, UK: Academic Press; 1997.

Pickles JO. *An Introduction to the Physiology of Hearing*. 2nd ed. London, UK: Academic Press; 1988.

Probst R, Lonsbury-Martin BL, Martin G. A review of otoacoustic emissions. *J Acoust Soc Am* 1991;89:2027–2067.

Shaw EAG. The external ear. In: Keidel WD, Neff WD, eds. *Handbook of Sensory Physiology*. Vol. 1. New York, NY: Springer Verlag; 1974:455–490.

von Bekesy G. *Experiments in Hearing*. New York, NY: McGraw-Hill; 1960.

Wever EG, Lawrence M. *Physiological Acoustics*. Princeton, NJ: Princeton University Press; 1954.

Yost WA. *Fundamentals of Hearing: An Introduction*. 4th ed. New York, NY: Academic Press; 2000.

Zemlin WR. *Speech and Hearing Science: Anatomy and Physiology*. 2nd ed. Englewood Cliffs, NJ: Prentice-Hall; 1988.

Zwicker E, Fastl H. *Psychoacoustics*. 2nd ed. Berlin, Germany: Springer-Verlag; 1999.

Audiology and Speech-Language Pathology as Professions

4

Audiology as a Profession

- To discuss the prevalence of hearing loss and the complications associated with hearing impairment;
- To define the profession of audiology;
- To appreciate the lineage of the profession of audiology;
- To describe the employment opportunities available to the audiologist;
- To understand the academic and clinical requirements needed to become an audiologist; and
- To appreciate the essential accreditations and professional affiliations important to clinical audiology.

- **Prevalence:** The total number of cases of a condition in a given population at a specific time.
- **Individuals with Disabilities Education Improvement Act (IDEIA, 2004):** The legislative provision to insure that all children with disabilities receive a free and appropriate education.
- **Inclusion:** The practice of placing children with disabilities in regular classrooms as opposed to special education classes.

Breaks in the communication chain can occur at a variety of places, sometimes in the sender or speaker, sometimes in the receiver or listener, and sometimes at the link between them, such as bad room acoustics or background noise. For those that occur in the speaker that are a result of a speech or expressive language disorder, most often a speech-language pathologist would be the professional involved in diagnosis and treatment of problems, at least those not requiring medical intervention. The focus in this book, however, is on the auditory aspects of the communication chain. As a result, the breaks in the chain considered here are most often in the receiver or listener. However, for severe breaks in the auditory portions of the communication chain resulting in substantial bilateral hearing loss, the speech of the person experiencing such a break may also be impaired (see Chapter 1). For breaks in the auditory portions of the communication chain, the professional involved in the measurement and treatment of hearing loss is most often an audiologist, at least for those disorders not amenable to medical intervention. This chapter describes the profession of audiology and gives the reader a glimpse of many aspects of this exciting profession. Chapter 5 provides a somewhat parallel description of the profession of speech-language pathology, with emphasis on the roles of these professionals in the management of hearing loss—especially in children.

The discussion in this chapter focuses on several areas. First, statistics on the total number of cases of hearing loss, or the prevalence of hearing loss, are reviewed. The impact of hearing loss on the well-being of the individual is also briefly described. These two areas are reviewed to give the reader some sense of the magnitude of the problem, both on a national scale and as it is experienced by the affected individuals themselves. Next, the definition and historical evolution of audiology are reviewed. Various employment opportunities in this health-related discipline are surveyed. The chapter concludes with a summary of typical graduate and professional training programs in audiology, a brief discussion of accreditation/licensure, and a description of some of the professional affiliations that audiologists find worthwhile.

PREVALENCE AND IMPACT OF HEARING LOSS

Before a discussion of audiology as a profession, it is helpful to develop some understanding of the nature of hearing loss in the United States. The estimated **prevalence**, or total number of existing cases of hearing loss, varies according to several factors. These factors include (a) how hearing loss was determined (i.e., questionnaire versus hearing test), (b) the criterion or formula used to define the presence of a hearing loss (severe versus mild hearing loss), and (c) the age of the individuals in the population sampled (adults versus children). Regardless of the methods used to determine prevalence, hearing loss is known to affect a large segment of the population in the United States. Studies focusing on the population under 18 years of age estimate that approximately 56,000 children under age 6 years are living with significant hearing loss in both ears. "Significant hearing loss" means that these children exhibit a hearing deficit in both ears, with the better ear exhibiting some difficulty in hearing and understanding speech. It has also been estimated that 2 to 3 of every 1,000 infants in the United States are born with a congenital hearing loss in the moderate to severe range. These data do not include children born with normal hearing who develop hearing loss later, a condition commonly referred to as progressive hearing loss. If young children with the milder forms of hearing loss are included, the prevalence rate is thought to involve significantly more children; estimates range from 120 in 1,000 to 150 in 1,000. Assuming a prevalence rate of 130 in 1,000 and a school-age population of 46 million (kindergarten through grade 12), the number of school-age children with some degree of hearing loss is approximately 3.5 million. These data should be viewed in light of the fact that elementary school enrollment is expected to increase as the baby boomlet continues to swell the school-age ranks.

Estimates of the prevalence of hearing loss for the adult population as a whole and for various age groups are summarized in Table 4.1. This table illustrates that based on figures from 2010, the total number of persons over 18 years of age with hearing loss in the United States is slightly more than 37 million. Also note that the prevalence rate for hearing loss increases with age. For example, in

TABLE

4.1

Prevalence and Prevalence Rates According to Age for Hearing Loss in the United States (18 y and over)

Age Group (y)	Prevalence (In Millions)	Prevalence Rate (Per Thousand)
All ages (total)	37.1	161.7
18–44	7.4	67.3
45–64	15.1	189.4
65–74	6.6	311.3
75+	7.8	451.2

Data were obtained from household interviews and reflect the prevalence of hearing loss in either one ear or both ears.
Adapted from Schiller, JS, Lucas, JW, Ward, BW, et al. Summary health statistics for US adults: National Health Interview Survey, 2010. National Center for Health Statistics. *Vital Health Stat 10* 2012;(252):1–207.

the age category of 18 to 44 years, the prevalence rate is 67.3 in 1,000, whereas for the age groups 65 to 74 years and 75 years and older, the prevalence rates are 311.3 in 1,000 and 451.2 in 1,000, respectively. These statistics confirm what many of us with living grandparents and great-grandparents already know: hearing loss is commonly associated with old age. This is particularly important when one considers the number of elderly persons in the United States and the projected growth rates of the aged population. The number of individuals older than 65 years exceeds 40 million, and that figure is expected to increase to more than 88 million by the year 2050. This substantial increase in longevity has stemmed in part from the medical profession's improved success in controlling infectious and chronic diseases.

The preceding paragraphs establish that many Americans of all ages have significant hearing problems. Although statistics such as these are important, they provide little insight into the devastating impact that a significant hearing loss can have on the individual. Children born with a severe or profound hearing loss experience the greatest hardship and under most circumstances exhibit a significant lag in educational progress. This is because the hearing loss interferes with the child's speech perception ability, which in turn may result in impairment of speech and language development, reduction in academic achievement, and disturbances in social and emotional development. Because the development of our language system depends heavily on auditory input, a reduction or elimination of auditory input drastically curtails the ability to learn speech and language. To illustrate, it has been noted that the average high-school graduate from a state school for the deaf has the equivalent of an eighth-grade education. Even children with hearing losses in only one ear or very mild losses in both ears may experience difficulties in speech or language development, speech recognition under adverse listening conditions (e.g., classroom noise), educational achievement, and psychosocial behavior. Although these communication and educational outcomes are likely to improve with recent advances in early identification and intervention for hearing loss, the definitive evidence to support this is still being accumulated by researchers.

Children are not the only ones affected negatively by significant hearing loss. Hearing loss in the adult can produce a number of psychosocial complications. For the elderly adult, the deterioration in hearing sensitivity and the associated problems with understanding speech are known to affect the quality of the individual's daily living. That is, the elderly who have hearing loss are more likely than those with normal hearing to have poor general health, reduced mobility, fewer excursions outside the home, fewer interpersonal contacts, more depression and anxiety, and increased tension.

Hearing loss also imposes a significant economic burden; relatively few deaf individuals are employed in professional, technical, and managerial positions. Moreover, the lifetime cost of deafness is substantial. The overall societal costs

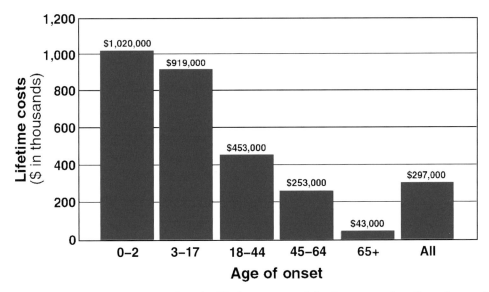

FIGURE 4.1 Bar graph illustrating the lifetime costs of deafness as a function of age of onset. (Adapted from Mohr PE, Feldman JJ, Dunbar JL. The societal costs of severe to profound hearing loss in the United States. *Int J Technol Assess Health Care* 2000; 16(4): 1120–1135. Project Hope Center for Health Affairs, Policy Analysis Brief, 2000.)

of deafness include such factors as diagnosis, periodic medical visits, audiologic evaluations, hearing aid fittings, assistive listening devices, special education, rehabilitation, and loss of potential income. As shown in Figure 4.1, the cost of deafness increases as age of onset decreases. For the child who is deaf before learning to talk, the lifetime cost exceeds $1 million, whereas lifetime cost is much less for individuals who acquire hearing loss later in life. Overall, the lifetime cost of deafness averages $297,000. Other less tangible costs borne by affected individuals and by their families derive from emotional stress, breakdowns in family communication, and isolation from peer and educational systems.

In summary, hearing loss occurs in large numbers of people and affects both children and adults. In addition, the prevalence rate of hearing loss increases markedly for the elderly population. Finally, the overall impact of hearing loss in both children and adults is significant, causing delays in the psychoeducational progress of children and producing serious psychosocial consequences for those who acquire hearing loss later in life.

AUDIOLOGY DEFINED

Audiology is typically subdivided into specialties according to the nature of the population served or the setting in which the audiologist is employed (Vignette 4.1). For example, a common area of specialization is pediatric audiology, in which the focus is placed on the identification, assessment, and management of the neonate,

VIGNETTE 4.1 • FURTHER DISCUSSION

Illustration of Various Specialty Areas in Audiology

Audiology is categorized into a number of specialty areas based on the population served or the employment setting. The pediatric audiologist concentrates on the audiologic management of children of all ages. The pediatric audiologist is often employed in a children's hospital or a health care facility primarily serving children. The medical audiologist works with patients of all ages and is more concerned with establishing the site and cause of a hearing problem. Medical audiologists are typically employed in hospitals as part of either a hearing and speech department or a department of otolaryngology (i.e., Ear, Nose, and Throat, or ENT). The rehabilitative or dispensing audiologist focuses on the management of children or adults with hearing loss. Rehabilitative audiologists are often seen in private practice and specialize in the direct dispensation of hearing aids. Rehabilitative audiologists are also employed by a variety of health care facilities (e.g., hospitals, nursing homes). The industrial audiologist provides consultative hearing conservation services to companies whose workers are exposed to high noise levels. The industrial audiologist may be in private practice or work on a part-time basis. Finally, the educational audiologist serves children in the schools and is employed or contracted by the educational system.

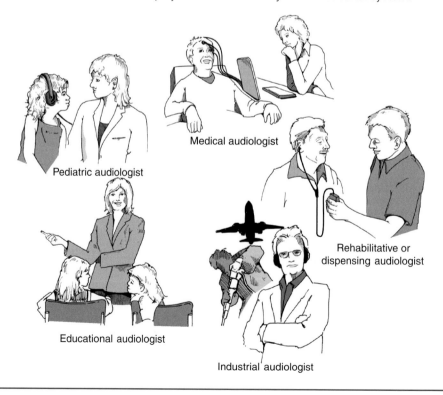

Pediatric audiologist

Medical audiologist

Rehabilitative or dispensing audiologist

Educational audiologist

Industrial audiologist

infant, and school-age child with hearing loss. The pediatric audiologist develops special knowledge in such areas as the causes of childhood deafness, the development of audition in children, child development, the audiologic screening and evaluation of children of different age groups, and parent counseling.

Another common specialty area is medical audiology. The medical audiologist is typically employed in a medical center to assist the physician in establishing an accurate diagnosis of an auditory disorder. Toward this end, the audiologist employs highly sophisticated and specialized tests to help pinpoint the location and cause of the hearing problem. The medical audiologist spends much of his or her time determining whether hearing loss is caused by a problem in the middle ear, the inner ear, or the higher centers of the auditory system within the brainstem and cortex.

Rehabilitative audiology is a third area of specialization that is gaining widespread popularity and acceptance. The rehabilitative audiologist is concerned with the appropriate management of an individual with a hearing deficit. It is common for the rehabilitative audiologist to specialize even further by limiting the service population to either adults or children. The rehabilitative audiologist is interested in fitting the individual with appropriate amplification, such as a personal hearing aid, to help compensate for the hearing loss. This specialist also provides the individual with information on the use and care of the hearing aid. Other services offered might include speechreading, speech remediation, auditory training, and individual and family counseling. If the audiologist specializes in the rehabilitation of children, his or her activities might also include conducting special parent-infant training programs, teaching speech and language, counseling parents, and readying the child for school.

Some audiologists practice exclusively in an industrial setting. These audiologists are referred to as industrial audiologists. Noise is a common by-product of our highly industrialized society. As we'll learn later, high levels of noise can produce permanent loss of hearing. Because many industries have work areas that produce high noise levels, audiologists are needed to develop programs that will protect employees from noise. Audiologists organize hearing conservation programs. These programs are designed to protect the worker from hearing loss by reducing the noise levels produced by noisy equipment, monitoring the hearing of employees, teaching employees about noise and its damaging effects, and providing ear protection to those who work in high-noise areas.

Finally, some audiologists specialize in educational audiology and are employed by public schools. Recall that the prevalence of hearing loss among school-age children is considerable. Educational audiologists are involved in identification, assessment, and monitoring of all school-age children with temporary or permanent hearing problems. The educational audiologist also selects and maintains hearing aids for children with hearing loss and assists regular teachers with educational programming.

HISTORICAL DEVELOPMENT OF AUDIOLOGY

Although instruments (audiometers) used to measure hearing date to the late 1800s, audiology as a discipline essentially evolved during World War II. During and following this war, many military personnel returned from combat with significant hearing loss resulting from exposure to the many and varied types of warfare noises. Interestingly, it was a prominent speech pathologist, Robert West, who called for his colleagues to expand their discipline to include audition. West (1936) stated: "Many workers in the field of speech correction do not realize that the time has come for those interested in this field to expand the subject so as to include … problems of those defective in the perception of speech. Our job should include … aiding the individual to hear what he ought to hear." Although a term had not yet been coined for this new field proposed by West, there was evidence that activity and interest in hearing disorders was present as early as 1936.

There has been considerable debate over who was responsible for coining the term *audiology*. Most sources credit Norton Canfield, an otolaryngologist (ear, nose, and throat physician), and Raymond Carhart, a speech-language pathologist, for coining the term independently of one another in 1945. Both of these men were intimately involved in planning and implementing programs in specialized aural rehabilitation hospitals established for military personnel during World War II. Today, Carhart is recognized by many as the Father of Audiology (Vignette 4.2).

VIGNETTE 4.2 • HISTORICAL NOTE

Raymond Carhart (1912–1975), Father of Audiology

The contributions of Dr. Raymond Carhart to the development of audiology from its earliest origins were so numerous and so significant that many think of him today as the Father of Audiology. A young professor in the School of Speech at Northwestern University when World War II broke out, he was commissioned as a captain in the army to head the Deshon General Hospital aural rehabilitation program for war-deafened military personnel at Butler, Pennsylvania. Deshon was named as one of three army general hospitals to receive, treat, and rehabilitate soldiers who incurred hearing loss as a result of their military service. These three hospitals, together with the Philadelphia Naval Hospital, admitted and served some 16,000 enlisted personnel and officers with hearing loss during the war.

This wartime mobilization effort served as the basis for the development of the new discipline that is now audiology. In 1945, Carhart and otologist Norton Canfield were credited with coining the word *audiology* to designate the science of hearing. From the outset, Carhart recognized that the strong interprofessional relationships between audiology and otology must be maintained. The military program was modeled on this concept, which determined its direction for the future. As a leader in the American Speech Correction Association, Carhart was instrumental in changing the name to the American Speech and Hearing Association soon after the close of World War II. Moreover, over the years he was one of the ASHA's most effective liaisons between audiology and otology when potentially divisive issues arose.

Returning to Northwestern as professor of audiology at the close of the war, Carhart set about immediately to develop a strong audiology graduate program and a clinical service center, placing Northwestern at the forefront of this field nationally. Many of his graduates became prominent in other universities across the country as teachers, research scientists, and clinical specialists. They, as well as his many professional associates in audiology and medicine, remember him for his brilliant and inquiring mind, which provided many of the research findings still undergirding the field today; for his scholarly publications; for his masterful teaching and speaking ability; and for his skill in the management of controversies within his national association, now the ASHA. But most of all, his former students and associates remember him as a warm human being and a mentor who was first of all a friend.

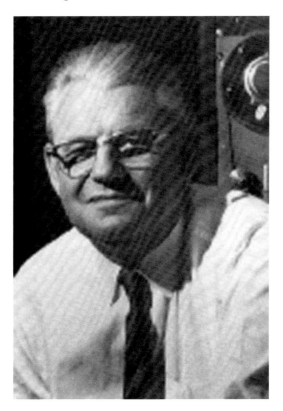

PROFESSIONAL OPPORTUNITIES

As shown in Figure 4.2, the modern-day audiologist has the opportunity to work within a wide variety of employment settings. The largest numbers of audiologists are employed in private audiology practices (30%), otolaryngology (ENT) practices (22%), clinics (12%), hospitals (11%), and colleges/universities (7%). Other work settings include schools, positions with hearing-aid manufacturers, Veterans Administration hospitals, and other federal agencies. The following discussion is a more detailed presentation of some of the more common professional opportunities in audiology.

Audiology as a Private Practice

Certainly the fastest-growing and perhaps most exciting employment setting is that of private practice. No other subgroup within the profession has shown such accelerated growth. In the 1970s, few audiologists were in private practice (Vignette 4.3). As noted earlier, 19% of today's audiologists are employed full-time in private practice. In fact, the private practice phenomenon has created an excellent market for professional opportunities in other areas of the profession. Many audiologists are leaving the traditional employment settings, attracted

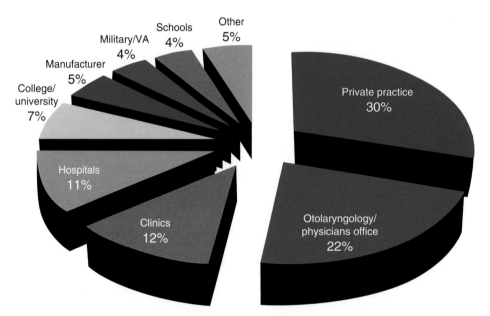

FIGURE 4.2 Distribution of employment settings for audiologists. Private practitioners are most typically seen in two employment settings, the physician's office (ENT) and the autonomous audiology office. (Adapted from American Academy of Audiology. *Audiology Demographic Profile*, 2012.)

VIGNETTE 4.3 • HISTORICAL NOTE

George S. Osborne (1940–2007), "Pioneer in Private Practice"

George S. Osborne, a pioneer, entrepreneur, visionary, and leader in the profession of audiology is perhaps best known for starting one of the very first successful private practices in the country. In the early 1970s, there were very few audiologists in private practice—most audiologists during this time worked in universities, hospitals, and community hearing and speech centers. Dr. Osborne, an audiologist and a dentist, saw the upside potential for private practice in audiology and launched the Oak Park Speech and Hearing Center in Oak Park, Illinois. The practice grew quickly and became one of the largest practices in the nation—in fact, the practice served as a model for many other audiologists to emulate. In addition to Oak Park, Dr. Osborne started two additional private practices in audiology—one in Minnesota and one in Pennsylvania. Today, private practice is one of the most popular and fastest-growing work settings in the profession of audiology.

   Dr. Osborne's enthusiasm for private practice led him to become an advocate for the profession, especially regarding the role of the private practitioner in audiology. He worked steadfastly to promote audiology to ensure that audiologists would achieve recognition and parity with other health care professionals. To this end, he actively promoted the doctorate in audiology (AuD) as the entry level degree for the profession and he developed a well-recognized AuD program at the Pennsylvania College of Optometry (School of Audiology), serving as its first Dean.

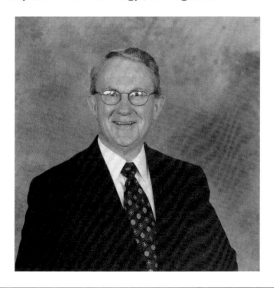

by the lure of a small business practice. The focus of these practices is on the sale of hearing aids, although many audiologists in private practice offer a wide array of audiologic services. Some audiologists may operate their businesses in medical clinics, hospitals, speech-language pathology offices, or otolaryngology practices; others may set up their own free-standing operation. There is, of course, a substantial risk involved in setting up a small business. The Small Business Administration estimates that about 60% of all new businesses fail during the first 5 years. Today, however, more and more successful businesses in audiology are started each year.

Why is it that private practice has become so popular, and why is it growing at such a fast pace? There are several reasons. First, small businesses provide an opportunity for financial independence and entrepreneurial expression and, perhaps most importantly, an opportunity to work for oneself. Second, private practice is growing because the opportunities it provides are becoming much more visible to those audiologists working in other settings. There is a dramatic increase in the memberships of organizations that are concerned with private practice and hearing aid dispensing and in the number of publications that serve the field. Third, the concept of franchises, or regional and national chains, in the hearing aid dispensing business has developed recently. Fourth, the sale of hearing aids has increased steadily over the past three decades, although with slower growth since the recession of 2008, yet, for adults, only approximately 20% of those who could benefit from hearing aids have purchased them. This suggests considerable potential and promise for future growth regarding the sale and delivery of hearing aids.

The sale of such devices remained relatively stable throughout the early and mid 1970s. From the late 1970s to the early 1990s, however, sales of hearing aids exhibited more than a threefold increase. During this same period, as noted previously, audiologists in private practice increased considerably in number. Since the early 1990s, however, annual hearing aid sales have increased at a much slower rate, most recently stabilizing at approximately 2 million instruments. Interestingly, the number of audiologists in private practice has increased over this same period.

Community and University Hospitals

Most hospitals in the United States employ audiologists. The demand for audiologic services in hospitals, long-term care facilities, and home health agencies is increasing steadily. The increased demand for audiologists in this type of setting, especially since the mid-1980s, may be attributed to several factors. First, there is a growing trend for hospitals to develop or enhance their rehabilitation programs, because the government's reimbursement systems (e.g., Medicare) now emphasize short-term hospital stays and subsequent outpatient rehabilitative services. Audiologic services are one form of outpatient rehabilitative service. Second, there is an increased awareness of the overall value of audiology and its contributions to health care. Third, most states are now mandating universal newborn hearing screening (see Chapter 8). Audiologists typically are employed by hospitals to coordinate those newborn screening programs. Finally, as was mentioned, the number of elderly individuals in the United States is growing, with at least one-third seeking health care, including audiologic services in many cases.

Predictably, the audiologic services provided in the hospital setting tend to be medically based. These audiologic services usually focus on providing information about the identification and location of an auditory disorder. The audiologist utilizes sophisticated auditory tests to evaluate the middle ear, the inner ear, the nerve pathways to the brain, and the auditory portions of the brain. This information is then pooled with diagnostic data obtained from other disciplines, such as otology (ear specialists), neurology, pediatrics, and psychology, to obtain a final diagnosis. In the hospital setting, the audiologist often works as part of a multidisciplinary team of medical and other professionals.

Assisting the team in determining the diagnosis, however, is not the only service the audiologist provides in the hospital environment. Other services include dispensing hearing aids, managing patients with unconventional hearing devices, screening, and monitoring the hearing of patients who are treated with drugs that could damage hearing.

Community-Based Clinics and Rehabilitation Centers

A common setting for the practice of audiology has been the private community-based clinics. Such practices can be implemented as a freestanding hearing and speech center or as a component of a larger rehabilitation center. Today, many metropolitan communities with populations greater than about 50,000 maintain community hearing and speech centers. These facilities provide comprehensive diagnostic and rehabilitative services to individuals with disorders of hearing, speech, or language. These centers receive much of their financial support from the community through individual contributions and through organizations such as the United Way and civic clubs. It is because of this type of support that such centers are able to serve substantial numbers of low-income patients. Audiologists are typically employed by these centers to provide a wide array of hearing services, such as hearing assessment, hearing aid selection and evaluation, hearing aid orientation, and aural rehabilitation for both children and adults with hearing loss. Some of the larger community-based hearing and speech centers in the United States are also involved in conducting hearing research and in training future professionals in audiology.

Audiology in the Schools

The passage in 1975 of the Education of All Handicapped Children Act (PL 94-142), a federal law designed to ensure all handicapped children a free and appropriate public school education, resulted in an increased awareness of the need for audiologic services in the schools. In 1990, this act became known as the Individuals with Disabilities Education Act (IDEA). In 1997, President Clinton signed the bill reauthorizing, updating, and expanding IDEA; the bill became known as public law 105-17. Finally, in 2004, President Bush signed a new bill, public law 108-446, now referred to as the **Individuals with Disabilities Education Improvement Act (IDEIA, 2004)**. In essence, IDEIA (2004) has brought unprecedented expansion of services to infants, toddlers, and preschool children with disabilities and their families. IDEIA (2004) retains the major provisions of the other federal laws, including a free and appropriate education to all children with disabilities. Part B of the law provides the rules and regulations for eligible children with disabilities aged 3 through 21. Part C helps states to develop and operate an early-intervention program for infants and toddlers with disabilities. This important bill specifies that local educational systems must provide, at no cost to the child, a wide range of audiologic services. These services included hearing evaluations, auditory training, speechreading, language training, and the selection and fitting of both personal and group amplification units. The fitting and management of cochlear implants are also covered under IDEIA (2004). Needless to say, such a mandate necessitates that audiologic services be offered in the schools. Additional factors, such as the policy of inclusion, have further increased the demand for educational audiology.

Within the context of audiology, **inclusion** refers to the practice of placing children with hearing loss in regular classrooms instead of in special classrooms containing only children with hearing loss. As more children with hearing loss are integrated into regular classroom settings, the need to provide these children with special audiologic assistance increases.

Another important variable has been the general recognition that many children with hearing loss in the schools are not being adequately served. It has been reported, for example, that fewer than 50% of children with hearing loss in the educational system are receiving adequate services. To be sure, the introduction of IDEIA (2004), along with inclusion and an awareness of the audiologic needs of a larger group of children, has created a market for educational audiology. It is expected that this market will continue to grow as audiology continues to demonstrate how it can contribute significantly to the needs of children with hearing loss in the schools.

The responsibilities of the school audiologist include many shared by most audiologists, such as hearing screening, hearing assessment, selection and evaluation of hearing aids, and direct provision of rehabilitative services. Additional services specific to the educational setting include maintenance of personal and group hearing aids; parent counseling; in-service education to teachers, special educators, and administrators; consulting for educational placement; and serving as a liaison to the community and other professional agencies.

Hearing-Aid Manufacturers

A growing employment opportunity for audiologists is with the manufacturers of hearing aids and audiologic equipment. In fact, virtually all hearing aid companies today employ audiologists to work in a variety of capacities. Clinical audiologists with good interpersonal communicative skills are always needed to provide expert services to audiologists who dispense a given manufacturer's hearing aid. Usually, such support services are related to fitting of the manufacturer's hearing aid, programming and installation of hearing aid fitting software, and general troubleshooting. Other opportunities for clinical audiologists might include positions that focus on administration, sales and marketing, and educational training. Similar positions are available with companies that manufacture audiologic equipment, although generally fewer such positions are available than with hearing-aid companies. Research audiologists can play an important role for the hearing aid manufacturer in the strategic planning, implementation, and reporting of research that leads to the development and enhancement of hearing instruments. Research audiologists in industry may also contract other research laboratories to assist the company in the development of data to support a new product or product strategy.

Department of Veterans Affairs Medical Centers and Other State and Federal Agencies

Most Department of Veterans Affairs (VA) medical centers/healthcare systems offer audiology and speech-language pathology services. In an effort to provide veterans with all of the patient services that might be needed, the VA has grouped medical centers, outpatient clinics, and community-based clinics into 21 Veterans Integrated Service Networks (VISNs) on the basis of geography, distribution of the veteran population, and availability of specialized services among medical centers in a VISN. A veteran patient may seek services in any of these VA settings with an audiology/speech-language pathology program; however, most veterans elect to receive care from the program nearest to where they reside. The VA is also expanding its telehealth capabilities to provide audiology and speech-language pathology services in remote settings where there are no professional personnel, including within the veteran's home.

The number of VA audiology programs has increased significantly during the past 5 years. The incidence and prevalence of hearing loss and tinnitus in the veteran population are greater than in the general population, probably as a result of noise exposure and the increasing age of the veteran population. Hearing loss and tinnitus are the two most common service-related disabilities in the VA in addition to providing audiology and speech-language pathology services, the VA, in association with affiliated universities, provides both funded and unfunded training programs for graduate students enrolled in doctor of philosophy (PhD) and doctor of audiology (AuD) programs. Moreover, the VA conducts a variety of basic and applied research in communication sciences and disorders.

A number of other federal and state agencies also employ audiologists. At the state level, there is typically a department responsible for ensuring the hearing health care needs of young children, usually associated with the department of public health. Departments of public health employ audiologists to perform the full range of audiologic services and to serve as advocates for children with hearing loss and their parents. Similarly, state departments of education and of vocational rehabilitation often employ audiologists to meet the audiologic needs of the populations that their agencies are charged with serving. At the federal level, most opportunities for audiologists are administrative and are not concerned with direct service delivery. Their function is usually to assist the states and regions in implementing or improving programs for hearing-handicapped citizens.

Military-Based Programs

Hearing health care services are available in all branches of the armed forces (army, navy, and air force). As noted earlier, the military services played a key role in the development of audiology as a profession. In fact, immediately after World War II, the army set up and staffed three hospitals, and the navy, one; each of these hospitals was devoted entirely to the rehabilitation and care of military personnel with hearing loss or other disorders of communication acquired in the military service.

Audiologic services are still an important and growing need in the armed forces. In 1975, it was reported that as many as 50% of service personnel assigned to combat arms jobs underwent measurable noise-induced hearing loss after 10 years of military service. Such documentation led to the recognition of great need for military audiologists. In 1967, the army employed only 11 audiologists, whereas in 1985, it employed more than 70. The resulting increased awareness of hearing conservation appears to have been successful.

A recent prevalence study of hearing loss among army combat arms personnel revealed that about 20% of these soldiers have measurable noise-induced hearing loss after a 20-year military career.

The most dramatic change over the past several years for the employment of audiologists in the military setting has been the rapid increase in the number of female audiologists. Presently, half of army audiology officers are women. The other branches of the military have similar percentages of female audiology officers.

Another dramatic recent change is the military audiologist's role in operational hearing conservation. Fifteen army audiologists served in Saudi Arabia during the first Gulf war, and six have served in Iraq and Afghanistan during the war on terrorism. That is, audiologists no longer work solely in clinical and research environments; today they are front-line contributors to survival and hearing health care wherever soldiers, sailors, marines, and airmen serve.

Because of the overall reduction of troop strength in the past several years, the number of active-duty officers in the military has been reduced significantly. Nevertheless, many audiologists have attained the prestigious rank of colonel and serve as commanders and administrators of large health care commands. In fact, several of today's prominent audiologists started their career in the military.

The military audiologist provides a full range of services. Typically, emphasis is placed on hearing conservation, screenings and assessments, diagnostic evaluations, hearing aid evaluations, and aural rehabilitation. Military hearing conservation programs include such components as identification of noise hazards, noise measurement analysis and noise reduction, selection and fitting of hearing protection devices, hearing health education, audiometric testing, and audiometric database management. Finally, the military audiologist has the opportunity to participate in research in hearing conservation, auditory perception and processing, and developing technology to increase soldiers' survivability and enhance their capability.

College and University Settings

A large number of major colleges and universities offer undergraduate and/or graduate training in audiology. Many audiologists with doctoral degrees assume academic positions in the university and become involved in teaching, service, and research. To train a clinical audiologist adequately, the university must offer appropriate clinical training. Accordingly, audiologists, many without doctoral degrees, are employed by the university to service patients with hearing loss from the community and to supervise students in training for a graduate degree in audiology. Audiologists working in this setting have frequent opportunities to participate in research and to train students.

EDUCATIONAL PREPARATION FOR AUDIOLOGY

For several decades, the entry-level degree required for the practice of clinical audiology was the master's degree. In 1993, however, the American Speech-Language-Hearing Association (for historical reasons, generally referred to as the ASHA instead of ASLHA), one of the primary accrediting bodies for training programs in audiology, endorsed the doctorate as the entry-level degree required for the practice of audiology. Accordingly, almost all residential master's degree programs in audiology have now been phased out. Presently, we have two doctoral degrees available, the clinical PhD, which has been in existence for many years, and a new professional doctorate, the AuD. In 1993, the first AuD program was established in the United States. Many others have been developed since then, and as of 2007, there were 71 such programs in the United States, including both traditional residential post-baccalaureate (3- or 4-year) programs and shorter distance-learning programs for those who already have a master's degree. The first quarter of this century will be a very significant period of transition in the type of education required to practice audiology, since entry level to the field has now moved from a master's degree to the doctoral degree.

Preparation for a career in audiology should begin at the undergraduate level with basic courses that provide a strong foundation for graduate or professional study. Courses in physics, biology, statistics, mathematics, computer science, anatomy and physiology, psychology, child development, human behavior, and education can provide meaningful preparation for graduate or professional study in audiology.

Students pursuing post-baccalaureate work in audiology come from a variety of backgrounds. In a typical large doctoral program (10 to 15 students per year), it is fairly common to find students with diverse undergraduate majors, including speech-language pathology, psychology, education, and special education. Students with undergraduate majors in the basic sciences and the humanities have been encountered less frequently. With the advent of the AuD, however, it is hoped that more students will come with undergraduate degrees in basic or life sciences, much like other preparatory professional health care disciplines (e.g., preparation for medicine, dentistry, and optometry).

What is a doctoral curriculum in audiology like? Table 4.2 details a training program for an audiology student enrolled in a 4-year post-baccalaureate doctoral program. Typically, AuD students complete a minimum of 75 semester credit hours of post-baccalaureate study. In the first year of study, most of the course work focuses on basic science and background information. The practicum during this first year is a mix of observation and limited participation. In the second year, introductory and intermediate applied courses are introduced, and the student becomes much more involved in practicum experience, especially in

TABLE
4.2

Sample Student Program for AuD

Semester	Course 1[a]	Course 2	Course 3	Course 4	Course 5
First Year					
Fall	Acoustics, calibration, and instrumentation	Anatomy and physiology of hearing mechanisms	Hereditary hearing loss	Measurement of hearing	Introduction to CCC[b]
Spring	Auditory clinical electro-physiology	Amplification I	Neuroscience	Psychoacoustics (3 h)	CCC
Summer	Principles of counseling (2 h)	Assessment of vestibular disorders (3 h)	CCC		
Second Year					
Fall	Pediatric audiology	Management of vestibular diseases	Amplification II	Pathology of auditory system	CCC
Spring	Aural rehab for children	Capstone I	Hearing loss and speech understanding	Microbiology and pharmacology for audiology	CCC
Summer	Hearing conservation	Hearing and aging	CCC		
Third Year					
Fall	Clinical research design	Professional issues and ethics (2 h)	Child language acquisition (2 h)	Capstone II	CCC
Spring	Cochlear implants	Business and financial management for audiologists (4 h)	Elective	Auditory prostheses	CCC
Fourth Year					
Externship (fourth-year placement)					

[a]All courses except CCC are 3 h unless otherwise specified.
[b]CCC, clinical case conference. All CCC courses are 1 h.

case management. During the third year, advanced clinical courses are required, and a series of short-term clinical rotations or externships are typically initiated to provide broader clinical experience. In years 2 and 3, students at many programs, such as the one illustrated here, may take Capstone I and II. The capstone is an independent project conducted by the student under the direction of a faculty member. It may involve a traditional research project, a literature review of a particular topic, or even development of a business or marketing plan. Finally, the fourth year is essentially full-time and quasi-independent clinical practice that may take place in residence or via an offsite clinical externship. The purpose of the externship, sometimes referred to as fourth-year placement, is to help the student make the transition from academic to professional life. Hence, it is seen that the program progresses from basic to applied science and that specialization increases during the later stages of the training program. Receiving an advanced degree in audiology is just the first step toward becoming a clinical audiologist certified by the ASHA or the American Academy of Audiology (AAA). For many audiologists, certification by the ASHA is still the desired clinical credential, since such certification is built into state requirements for professional licensure. In the master's-based educational model, once the student received the master's degree, the second step toward certification was to complete an internship known as the clinical fellowship year (CFY). This meant that the student had to spend the first year of salaried practice under the supervision of an experienced and certified audiologist. Doctoral programs have essentially built this internship into the final year, so that an additional CFY is not required. The third step toward certification by the ASHA or the AAA, which can be completed at any time, is passing a national written examination in audiology.

Some students prefer to continue their study of audiology and obtain a doctoral degree in research, the PhD. This program usually takes at least 3 years beyond the AuD, and the student concentrates on theoretical and research aspects of the profession. Common employment opportunities for the PhD include college and university teaching, research, and administration.

PROFESSIONAL LICENSURE AND CERTIFICATION

All professional organizations license their practitioners through minimum standards, rules, and regulations. Such a practice helps to ensure that services are being provided in a manner that meets professional standards for practice. Regulation of audiology began in the 1950s, and all but three states now regulate the AuD. Typically, the professional license is issued by a government agency and grants an individual the right to practice a given profession. Most states model their regulatory rules in audiology after the ASHA standards for the certificate of clinical competence. The ASHA certification program began in

1952 and continues as the primary certification venue for audiologists. In 1999, AAA developed its own certification program, and more and more audiologists are now using AAA for their professional certification. In 2012, about 14,000 individuals were certified in audiology through ASHA and about 1,400 were board certified by AAA.

PROFESSIONAL AFFILIATIONS

Like all professionals, audiologists should maintain affiliations with their professional organizations. The AAA, founded by James Jerger in 1988, is the world's largest professional organization of, by, and for audiologists (Vignette 4.4).

The academy, with just under 12,000 members, is dedicated to providing quality hearing care to the public. It is also committed to enhancing the ability of its members to achieve career and practice objectives through professional development, education, research, increased awareness of hearing disorders, and audiologic services. The academy typically focuses on issues related to the practice of audiology, such as standards and ethics, publications, training, standardization of methods, professional meetings, and professional scope. As noted earlier, the AAA offers clinical certification to members interested in and eligible for such certification. This is separate from the clinical certification offered by the ASHA. The AAA also publishes a professional and a scientific journal, public information material, and position statements.

Another important professional organization for the audiologist is the ASHA. Similar to AAA, the ASHA decides on standards of competence for

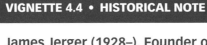

VIGNETTE 4.4 • HISTORICAL NOTE

James Jerger (1928–), Founder of the American Academy of Audiology

Dr. James Jerger is widely recognized as the founder and driving force of the AAA. In 1987, at the ASHA convention, five well-known audiologists were recruited to discuss the future of audiology. During this session, Jerger noted that it was time for a new professional organization of, by, and for audiologists. Jerger's comments were met with an overwhelmingly enthusiastic response. As a follow-up to the ASHA session, Jerger invited 32 audiology leaders to Houston, Texas, in early 1988. The purpose of the study group was to establish an independent, freestanding national organization for audiologists. The group voted unanimously to develop a new organization for audiologists, to be called the American College of Audiology, and the first national office was established in Baylor College of Medicine. In addition, an ad hoc steering committee was appointed to develop bylaws.

In the few short months to follow, remarkable progress was made. Bylaws for the organization were approved, and the organization was renamed the American Academy of Audiology. The academy was incorporated, an organizational structure was established and officers elected, and dues were established. Committee assignments were made, dates for the first annual meeting were determined, and a major membership drive was launched. In 1989, the first AAA convention was held in Kiawah Island, South Carolina, and the response exceeded all expectations. Close to 600 participants attended the meeting and overflowed the conference facilities. Since 1989, the AAA has undergone significant growth in membership and development. By 1993, the AAA had reached a point in membership size and fiscal responsibilities that it became necessary to move the national office to Washington, D.C., and contract staff to assist in the organization's management. Today, the AAA national office is in Reston, Virginia. Unquestionably, without the far-reaching vision and the extraordinary leadership capabilities of James Jerger, the creation of the AAA would not have been possible. Jerger will always be remembered not only for his extraordinary contributions to the research literature in audiology but also for the role that he played in furthering the cause of the profession of audiology through the development of the AAA.

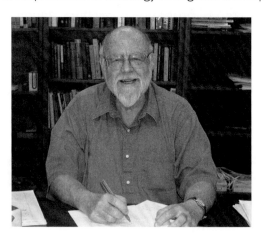

the certification of individuals in the area of audiology (also speech-language pathology). The ASHA also conducts accreditation programs for colleges and universities with degree programs in speech-language pathology and audiology and for agencies that provide clinical services to the public. Among the many services that the ASHA offers its more than 145,000 members, of whom approximately 13,000 are audiologists, is an extensive program of continuing education. This program includes an annual national convention, national and regional conferences, institutes, and workshops. The ASHA also publishes professional and scientific journals, public information material, reports and position statements, monographs, and many other special publications.

Another professional affiliation for the audiologist is the American Auditory Society, an organization encompassing numerous disciplines concerned with hearing and deafness. The membership roster includes practitioners of such professions as audiology, otolaryngology, education of those with hearing loss, pediatric medicine, and psychology, as well as members of the hearing aid industry. The society sponsors an annual convention and publishes a scientific journal.

The Academy of Doctors of Audiology (ADA), previously known as the Academy of Dispensing Audiologists, is an organization of approximately 1,000 members designed to meet the professional needs of audiologists in private practice, especially those who directly dispense hearing aids. Most members of the ADA also hold membership in the AAA; in fact, the two organizations occasionally collaborate on a number of activities of mutual interest. Similar to other professional organizations, the ADA publishes a professional journal, sponsors an annual meeting, offers continuing education, and promotes public awareness of hearing loss.

Audiologists may associate with many other professional organizations depending on their areas of interest and specialization. There are professional organizations for the pediatric audiologist, the rehabilitative audiologist, the military audiologist, and the audiologist employed in the educational setting.

SUMMARY

Hearing loss affects a large segment of the population of the United States, and this figure is expected to grow over the next several years. Furthermore, hearing loss in both children and adults can be a significant handicapping condition. The profession of audiology evolved in an attempt to help individuals with hearing loss overcome these handicaps. Audiology has been described as a profession that is concerned with the prevention of hearing loss and the identification, evaluation, and rehabilitation of children and adults with hearing loss. The audiologist has numerous employment opportunities and can work in a variety of employment settings. Audiology is a young, dynamic, and challenging profession that provides a wide range of exciting opportunities for a rewarding career.

CHAPTER REVIEW QUESTIONS

1. Describe some of the different employment opportunities of audiologists.
2. What is the legislative provision IDEIA? Why is it important for children with hearing loss?
3. Briefly describe the educational preparation necessary for becoming an audiologist.

REFERENCES AND SUGGESTED READINGS

American Academy of Audiology. Position Statement regarding the professional doctorate. *Audiology Today* 1990;2(5):10.

Bess FH. Prevalence of unilateral and mild hearing loss in school-age children. *Workshop Proceedings: National Workshop on Mild and Unilateral Hearing Loss, Centers for Disease Control and Prevention and the Marion Downs Hearing Center*; 2005.

Bess FH, Dodd JD, Parker RA. Children with minimal sensorineural hearing loss: Prevalence, educational performance and functional health status. *Ear Hear* 1998;19:339–354.

Bess FH, Gravel JS. *Foundations of Pediatric Audiology: A Book of Readings*. San Diego, CA: Plural; 2006.

Bunch CC. *Clinical Audiometry*. St Louis, MO: Mosby; 1943.

Hale ST, Bess FH. Professional Organizations. In: Lubinski R, Frattali CM, eds. *Professional Issues in Speech-Language Pathology and Audiology*. 3rd ed. Clifton Park, NY: Thomson Delmar Learning; 2006.

Herbst KRG. Psychosocial consequences of disorders of hearing in the elderly. In: Hinchcliffe R, ed. *Hearing and Balance in the Elderly*. Edinburgh, UK: Churchill Livingstone; 1983.

Humes LE, Diefendorf AO. Chaos or order? Some thoughts on the transition to a professional doctorate in audiology. *Am J Audiol* 1993;2:7–16.

Humes LE, Joellenbeck LM, Durch JS, eds. *Noise and Military Service: Implications for Hearing Loss and Tinnitus*. Washington, DC: National Academies Press; 2006.

Individuals with Disabilities Education Improvement Act of 2004. 20 U.S.C. § 1400 et seq. (reauthorization of the Individuals with Disabilities Education Act of 1990), 2004.

Jerger J. *Audiology in the USA*. San Diego, CA: Plural Publishing; 2009.

Kochkin S. MarkeTrak III: Why 20 million in U.S. don't use hearing aids for their hearing loss. *Hearing J* 1993;46(1):20–27;46(2):26–31;46(4):36–37.

Kupper L. The IDEA Amendments of 1997. National Information Center for Children and Youth with Disabilities. *News Digest* 1997;26.

Matkin ND. Early recognition and referral of hearing impaired children. *Pediatr Rev* 1984;6:151–158.

Niskar AS, Kieszah SM, Holmes A, et al. Prevalence and hearing loss among children 6 to 19 years-of-age. Third National Health and Nutrition Examination Survey. *JAMA* 1988;279:1070–1075.

Northern JL, Downs MP. *Hearing in Children*. 5th ed. Baltimore, MD: Lippincott Williams & Wilkins; 2001.

Schiller JS, Lucas JW, Ward BW, et al; National Center for Health Statistics. Summary health statistics for US adults: National Health Interview Survey, 2010. *Vital health Stat 10* 2012;(252):1–207.

Strom KE. Rapid product changes mark the new mature digital market. *Hear Rev* 2006;13(5):70–74.

Walden B, Prosek R, Worthington D. The Prevalence of hearing loss within selected U.S. army branches. *Interagency No. 1A04745*. Washington, DC: Army Medical Research and Development Command; 1975.

West R. The mechanical ear. *Volta Rev* 1936;38:345–346.

WEBSITES

American Speech-Language-Hearing Association: www.asha.org

American Academy of Audiology: www.audiology.org

American Auditory Society: www.amauditorysoc.org

Academy of Doctors of Audiology: www.audiologist.org

PL 94–142 (1975): www.ed.gov/policy/speced/leg/idea/history.html

5

The Profession of Speech-Language Pathology

- To discuss the prevalence and impact of speech-language disorders;
- To define the profession of speech-language pathology (SLP);
- To appreciate the historical development of the profession;
- To understand the specialized roles of SLP for serving the hearing impaired;
- To understand the academic and clinical requirements required for SLP; and
- To appreciate certification/licensure standards and professional affiliations important to SLP.

- **Autism spectrum disorders:** A disorder that compromises normal language and development.
- **Cochlear implant:** A cochlear implant is a small, complex electronic device that can help to provide a sense of sound to a person who is profoundly deaf or severely hard of hearing. The implant consists of an external portion that sits behind the ear and a second portion that is surgically placed under the skin.
- **National Institute on Deafness and Other Communication Disorders (NIDCD):** A separate institute within the National Institutes of Health (NIH) that supports research and research training in communication disorders.
- **Aphasia:** A language disorder due to damage to the brain.

The purpose of this chapter is to provide a brief overview of the profession of speech-language pathology (SLP), with a special emphasis on the speech-language pathologist's role in the management of children with hearing loss. SLP profession-als are key members of multidisciplinary teams helping individuals who have expe-rienced breaks in the communication chain, including those with breaks primarily impacting the listener or receiver. First, the discussion reviews the prevalence and impact of speech-language disorders, the definition and historical overview of SLP, and the role of the speech-language pathologist in serving young children with hearing loss. Indeed, the needs of children with hearing loss require the integrated efforts of both medical and nonmedical specialists representing such disciplines as audiology, SLP, otolaryngology, education of the deaf, pediatrics, and psychology. Such a multidisciplinary approach is essential if we hope to adequately address the overall perplexities of hearing loss and seek out newer and better ways to serve children and adults with breaks in the auditory portions of the communication chain. To be sure, the speech-language pathologist plays an integral role in the ef-fective management of the hearing impaired—their unique skills in such areas as listening, speaking, reading, writing, and cognition contribute significantly to the overall development of communicative competence in children with hearing loss. In fact, with the advent of universal newborn hearing screening and improved hearing technologies, the roles of the speech-language pathologist for serving the hearing impaired have expanded. The chapter concludes with a summary of the educational preparation for SLP, a brief discussion of certification/licensure, and a description of some of the professional affiliations of speech-language pathologists.

PREVALENCE AND IMPACT OF SPEECH-LANGUAGE DISORDERS

Effective communication is considered essential to our life quality and, ultimately, our success in modern day society. Yet, we find that about one in every six Americans experiences some form of communication disorder. Unfortunately, because of the lack of published data, it is difficult to estimate with any degree of precision the combined prevalence of speech, hearing, lan-guage, voice, and swallowing disorders in the United States. We do know that the prevalence of communication disorders is substantial affecting large numbers of children and adults. The prevalence of hearing loss was discussed in Chapter 4. With regard to the prevalence of persons with speech, language, voice, and swallowing disorders, consider the following statistics proffered by the **National Institute on Deafness and Other Communication Disorders (NIDCD)**, a separate institute within the National Institutes of Health (NIH) that supports research and research training in deafness and other communication disorders:

Children

- About 8% of kindergarten children in the United States have specific language impairment (SLI)—these children experience difficulty in developing and using language. Moreover, SLI not only affects speaking but reading and writing tasks as well.
- Approximately 1 out of every 200 American children is diagnosed with **autism spectrum disorders**—a disorder that compromises normal language and development.
- About 1 million American children stutter.
- About 5% of children in the United States entering first grade exhibit speech (phonologic) disorders.

Adults

- Nearly 1 million US adults have **aphasia**, a language disorder due to damage to the brain following a stroke or other injury to the brain.
- More than 6 million adults over the age of 60 years experience swallowing problems.
- Fifty-five thousand Americans are affected annually with cancer of the head and neck.

Hence, the prevalence numbers are substantial. Importantly, it is conjectured that as the population ages and chances for survival increase, the number of Americans with communication disorders will also increase during the next century.

It is also important to recognize that the impact of these communicative disorders can affect life quality—that is, communication disorders can compromise social, recreational, emotional, educational, and vocational aspects of one's life. The cost in terms of unrealized potential is also significant. Data suggest that people with severe speech disabilities are more often found to be unemployed or in a lower economic class than people with other less severe disabilities. Indeed, communication disorders may cost the United States from $154 billion to $186 billion per year—figures equal to 2.5% to 3% of the gross national product.

The prevalence and impact of speech, language, voice, and swallowing disorders illustrates clearly the needs of this population and the important role that the speech-language pathologist can play in the identification and management of communication disorders. Speech-language pathologists diagnose the nature and extent of the communication problem and, based on the diagnosis, develop and implement evidence-based treatment strategies for the effective management of the communication disorder.

SPEECH-LANGUAGE PATHOLOGY DEFINED

SLP is defined as the study of disorders that affect a person's speech, language, cognition, voice, or swallowing and includes the diagnosis and habilitation or rehabilitation of communication problems and/or swallowing difficulties. Speech-language pathologists, sometimes referred to as speech therapists, are concerned with both typical and atypical human communication in such areas as speech (articulation, intonation, rate, intensity, voice, fluency), language (phonology, morphology, syntax, semantics, and pragmatics), cognition (attention, memory, sequencing, problem solving), and feeding and swallowing. Some of the potential causes of speech, language, and swallowing disorders might include neonatal problems (e.g., low birth weight); developmental disabilities such as SLI, learning disabilities, and autism spectrum disorders; laryngeal complications; neurological disease or complications such as traumatic brain injury, cerebral palsy, Parkinson disease, and amyotrophic lateral sclerosis (Lou Gehrig disease); genetic disorders (e.g., Down syndrome, fragile X syndrome); and auditory disorders—a topic that is discussed in more detail later in this chapter and in Chapter 10 of this book.

Similar to audiologists, speech-language pathologists work in a variety of settings (see Fig. 5.1). The vast majority of speech-language pathologists work in the schools (54%), followed by hospitals (13%), skilled nursing facilities (9%), home health care facilities (6%), SLP/Audiology (AUD) offices (4%),

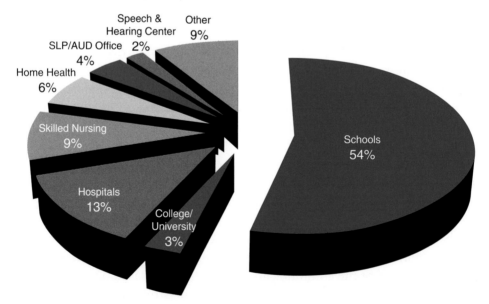

FIGURE 5.1 Practice setting of speech-language pathologists.

colleges and universities (3%), and speech and hearing centers (2%). The "other" category (9%) includes such settings as physician's offices, other residential facilities, and other nonresidential facilities. It is of interest to contrast the practice settings of SLP to audiology, the latter shown in Figure 4.1 in Chapter 4. While more than one-half of speech-language pathologists are employed in the schools, only 4% of audiologists practice in the school setting. By far, the largest employment settings in audiology are private practice (30%) and otolaryngology/physicians' offices (22%), a setting that might also be considered a form of private practice, with relatively few SLPs working in similar settings.

HISTORICAL DEVELOPMENT OF SPEECH-LANGUAGE PATHOLOGY

Although the history of SLP begins long before the twentieth century, most relate the beginning of contemporary SLP with the founding of the American Speech-Language-Hearing Association (ASHA)—the nation's leading professional organization for SLP and an organization that continues to be of interest to many audiologists (see Chapter 4). In the early 1900s, there were two special interest groups in speech correction that evolved—one was affiliated with the National Education Association (NEA), a professional group of teachers. The interest group, known as the National Society for the Study and Correction of Speech Disorders, was a subgroup of NEA in 1918 and continued until 1939. The second group, which eventually became the ASHA, was led by Carl Seashore, a professor of psychology at Iowa State University. Seashore recognized the need for a professional organization that focused only on speech and language disorders. In 1925, Seashore assembled a meeting in the home of Lee Edward Travis, a professor at the University of Iowa who was keenly interested in the problem of stuttering. There were fewer than 25 individuals at that first meeting, and they came together because they all possessed a common interest in communication disorders. Seashore proposed the possibility of creating a professional organization of "speech correction"—an organization independent of the National Association of Teachers of Speech (NATS). NATS was the principal organization for individuals interested in interpersonal communication and public address. Although NATS had almost no interest in communication disorders, it was the only organization that offered opportunities for those interested in this area to publish scholarly works in speech disorders and to vet with colleagues on topics of mutual interest at the annual convention. In December of 1925, the American Academy of Speech Correction (ASHA's predecessor) was established. The association went through a number of name changes throughout their history, but finally settled on American Speech-Language Hearing Association in 1978.

Although Seashore is credited for recognizing the need for a professional organization in communication disorders, it was actually Robert West who led the effort to break from NATS and formally organize the American Academy of Speech Correction. Consequently, by most accounts Robert West is considered the founding father of SLP (see Vignette 5.1).

To be sure, the profession of SLP has undergone significant change and growth since those early founding years. In particular, a dramatic expansion in scope of practice has taken place with the increased emphasis on early identification and intervention of children with speech, language, and hearing disorders; changes in federal laws that guarantee special education and related services to children with disabilities; and the dramatic increase in the aged population—a group prone to medical conditions that lead to speech, language, and swallowing disorders. These changes and others have also resulted in the expansion of employment opportunities for the speech-language pathologist—in fact, for those speech-language pathologists interested in serving children with hearing loss, employment opportunities appear to be growing in such settings as schools, private practice, and hospitals/medical centers.

VIGNETTE 5.1 • HISTORICAL NOTE

Robert William West (1892–1968), Father of Speech-Language Pathology

Most leading authorities recognize Robert West as the founding father of contemporary SLP. His reputation was built upon his outstanding contributions to the organization of ASHA and his scholarly writings. In the words of Charles Van Riper, a renowned speech-language pathologist and pioneer in the profession, "If any one individual could be singled out as the father of the field, it would have to be West, for he not only participated in its birth but nurtured it in its early precarious years and lived long enough to enjoy its maturity."

West began his professional career as a high school teacher in Wisconsin and taught for 17 years before he entered college, receiving a BA in 1916 from West Virginia College. He served in the medical corps during World War I (WWI). After WWI, West obtained a master's degree and a Ph.D. from the University of Wisconsin—he was only the second person in the United States to obtain Ph.D. in the field of speech disorders. After receiving his doctorate, West became director of the Speech Clinic at the University of Wisconsin serving in that capacity from 1928 to 1950.

By most accounts, Robert West was considered a remarkable man—a private person, he was nevertheless exceptionally bright, hardworking, and intolerant of mediocrity. Graduate students were reportedly left terrified, shaking, and humbled following his critiques of their class presentations. He was very active in organizational affairs, serving as president of the Speech Association of America in 1943 and as a charter member of ASHA (1925) (American Academy of Speech Correction). He was also the first president of ASHA (1925–1928). In 1936, West called for the American Academy of Speech Correction to include hearing as part of their scope of practice. To recognize West's many contributions to the profession, ASHA awarded him honors of the association in 1947.

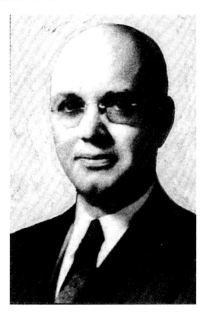

ROLES OF THE SPEECH-LANGUAGE PATHOLOGIST IN SERVING THE HEARING IMPAIRED

We noted at the beginning of this chapter that SLP plays an important role in the management of individuals with hearing loss. Speech-language pathologists possess unique knowledge and skills in several areas essential for linguistic competence including normal communicative development and the effect of hearing loss on communicative development, the assessment of communicative skills and intervention with individuals with hearing loss, and the prevention of communicative disorders. Although speech-language pathologists work with both children and adults with hearing loss, the vast majority focus their efforts on children—this may be because so many speech-language pathologists work in the schools. This section briefly reviews some of the responsibilities of the speech-language pathologist in the management of children with hearing loss.

It is well recognized that mild-to-profound permanent hearing loss compromises auditory, language, speech, academic, and social-emotional development. Speech-language pathologists are trained to evaluate a child's speech and language competence and, based on the outcome of that evaluation, develop and implement an effective intervention plan. ASHA estimates that close to 50% of all speech-language pathologists working in the schools serve children with hearing loss. Some speech-language pathologists, especially those working in medical or private practice settings, concentrate their entire practice on children with hearing loss and their families. When working with children with hearing loss, the speech-language pathologist may perform any of the following functions (Tye-Murray, 2009):

- Evaluate speech and language performance.
- Evaluate preliteracy and literacy skills, including phonological awareness.
- Evaluate speechreading skills.
- Perform visual inspection and listening check of amplification systems.
- Collaborate in the assessment of central auditory processing disorders.
- Provide speech and language therapy.
- Consult with parents and classroom teachers.
- Provide instruction in sign language to child, classroom teacher, and parents if appropriate.
- Maintain bridges of communication between clinical setting and home, and ensure that therapy objectives are reinforced informally throughout a child's day.
- Advise audiologist's about appropriate language levels for audiological tests.
- Provide speech perception testing.

Some speech-language pathologists choose to focus on developing communicative competence in infants and toddler with hearing loss; others prefer to work with school-age children. Ideally, the speech-language pathologist becomes involved in the case management of children with hearing loss shortly after the hearing loss has been identified. However, sometimes the speech-language pathologist is the first to see the child—that is, the child may be referred to a speech-language pathologist because of developmental delays in speech and/or language. At the infant and toddler stage, strategies of the speech-language pathologist center on managing the acoustic environment by making sure that parents and teachers fully understand and appreciate the importance of troubleshooting and daily checking of hearing aids, as well as working with parents to become involved in the enhancement of their child's speech and language development (see Chapter 10).

At the school-age level, speech-language pathologists assess communication skills of children with hearing loss in the appropriate communication modality of the child (total communication, manual, spoken language) and with the appropriate sensory aids (hearing aids, cochlear implants). In general, this evaluation focuses on receptive and expressive language in oral, signed, or written modalities and the perception or production of speech and voice characteristics, speechreading, listening, and communication strategies. The speech-language pathologist may also provide advice/consultation to members of the team working with the child and the child's family (e.g., audiologist, social worker, teacher, and psychologist). For example, it may be helpful to share information concerning the child's communication skills and to provide the team with a better understanding of how those skills differ from normal hearing peers. It also may be of value to provide the team with a realistic perspective of the child's expected progress for speech-language development. The speech-language pathologist can also work with parents and teachers—to provide them with suggestions on how best to integrate speech and language practice into the daily routine at home and in the classroom. Finally, after the child receives a new device, such as a cochlear implant or FM system (a microphone transmitter is worn by the teacher and a signal is broadcast to an FM receiver worn by the child), the speech-language pathologist, along with an audiologist, works with the child and family to achieve the full potential benefit of the devices by working to improve listening and speaking skills. Most certainly, the ongoing evaluation of amplification devices used in the classroom environment is essential. A summary of some of the treatment areas usually coordinated by speech-language pathologists in the management of children with hearing loss is shown in Table 5.1.

EDUCATIONAL PREPARATION FOR SPEECH-LANGUAGE PATHOLOGY

What type of educational training is needed to become a speech-language pathologist? The entry-level degree for practicing SLP is a 2-year master's degree program from an accredited academic institution. Similar to audiology, preparation for graduate study begins at the undergraduate level with basic courses that provide a foundation for professional study. Courses in human communication, biology, psychology, anatomy and physiology, statistics, child development, and education are examples of course work that will provide a strong preparation for graduate study in SLP. Graduate students in SLP receive a broad-based education and training leading to knowledge and skills across numerous areas of clinical practice including articulation, fluency, voice and resonance, expressive and receptive language, hearing, swallowing, cognitive aspects of communication, social aspects of communication, and communication modalities. Students receive a rigorous academic program of course

TABLE

5.1

Treatment Areas Coordinated by Speech-Language Pathologists in the Management of Children with Hearing Loss

Treatment Area	Treatment Goal
Language development	Enhancing parent-child communication in the chosen communication modality/language Developing understanding of increasingly complex concepts and units of discourse Supporting acquisition of vocabulary networks and word knowledge Enhancing self-expression and acquisition of pragmatic, syntactic, and semantic rules Developing narrative skills (spoken, signed, or written)
Speech-production skill development	Increasing vocalization with appropriate timing and vocal tract space characteristics Increasing phonetic and phonemic repertoires Establishing links between perception and production Improving voice and prosody Improving speech intelligibility
Academic performance	Increasing reading and literacy skills Optimizing overall education achievement with a language base
Social-emotional growth	Establishing acceptance of hearing loss

Adapted from Carney AE, Moeller MP. Treatment efficacy: Hearing loss in children. *JSLHR 1998;*41:S61–S84.

work and at least four semesters of clinical practicum usually from a variety of clinics, schools, and hospitals. In the final semester of study, students complete a full-time 10-week externship—a time in which they spend 40 hours per week honing their clinical skills in a "real-world" clinical setting. Although most students who enter graduate study majored in communication disorders at the undergraduate level, it is common to find students with undergraduate majors in such disciplines as psychology, education, linguistics, and special education.

It is important to note at this point that the need for well-qualified speech-language pathologists to serve the growing needs of young children with hearing loss has never been greater. As the age of the identification for children with hearing loss decreases and improved technologies become readily available, the educational choices parents are making for their children are also changing. Moreover, evidence suggests that children who benefit from early identification, improved technology, and quality intervention achieve at levels similar to their normal hearing peers. Hence, it is not surprising to learn that more and more parents are opting for programs that focus on listening and speaking rather than using language-based signs. One program contrasted the modality choices of parents of children with hearing loss over a 10-year span—in 1995, 40% of the families chose spoken-language options, compared to 60% who chose sign language options; conversely, in 2005, 85% of the families with hearing chose spoken-language options, while only 15% opted for sign language programs. Importantly, although many parents are choosing spoken-language programs, we continue to find that the vast majority of graduate programs for training teachers of the deaf and related professionals focus on sign language-based options. Moreover, to be certified by ASHA, speech-language pathologists only need to take one course in audiology—a basic course in aural habilitation/rehabilitation is no longer required for certification. Indeed, a shortage of well-trained speech-language pathologists may well preclude some children from reaching their full educational potential. Fortunately, a few university-based graduate programs are beginning to offer students in SLP specialized training for serving the needs of young children with hearing loss and their families. An example of a curriculum for SLP that includes a specialty track in young children with hearing loss is shown in Table 5.2. In addition to many of the traditional courses offered in SLP, this specialized program includes 13 hours of course work and associated practicum dealing with young hearing impaired children. Hopefully, similar programs will be implemented at other institutions—this is critical if we expect to meet the changing needs of the hearing-impaired population.

PROFESSIONAL CERTIFICATION AND LICENSURE

To be "certified" in SLP means holding the Certificate of Clinical Competence (CCC), a nationally recognized professional credential that represents a level of excellence. Those who have achieved the CCC—ASHA certification—have voluntarily met rigorous academic and professional standards, typically going beyond the minimum requirements for state licensure. They have the knowledge, skills, and expertise to provide high-quality clinical services, and they actively engage in ongoing professional development to keep their certification current.

The standards for certification for SLP are established by speech-language pathologists, who are members of ASHA. These certification standards are based on skills validation studies and practice analyses involving employers,

TABLE
5.2

Specialty Track Curriculum Focusing on Hearing Loss in Young Children for SLP

Year One

Fall 1 (15 h)	Neurology 3 h	Child language impairments I: nature 2 h	Child language impairments II: assessment 2 h	Clinical principles and procedures 2 h	Articulation disorders and procedures 3 h	Teaching children with hearing loss to listen and speak (development) 2 h	Practicum and clinical case conference 1 h			
Spring 1 (20 h)	Aural rehabilitation for children 3 h	Aphasia 3 h	Dysphagia 3 h	Child language impairments III: intervention 2 h	Cochlear implants in infants and children 2 h	Research methods 1 h	Motor speech disorders 2 h	Independent study 1 h Note: ends early February	Teaching children with hearing loss to listen and speak (assessment) 2 h	Practicum and clinical case conference 1 h
Summer 1 (12 h)	Language and literacy in deaf children 3 h	Traumatic brain injury 2 h	Teaching children with hearing loss to listen and speak (intervention) 1 h	Craniofacial anomalies 2 h	Voice disorders 2 h	Internship/externship in deaf education 2 h	Practicum and clinical case conference 1 h			

Year Two

Semester					
Fall 2 (11 h)	Introduction to amplification for infants and children 2 h	Augmentative and alternative communication 2 h	Stuttering 3 h (incoming students from 2012)	Acoustics and perception 3 h	Practicum and clinical case conference 1 h
Spring 2 (8–9 h)	Family-centered counseling and interview 1 h	Professional issues 1 h	Optional: feeding and swallowing disorders 1 h	7-wk externship 6 h	

leaders in the discipline of communication sciences and disorders, and practitioners in the professions of SLP. Certificate holders are expected to uphold these standards and abide by ASHA's code of ethics. More than 140,000 professionals currently hold ASHA certification. ASHA is the nation's leading professional, credentialing, and scientific organization for speech-language pathologists and speech/language scientists. Importantly, ASHA certification is not contingent upon membership in any professional organization.

Most professions, including SLP, are also regulated by state government in order to serve, safeguard, and promote the health, safety, and welfare of the public. This is done by ensuring that licensure qualifications and standards for professional practice are properly evaluated, applied, and enforced. In many states, the ASHA CCC's are used as the gold standard for verifying appropriate qualifications for speech-language pathologists.

PROFESSIONAL AFFILIATIONS

As noted earlier, ASHA is the primary scientific and professional organization representing the profession of SLP. The association maintains national standards for graduate training program accreditation and credentialing of service providers. Throughout its history, the association has been characterized by enormous growth in membership and a corresponding need for greater staff support. Presently, there are about 250 staff members who work in the ASHA national office. The purposes of ASHA, as stated in its bylaws (ASHA, 2008), are:

1. To encourage basic scientific study of the processes of individual human communication with special reference to speech, language, hearing, and related disorders
2. To promote high standards and ethics for the academic and clinical preparation of individuals entering the discipline of human communication sciences and disorders
3. To promote the acquisition of new knowledge and skills for those within the discipline
4. To promote investigation, prevention, and the diagnosis and treatment of disorders of human communication and related disorders
5. To foster improvement of clinical services and intervention procedures concerning such disorders
6. To stimulate exchange of information among persons and organizations, and to disseminate such information
7. To inform the public about communication sciences and disorders, related disorders, and the professionals who provide services

8. To advocate on behalf of persons with communication and related disorders
9. To promote the individual and collective professional interests of the members of the association (Article II)

The ASHA bylaws address many other issues and serve to provide information about all aspects of the operation and mission of the association, including governance, standards, the code of ethics, publications, and other key organizational components. ASHA membership currently exceeds 145,000 speech-language pathologists and about 13,000 audiologists. Approximately 1,200 ASHA members hold certification in both SLP and audiology.

Like all professional organizations ASHA offers a variety of services to its membership such as educational programs and materials, career opportunities, publications, an annual convention, legislative provisions, marketing and public information, and supplemental benefits (i.e., insurance). An important educational benefit of membership is the opportunity to participate in special interest groups (SIGs). SIGs were established within ASHA to promote knowledge and skills in specialized areas. ASHA members may join one or more of the SIGs and have access to educational programs, research, publications, and dialogue with members that possess similar interests. SIGs have the opportunity to determine what programs and issues are most germane to the members of the group at any given time. SIGs that may be of interest to speech-language pathologists interested in serving children with hearing loss include hearing and hearing disorders in childhood, school-based issues, and language learning and education.

Another important organization for speech-language pathologists who are interested in working with deafness is the Alexander Graham Bell Association for the Deaf and Hard of Hearing, sometimes referred to as AG Bell. AG Bell, a not for profit corporation, is committed to helping families, health care providers, and education professionals to understand childhood hearing loss and the importance of early diagnosis and intervention. Through advocacy, education, research, and financial aid, AG Bell helps to ensure that every child and adult with hearing loss has the opportunity to listen, talk, and thrive in mainstream society. An independent subsidiary of AG Bell is the AG Bell Academy for Listening and Spoken Language. The Academy was established in 2005 and envisions a future where individuals and families will have qualified listening and spoken-language professionals available in their immediate geographic area. The Academy is uniquely positioned to advance the revolutionary global opportunity for deaf or hard of hearing individuals to listen and talk via proven technologies and with guidance and education from certified professionals such as the speech-language pathologist.

Other organizations of possible interest to speech-language pathologists serving individuals with impaired hearing may include Educational

Audiology Association, an international organization of audiologists and related professionals (including speech-language pathologists) who deliver a full spectrum of hearing services to all children, particularly those in educational settings; and the American Society for Deaf Children (ASDC), a national organization of families and professionals committed to educating, empowering, and supporting parents and families of children who are deaf or hard of hearing. The ASDC helps families find meaningful communication options, particularly through the competent use of sign language, in their home, school, and community; and National Association of the Deaf (NAD)—the nation's largest consumer organization safeguarding the accessibility and civil rights of 28 million deaf and hard of hearing Americans in education, employment, health care, and telecommunications. The NAD focuses on grassroots advocacy and empowerment, captioned media, deafness-related information and publications, legal assistance, policy development and research, public awareness, certification of interpreters, and youth leadership development.

SUMMARY

Contemporary SLP began in the 1920s and was a spin-off from traditional programs in interpersonal communication and public address, psychology, and linguistics. As our society became more aware of the vast numbers of children and adults with communication disorders, the profession of SLP evolved in an effort to better understand the complicated issues associated with communication problems and to help individuals afflicted by speech-language disorders overcome their debilitating handicaps. SLP is described as the study of disorders that affect a person's speech, language, cognition, voice, or swallowing and includes the diagnosis and habilitation or rehabilitation of communication problems and/or swallowing difficulties. The speech-language pathologist has numerous employment opportunities one of which is serving children and adults with hearing loss—especially young children.

CHAPTER REVIEW QUESTIONS

1. Why is the speech-language pathologist uniquely qualified to participate in the management of children with hearing loss?
2. Describe some of the responsibilities of a speech-language pathologist in the management of school-age children with hearing loss.
3. The need for qualified speech-language pathologists to work with hearing-impaired children has never been greater. Why?

REFERENCES AND SUGGESTED READINGS

American Speech-Language-Hearing Association. *Scope of Practice in Speech-Language Pathology* [*Scope of Practice*]. Available from http://www.asha.org/policy; 2007.

American Speech-Language-Hearing Association. Roles of speech-language pathologists and teachers of children who are deaf and hard of hearing in the development of communicative and linguistic competence [Position Statement]. Available from www.asha.org/policy; 2004.

American Speech-Language-Hearing Association. *Bylaws of the American Speech-Language-hearing Association* [*Bylaws*]. Available from www.asha.org/policy; 2012.

Carney AE, Moeller MP. Treatment efficacy: Hearing loss in children. *J Speech Lang Hear Res* 1998;41:S61–S84.

Hale ST, Bess FH. Professional organizations. In: Lubinski R, and Hudson MW., *Professional Issues in Speech-Language Pathology and Audiology*. 4th ed. Clifton Park, NY: Delmar Cengage Learning.

Houston KT, Perigoe CB, eds. *Professional preparation for listening and spoken language practitioners*. *Volta Rev* 2010;110(2):85–354.

National Institute on Deafness and Other Communication Disorders. *Strategic Plan: 2006–2008*. http://www.nidcd.nih.gov/StaticResources/about/Plans/stratetic/strategic06-08.pdf

Seewald R, Tharpe AM. *Comprehensive Handbook of Pediatric Audiology*. San Diego, CA: Plural Publishing; 2011.

Tye-Murray N. *Foundations of Aural Rehabilitation, Children Adults, and Their Family Members*. 3rd ed. Clifton Park, NY: Delmar Learning; 2009.

Detecting Breaks in the Communication Chain

6

Auditory Disorders

Chapter Objectives

- To understand various classification systems for disorders of the auditory system;
- To appreciate the strong role played by genetics in many auditory disorders;
- To learn how otitis media develops and its potential consequences for communication; and
- To become familiar with several of the more prevalent or more severe disorders affecting the cochlea and their consequences for communication.

Key Terms and Definitions

- **Endogenous:** A trait or disorder that arises from the individual's genes.
- **Exogenous:** A trait or disorder that is not attributable to genetic causes.
- **Congenital:** A trait or disorder that is present at birth but may or may not be of genetic origin.
- **Otitis media:** An inflammation of the mucosal lining of the middle ear cavity that may include the accumulation of fluid in the cavity.
- **Presbycusis:** Loss of hearing that occurs with advancing age, especially beyond the age of 50 or 60 years.
- **Retrocochlear pathology:** A disease or disorder of the auditory system that impacts structures located from the auditory nerve through the auditory cortex (i.e., "beyond the cochlea").

A variety of disorders, both congenital and acquired, directly affects the auditory system and can result in breaks in the communication chain. These disorders can occur at the level of the external ear, the external auditory canal, the tympanic membrane, the middle ear space, the cochlea, the auditory central nervous system, or any combination of these sites. The following review offers a discussion of some of the more commonly seen disorders that can impair the auditory system.

CLASSIFICATION OF AUDITORY DISORDERS

There are a variety of ways in which auditory disorders may be classified, such as by the portion(s) of the auditory system impacted by the disorder (outer ear, middle ear, inner ear, etc.) or whether the disorder is genetic or nongenetic, that is, **endogenous** or **exogenous**. Exogenous ("outside the genes") hearing disorders are those caused by inflammatory disease, toxicity, noise, accident, or injury that inflicts damage on any part of the auditory system. Endogenous ("in the genes") conditions originate in the genetic characteristics of an individual. An endogenous auditory defect is transmitted from the parents to the child as an inherited trait. However, not all **congenital** hearing disorders are hereditary, nor are all hereditary disorders congenital. For example, the child whose hearing mechanism is damaged in utero by maternal rubella is born with a hearing loss. This hearing loss is congenital but not hereditary. On the other hand, some hereditary defects of hearing may not manifest themselves until adulthood. A breakdown of the estimated percentage of individuals with exogenous and endogenous types of hearing loss is shown in Figure 6.1.

Genetic Transmission of Hearing Loss

As Figure 6.1 shows, hearing loss resulting from hereditary factors is thought to make up approximately 50% of all auditory disorders. It is estimated that there are more than 400 different genetic syndromes in which hearing loss is a regular or occasional feature (see Table 6.1). This is referred to as syndromic hearing loss since it is one symptom of several comprising a genetic syndrome. In addition, there are at least 35 types of genetic deafness that are known to occur without any other associated anomalies. This is referred to as nonsyndromic hearing loss, and hearing loss is the only symptom or feature of the genetic disorder. Of all cases of genetic hearing loss, about 20% to 30% are syndromic and 70% to 80% are nonsyndromic. Vignette 6.1 provides information about one of the more common syndromic forms of hearing loss, Usher syndrome.

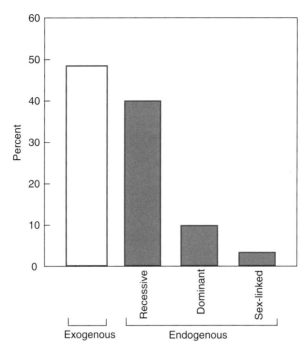

FIGURE 6.1 Percentage of individuals who exhibit exogenous and endogenous types of hearing loss.

Whether occurring as one manifestation of a particular syndrome (group of signs/symptoms that characterize a disorder or condition) or with no other abnormalities, hereditary hearing loss is usually governed by the mendelian laws of inheritance. According to these genetic laws, genetic traits may be dominant or recessive. Genes are located on the chromosomes, and, with the exception of those genes that are located on the sex chromosomes of males (Y chromosome), they come in pairs. One member of each gene pair (and the corresponding member of a chromosome pair) is inherited from each parent. Humans have 22 pairs of autosomes, or non–sex-determining chromosomes, and one pair of sex-determining (X, Y) chromosomes. The sex chromosome pair for females consists of two X chromosomes, and for males, one X and one Y chromosome. In the process of human reproduction, each egg and each sperm cell carries one-half of the chromosomes of each parent. When the egg is fertilized, the full complement of chromosomes is restored, so that half of a child's genes are from the mother and half are from the father.

Most genes are located in the nucleus of a cell, but genetic material can also be found in the cell's mitochondria. Mitochondria are semiautonomous structures that reside in the cytoplasm of cells (the material within the cell's membrane, but outside the cell's nucleus) and are the "power supplies" for

TABLE
6.1

Examples of Autosomal Dominant, Recessive, and Sex-Linked Syndromic Forms of Hereditary Hearing Loss

Mode of Transmission/ Disorder	Prevalence	Clinical Characteristics	Hearing Loss
Autosomal Dominant			
Waardenburg syndrome	1/4,000; 3% of childhood hearing loss	Pigmentary anomalies (white forelock, blue irises, premature graying, partial albinism) craniofacial anomalies—hypertelorism, high nasal bridge, synophrys	20%–50% exhibit SNHL depending on expression of syndrome.
Branchio-oto-renal syndrome	1/40,000; 2% of children with profound hearing loss	Branchial abnormalities—ear pits and tags, cysts and fistula; renal abnormalities	75% exhibit hearing loss; 30% conductive, 20% SNHL, 50% mixed
Treacher Collins syndrome	Unknown	Craniofacial anomalies: poorly developed malar bones, notching of eyelids, malformations of the external ear or canal, micrognathia, cleft palate	30% exhibit conductive hearing loss; SNHL may be present.

Recessive

Usher syndrome	3.5/100,000; 10% of childhood hearing loss	SNHL and retinitis pigmentosa	Type 1: congenital bilateral profound hearing loss and absent vestibular function; Type 2: moderate bilateral SNHL and normal vestibular function; Type 3: progressive bilateral SNHL, variable vestibular dysfunction—found primarily in Norwegian population
Pendred syndrome	Unknown; 5% of congenital childhood hearing loss	Thyroid goiter and SNHL	Severe-to-profound SNHL; 15% may be progressive.
Jervell and Lange-Nielsen syndrome	Unknown (rare)	SNHL and syncopal episodes	Profound bilateral SNHL

Sex-Linked

Norrie syndrome	Unknown	SNHL, congenital or rapidly progressive blindness, pseudoglioma, opacification, and ocular degeneration	One-third exhibit progressive SNHL beginning in second or third decade of life
Alport syndrome	Unknown (predilection for males)	SNHL and nephritis	Bilateral progressive SNHL

SNHL, sensorineural hearing loss.

VIGNETTE 6.1 • FURTHER DISCUSSION

Usher Syndrome: A Description

Usher syndrome represents one of the most common forms of genetic syndromic hearing loss. About 4 of every 100,000 babies born in the United States will have Usher syndrome. According to the National Institute on Deafness and other Communication Disorders (NIDCD; http://www.nidcd.nih.gov/health/hearing/pages/usher.aspx), Usher syndrome "is the most common condition affecting both hearing and vision." The two most common symptoms are hearing loss and a visual disorder known as retinitis pigmentosa, which impacts the primary sensory organ for vision, the retina. Those with Usher syndrome can have varying degrees of hearing loss and varying degrees of vision problems. Usher syndrome is an autosomal recessive genetic disorder (see text).

There are three types of Usher syndrome, Type 1, Type 2, and Type 3, with the vast majority of the cases in the United States being the first two types. In general, the severity and onset of the hearing and vision problems decreases with advancing type such that the Type 1 cases often have profound hearing loss in both ears from birth, decreased night vision as a child, progressing rapidly to tunnel vision or total blindness in their 20s, and balance problems from birth. Type 3 cases, on the other hand, have normal hearing at birth, but hearing loss develops in childhood or early teens reaching a severity requiring the use of hearing aids in adulthood. Type 3 cases also have night vision problems that vary in degree initially, often starting in the teens and then progressing slowly with advancing age to tunnel vision or total blindness as an adult in their 20s or 30s. Type 3 cases are less likely to have vestibular problems. Type 2 cases, then, are somewhere between Type 1 and Type 3 in severity and progression of auditory and visual symptoms.

Recall that in our discussion of the communication chain in Chapter 1, it was critical to get important sensory input to the brain's language centers at an early age. For Type 1 Usher syndrome cases, given the presence of deafness at birth in both ears, providing input to the language centers of the brain is challenging. Early diagnosis and intervention with cochlear implants to provide auditory input is increasingly common in such cases. This is often supplemented by delivery of information through the eyes via sign language or other visual language systems at an early age. Given the rapid progression of the visual impairment in childhood, early training in the use of supplementary visual information is critical.

cells. Mitochondria are transmitted to each of the offspring exclusively via the mother's egg. Some forms of genetic hearing loss have been associated with defects in the mitochondria. If the mother has such a genetic defect, she will pass the hearing loss to all of her offspring.

Autosomal Dominant Inheritance

In autosomal dominant inheritance, the trait is carried from one generation to another. The term "autosomal" implies that the abnormal gene is not located on one of the two sex chromosomes. Typically, one parent exhibits the inherited trait, which may be transmitted to 50% of the offspring. This does not mean that half the children in a given family will necessarily be affected. Statistically, there is a 50% chance that any given child, whether male or female, will be affected (Vignette 6.2). Autosomal dominant inheritance is believed to account for approximately 20% of cases of genetically caused (endogenous) deafness. Because of the interaction of a number of genes, some traits may manifest themselves only partially; for example, only a very mild hearing loss may be observed despite a genetic structure indicating profound hearing loss.

Autosomal Recessive Inheritance

In contrast to autosomal dominant inheritance, both parents of a child with hearing loss of the autosomal recessive type are clinically normal. Appearance of the trait in the offspring requires that an individual possess two similar abnormal genes, one from each parent. The parents themselves are often *heterozygous* carriers of a single abnormal recessive gene. This means that each carries two different genes, one normal and one abnormal with respect to a particular gene pair. Offspring carrying two of either the normal or the abnormal type of gene are termed "homozygotes." Offspring may also be heterozygotes like their parents, carrying one of each gene type. If no abnormal gene is transmitted, the offspring is normal for that trait. If there is one abnormal gene, the child becomes a *carrier* for the trait. Finally, if two abnormal genes, one from each parent, are transmitted, the offspring is affected and becomes a homozygous carrier. The probability that heterozygote parents will bear an affected, homozygous child is 25% in each pregnancy on the basis that each child would inherit the abnormal gene from both the father (50% chance) and the mother (50% chance). Because the laws of probability permit this type of hearing loss to be transmitted without manifestation through several generations, the detection of the true origin is often quite difficult. Recessive genes account for the majority of cases of genetic hearing loss and can account for as much as 80% of childhood deafness.

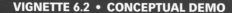

VIGNETTE 6.2 • CONCEPTUAL DEMO

#5

Illustration of Mendelian Law

For this demonstration, you will need two paper cups and five poker chips or checkers (three chips of one color and two of another). For the first illustration, select one chip of one color and three of the other color. We will assume that you have one black chip and three white ones. Divide the four chips into two pairs, each pair representing a parent. The black chip represents a dominant gene for deafness. Whenever it is paired with another black chip or a white chip, it dominates the trait for hearing, resulting in deafness in the person with the gene. In this example, we have one deaf parent (one black chip, one white chip) and one normal-hearing parent (two white chips).

Each parent contributes one gene for hearing status to each offspring. When the deaf parent contributes the gene for deafness (black chip), the offspring will always be deaf. This is because the normal-hearing parent has only recessive genes for normal hearing (white chips) to contribute to the offspring. Separate the black chip from the deaf parent and slide it toward you. Slide each of the white chips from the other parent toward you, one at a time. For both of these possible offspring, the child will be deaf (a black chip paired with a white one). Now return the chips to the parents and slide the white chip from the deaf parent close to you. Slide each of the white chips from the normal parent closer to you, one after the other. Notice that when the deaf parent contributes a gene for normal hearing (white chip), the offspring will have normal hearing. This is true for pairings of each gene from the normal-hearing parent. For these two possible gene pairings, the offspring would have normal hearing.

In total, there were four possible gene pairings for the offspring. Of these, two were predicted to produce deafness and two were predicted to result in normal hearing. In this illustration of autosomal dominant deafness, the odds are that 50%, or one-half, of the offspring from these two parents will be deaf.

Now, remove one of the white chips and replace it with a black one. Form two pairs of chips in front of you, each having one black and one white chip. In this case, the black chip represents the gene for deafness again, but it is recessive. The gene for normal hearing (white chip) is dominant. There will again be four possible pairings of the chips in the offspring, one from each parent. Examine the various combinations of genes by first sliding one chip closer to you from the parent on the left. Examine two possible pairings for each gene from the parent on the right. Now repeat this process by sliding the other chip from the parent on the left closer to you. When you have finished, you should have observed the following four pairs of chips for the offspring (black-white, black-black, white-black, and white-white). In this case of autosomal recessive deafness, only one of the possible combinations would produce a deaf offspring (black-black). The probability of a deaf child is one in four, or 25%. Two of the three normal-hearing offspring, however, will carry a gene for deafness (black-white chip pairs). These offspring are referred to as "carriers" of the trait.

It is sometimes difficult to understand that the mendelian laws of hearing are only probabilities. In the case of autosomal recessive deafness, for example, one might think that if the parents had four offspring, then they would have one deaf child. That is only the probability. They could very well have four normal-hearing children or four deaf children. To see how this occurs, place one black and one white chip in each of the two paper cups. Shake up the left cup and draw a chip. Repeat the process with the right cup. Examine the two chips (genes) selected, one from each cup (parent). Record the outcome (deaf or normal hearing) and replace chips in the cups. Do this 20 times, representing five families of four offspring each. When you're finished, you will likely find some families of four that had two, three, or four deaf offspring. If you did this an infinite number of times, however, 25% of the offspring would be deaf, as predicted by mendelian laws for autosomal recessive deafness.

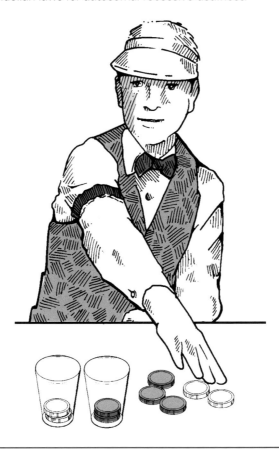

X-Linked Inheritance

In the X-linked or sex-linked type of deafness, inherited traits are determined by genes located on the X chromosome. As noted earlier, normal females have two X chromosomes, whereas males possess one X and one Y chromosome. Sons receive their Y chromosomes from their fathers; their X chromosomes are inherited from their mothers. Daughters, on the other hand, receive one X chromosome from their fathers and the other from their mothers. Approximately 2% to 3% of deafness occurs as a result of X-linked inheritance. Examples of autosomal dominant, recessive, and sex-linked syndromic forms of hereditary deafness are shown in Table 6.1.

Advances in Hereditary Deafness

The progress made in genetic research during the past 25 years has been truly remarkable and, subsequently, is continually changing our current understanding of hereditary deafness. Through gene mapping (identifying the chromosomal location of the gene) and localization (isolating the gene responsible for a disorder), it is now possible to identify genes responsible for deafness. Currently, the chromosomal locations of approximately 80 genes for syndromic and nonsyndromic hearing loss have been mapped. Figure 6.2 illustrates the locations of each of these genes for hearing loss on the 22 chromosome pairs, as well as the X and Y chromosomes. For example, in 1997, a specific gene (GJB2 or connexin 26; see chromosome pair #13 in Fig. 6.2) was identified that appears to be the cause of sensorineural hearing loss in many individuals. By testing for this gene alone, it is possible to identify the cause of deafness in as many as 40% of individuals in whom the cause of deafness was previously unknown. Identifying the genes that cause hearing loss may ultimately lead to therapeutic or preventive intervention in persons who exhibit genetic hearing impairment. Moreover, the possibility of genetic screening to determine the diagnosis after identification of hearing loss is now a topic of widespread discussion. Genetic screening may have important benefits for both the child and the child's parents. Genetic testing and counseling can assist families, enabling them to learn more about the cause of hearing loss, to determine the probability of recurring risks, and to accept a diagnosis of deafness.

Site of Lesion

Also important in the classification of an auditory disorder is the location of the lesion in the auditory portion of the communication chain. Disorders of the outer or middle ear cause a type of hearing loss, known as *conductive* hearing loss (see Chapter 7), that is frequently amenable to medical treatment. If damage occurs to the nerve endings or to the hair cells in the inner ear, the hearing loss

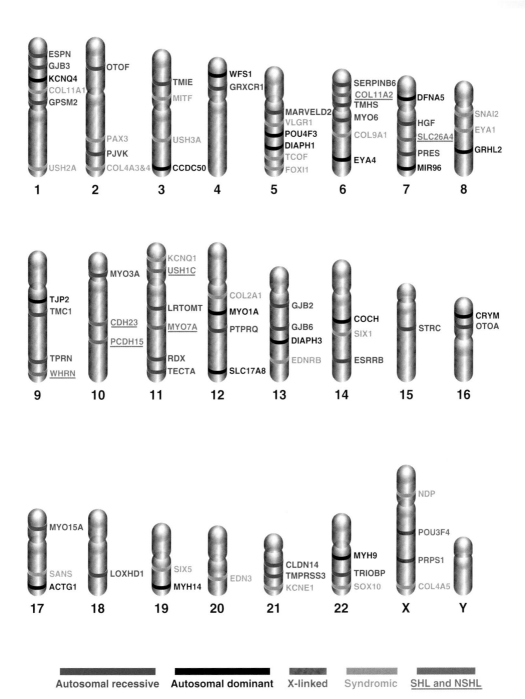

FIGURE 6.2 The locations of genes with mutations causing hearing loss on various chromosomes (pairs 1 to 22, plus the X and Y chromosome). (From Dror AA, Avraham KB. Hearing impairment: A panoply of genes and functions. *Neuron* 2010;68:293–308.)

is termed *sensorineural* (Chapter 7). Hearing losses resulting from damage to the auditory nerve after it leaves the cochlea are sometimes designated neural or *retrocochlear*. When damage occurs to the nerve pathways within the auditory central nervous system (see Chapter 3), the resulting condition is often known as *central* auditory impairment. So, the label used to describe the type of hearing loss, such as "conductive," "sensorineural," "retrocochlear," or "central," identifies the general location in the auditory portion of the communication chain where the break or lesion occurs.

Outer ear and middle ear disorders do not pose as serious a threat to the development and use of the communication chain as disorders located in the inner ear. This is basically because most outer ear and middle ear disorders are medically treatable, once diagnosed, and do not result in long-term loss of input to the higher centers of the communication chain. Moreover, the hearing impairments associated with middle ear problems, in general, tend to be less severe, often mild in degree, and this, together with the loss typically being temporary, poses a less serious threat to the communication chain. As a result, the disorders reviewed in this chapter primarily involve the cochlea and result in permanent sensorineural hearing loss of varying degrees. One clear exception to this, however, involves a middle ear disorder known as **otitis media**. This is a very prevalent disorder among young children and, despite diagnosis and medical treatment, can be a persistent hearing problem. As a result, this chapter begins with a description of this middle ear disease and then moves on to those disorders resulting in sensorineural hearing loss.

THE PROBLEM OF OTITIS MEDIA

An important middle ear disorder frequently seen by the clinician is otitis media, one of the most common diseases in childhood. Otitis media refers to inflammation of the middle ear cavity. It is considered an important economic and health problem because of its prevalence, the cost of its treatment, the potential for secondary medical complications, and the possibility of long-term nonmedical consequences. The clinician must be familiar with this middle ear disorder and have a grasp of such important topics as the classification of otitis media, its natural history and epidemiology, its cause, its management, and its potential complications.

Classification of Otitis Media

Otitis media is often classified on the basis of the temporal sequence of the disease. In other words, the disease is categorized according to the duration of the disease process. For example, acute otitis media typically will run its full course within a 3-week period. The disease begins with a rapid onset, persists for a week to 10 days, and then resolves rapidly. Some of the more common symptoms associated with acute otitis media include a bulging, reddened tympanic membrane, pain, and upper respiratory infection. If the disease has a slow onset and persists for 3 months or more, it is referred to as chronic otitis media (COM). Symptoms associated with COM may include a large central perforation in the eardrum and discharge of fluid through the perforation.

Otitis media is also classified according to the type of fluid that is observed by the physician in the middle ear cavity. A clear fluid that is free of cellular debris and bacteria is described as serous, and the term serous otitis media is used to describe this condition. If the fluid is purulent or suppurative, like the fluid found most often in acute otitis media, it will contain white blood cells, some cellular debris, and many bacteria. Acute otitis media is sometimes referred to as acute suppurative otitis media or acute purulent otitis media. Sometimes the fluid is mucoid because it has been secreted from the mucosal lining of the middle ear. This fluid is thick in substance and contains white blood cells, few bacteria, and some cellular debris. When mucoid fluid is present, the disease may be referred to as mucoid otitis media, or secretory otitis media. Figure 6.3 illustrates a normal tympanic membrane along with several pathologic conditions including serous otitis media, otitis media with bubbles in the fluid, and acute otitis media.

Natural History and Epidemiology of Otitis Media

To understand fully the nature of otitis media, one must appreciate the natural history and epidemiology of the disease. Natural history and epidemiology are terms used to denote the study of the relationships of various factors that determine the natural frequency and distribution of a disease. It has already been stated that otitis media with effusion is one of the most prevalent diseases in childhood (Vignette 6.3). Depending on the study reviewed, 76% to 95% of all children have at least one episode of otitis media by 6 years of age. In addition, the prevalence of the disease peaks during the early years of life. The prevalence of otitis media is typically greatest during the first 2 years of life and then decreases with increasing age. Importantly, there appears to be a relationship between the age of onset and the probability of repeated episodes. Children who appear to be prone to middle ear disease and experience five to six bouts within the first several years of life have usually experienced their first episode of the disease during the first 18 months of life. Seldom does a child become otitis prone if the first episode occurred after 18 months of age.

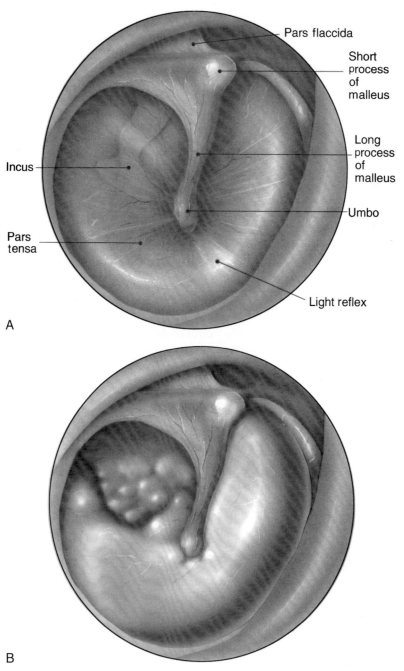

FIGURE 6.3 Normal tympanic membrane *(A)* and three pathologic conditions: *B*, serous otitis media;

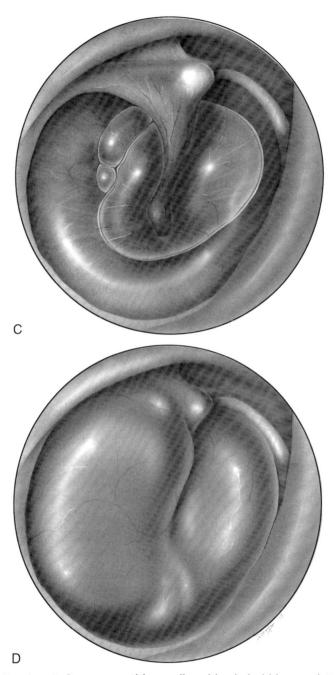

C

D

FIGURE 6.3 *(Continued) C*, serous otitis media with air bubbles; and *D*, acute otitis media. (From English GM. *Otolaryngology*. Hagerstown, MD: Harper & Row; 1976.)

VIGNETTE 6.3 • FURTHER DISCUSSION

Prevalence of Middle Ear Disease in Children

The prevalence of middle ear disease has reached epidemic proportions. Three out of four children experience otitis media by the time they reach 3 years. For children below the age of 6 years, otitis media is the most common reason for a doctor visit. It is estimated that one visit in three that is made for illness results in the diagnosis of middle ear disease. According to the National Center for Health Statistics, ear infection diagnoses increased 150% between 1975 and 1990. Moreover, in 1975, there were 10 million doctor visits for earaches; by 1990, there were 24.5 million visits, costing more than $1 billion annually. Nine out of every ten children will have at least one ear infection; most will have at least one acute ear infection by age 3, and more than one-third of all children will have three acute infections. Why is the prevalence of ear infections increasing? Many authorities believe that childcare is a significant factor. Children in day care facilities experience a much higher prevalence of upper respiratory infections and, subsequently, ear infections.

The extent of the management for ear infections is also substantial. For example, the most common surgery on children is myringotomy with insertion tubes (see Figs. 6.4 and 6.5), a procedure used to drain fluid and restore hearing. In addition, the cost of antibiotics commonly prescribed for ear infections amounts to several billion dollars in annual worldwide sales. Clearly, middle ear disease has become one of the major health care problems among children in the United States.

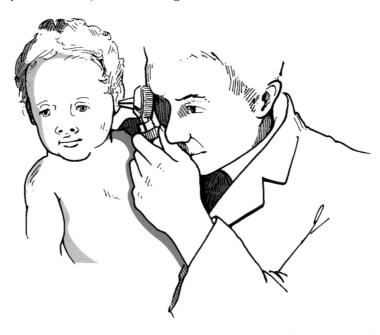

Otitis media varies slightly with gender, with more cases seen in males than in females. There is seasonal variation in otitis media, with higher occurrence during winter and spring. Some groups are more at risk for middle ear disease than others. Some of the groups considered more at risk for otitis media are children with cleft palate and other craniofacial disorders, those with Down syndrome, and those with learning disabilities. Children who reside in the inner city and children who attend daycare centers are also prone to suffer from middle ear disease, as are Native Americans.

Cause of Otitis Media

It is commonly believed that otitis media develops because of eustachian tube obstruction. As mentioned in Chapter 3, the eustachian tube is important to a healthy middle ear because it provides for pressure equalization and fluid drainage. If the pressure equalization system is obstructed, a negative pressure can develop in the middle ear cavity. The negative pressure literally sucks the fluid from the membranous lining of the middle ear canal. The fluid that has accumulated from the mucosal lining of the middle ear has no place to escape because the eustachian tube is blocked. Vignette 6.4 shows a representation of this general process. A number of factors may produce eustachian tube obstruction, including large adenoid tissue in the nasopharyngeal area and inflammation of the mucous lining of the tube. It is also important to note that the muscular opening function of the eustachian tube is poor in children with otitis media and in children with histories of middle ear disease. In fact, in general, the muscle responsible for opening and closing the tube (tensor veli palatini) is less efficient among young infants and children. Moreover, the position of the eustachian tube in children lies at an angle of only 10 degrees in relation to the horizontal plane, whereas in adults this angle is 45 degrees (Fig. 6.4). Further, the tube is much shorter in infants. Because of the angle and shortness of the tube in children, fluid, such as milk, is able to reach the middle ear from the nasopharyngeal area with greater ease and has greater difficulty escaping from the middle ear cavity.

Hearing loss is considered the most common complication of otitis media. Although the type of the loss is usually conductive because the problem is located in the middle ear, sensorineural or inner ear involvement can also occur, especially in long-standing cases of otitis media. The hearing loss is usually flat, affecting all frequencies equally, and is mild in degree, usually around a 25-dB hearing loss for midfrequency pure tones (500 to 2,000 Hz). The degree of hearing loss in individual cases, though, can range from normal sensitivity to hearing losses as great as 50 dB. In general, the prevalence rate for hearing loss associated with otitis media depends on the criteria used to define hearing loss.

VIGNETTE 6.4 • FURTHER DISCUSSION

Development of Acute Otitis Media

The drawings that accompany this vignette illustrate the general pattern of events that can occur in acute otitis media. Panel A shows the landmarks of a normal middle ear system. Note also the appearance of the eustachian tube, especially at the opening in the nasopharyngeal area. Panel B shows that the pharyngeal end of the eustachian tube has been closed off by swelling because of pharyngeal infection

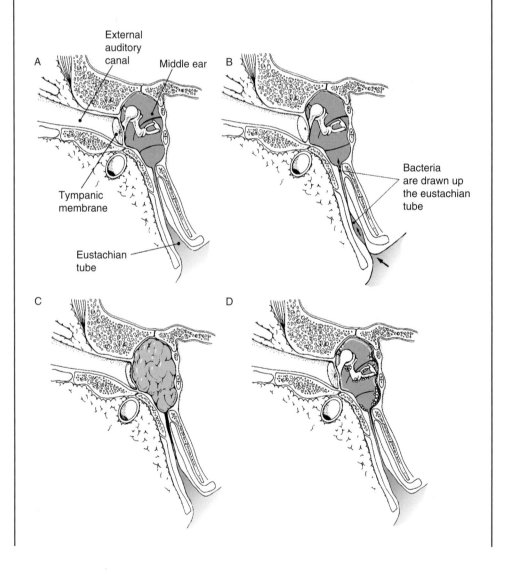

or possibly an allergy. More specifically, the upper respiratory infection produces a congestion of the mucosa in the nasopharyngeal area, the eustachian tube, and the middle ear. The congestion of the mucosa of the tube produces an obstruction that prevents ventilation of the middle ear space. Also, the tympanic membrane is retracted inward because of negative pressure caused by absorption from the middle ear. Finally, bacteria from the oral pharyngeal area are drawn up the eustachian tube to the middle ear space. Panel C illustrates a full-blown condition of acute otitis media. Fluid secretions from the goblet cells of the mucosal lining of the middle ear are now trapped and have no way to leave the middle ear cavity. The bacteria drawn from the eustachian tube proliferate in the secretions, forming a viscous pus. Observe also that the tympanic membrane is no longer retracted but is bulging.

Panel D shows a condition that may well result after antimicrobial treatment. The bacteria have been killed by the antibiotics, and a thin or mucoid-type fluid remains (represented in the drawing by bubbles around the perimeter of the middle-ear cavity). Other possible outcomes after medical treatment might be the return to a completely normal middle ear, as in A, or a condition like the one shown in B.

The onset of otitis media with effusion, although asymptomatic, would follow a similar pattern of events. Recurrent episodes of acute otitis media or middle ear disease with effusion are probably a result of abnormal anatomy or physiology of the eustachian tube.

Unfortunately, prevalence data are difficult to determine because of the lack of well-controlled studies in this area.

Another complication that may result from long-standing middle ear disease with effusion is deficiency in psychoeducational and/or communicative skills. It is widely suspected that otitis-prone children are more susceptible to delays in speech, language, and cognitive development, and in education. The research findings in this area, however, are inconclusive, and a cause-effect relationship cannot be assumed at the present time. Clearly, given our understanding of the development of the communication chain, if COM resulted in a mild or mild-to-moderate hearing loss of 25 to 50 dB that developed at an early age (<18 months) and the hearing loss persisted for many months, a negative effect on the development of communication skills *could* occur. As a result, the key is the identification and treatment of otitis media early in the development of the disease.

Medical Complications Associated with Otitis Media

A number of medical complications are associated with otitis media. The most common medical complications are COM with associated cholesteatoma, perforations or retraction pockets of the tympanic membrane, tympanosclerosis, adhesive otitis media, and facial paralysis.

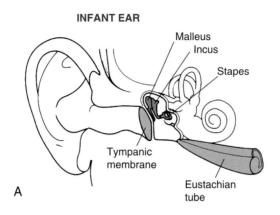

INFANT EAR

Malleus
Incus
Stapes
Tympanic
membrane
Eustachian
tube

A

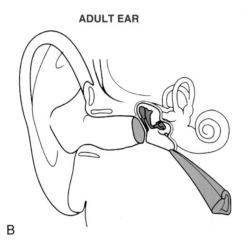

ADULT EAR

B

FIGURE 6.4 Anatomic illustration of the eustachian tube in an infant ear compared with that of the adult ear. Note that the tube of an infant lies more on a horizontal plane.

COM and Associated Cholesteatoma   Cholesteatoma refers to the accumulation of cellular debris developed from perforations of the tympanic membrane. Sometimes this pseudotumor becomes infected and causes some erosion of the ossicles. No typical pattern of hearing loss is associated with cholesteatomas, and the loss may vary in severity from slight to moderate.

Perforation of the Tympanic Membrane   Spontaneous perforations or holes in the eardrum usually occur subsequent to acute infections, but may also be associated with COM. Perforations of the tympanic membrane produce hearing

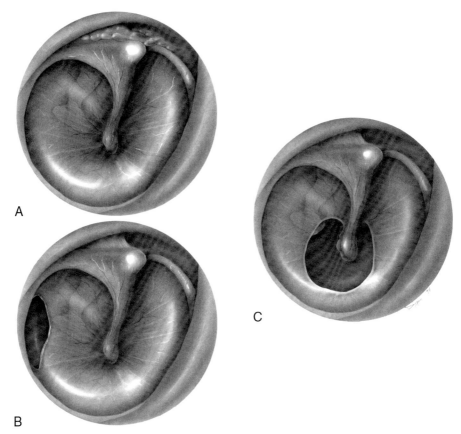

FIGURE 6.5 Perforations in three tympanic membranes. *A:* Attic perforation and associated cholesteatoma. *B:* Marginal perforation. *C:* Large central perforation. (Adapted from English GM. *Otolaryngology*. Hagerstown, MD: Harper & Row; 1976.) (4E, Figure 5.9)

deficits in the mild-to-moderate category, provided there are no ossicular defects. The hearing loss is a result of reduction in the areal ratio between the tympanic membrane and oval window and the direct coupling of sound waves to the round window (see Chapter 3 for a discussion of these mechanisms). Figure 6.5 illustrates several different perforations of the tympanic membrane.

Tympanosclerosis Tympanosclerosis is characterized by white shale-like plaques on the tympanic membrane and deposits on the ossicles. It occurs most often after COM, which, when resolved, leaves behind a residual material. The shale-like plaques create a stiffening effect on the tympanic membrane and the ossicular chain, producing conductive hearing loss in the low frequencies.

Adhesive Otitis Media   Adhesive otitis media is a thickening of the mucous membrane lining the middle ear cavity. It can cause fixation of the ossicles and subsequent hearing loss.

Facial Paralysis   Facial paralysis may occur in the course of acute or COM. The facial nerve passes through the middle ear area in a bony tube called the fallopian canal. It is possible for the fallopian canal to become eroded and expose the facial nerve to the toxic effects of the infection.

Management of Otitis Media

A common means of treating acute otitis media is the routine administration of antimicrobial agents. These antibiotics are designed to combat the various pathogens thought to exist within the middle ear fluid. Pharmaceutical agents, such as ampicillin, amoxicillin, erythromycin, and amoxicillin/clavulanic (Augmentin), are frequently administered in the management of acute otitis media. Unfortunately, the overall effectiveness of antibiotic therapy in the treatment of ear disease has not been clearly established. Even when appropriate antimicrobial agents have been prescribed and the fluid is sterilized, the effusion may persist for 2 weeks to 3 months. Also, antibiotic medications can produce adverse side effects such as diarrhea, nausea, vomiting, skin rash, and malaise. Finally, antihistamines and decongestants have also been used in the treatment of middle ear disease; however, this form of treatment has been shown to be ineffective.

A common surgical approach to the management of both suppurative and nonsuppurative otitis media is a myringotomy. Myringotomy is a surgical procedure that involves making an incision in one of the inferior quadrants of the tympanic membrane, as shown in Figure 6.6. In the acute forms of the disease, a myringotomy is performed when there is severe pain or toxicity, high fever, failure to respond to antimicrobial therapy, or some serious secondary medical complication. In secretory otitis media, a myringotomy is more commonly performed, usually to remove fluid and restore hearing sensitivity. This surgical procedure is performed in cases where the disease has persisted for at least 3 months. The eardrum incision can heal quickly, however, and the fluid reappears. To avoid this possibility and to ensure sustained middle ear aeration, ventilating tubes or grommets are often inserted into the eardrum (Fig. 6.7).

Tonsillectomy and adenoidectomy are also considered as a management approach to otitis media. Although tonsillectomy does not seem to be an effective treatment protocol, adenoidectomy is a common surgical procedure for the management of bilateral otitis media in children 4 years of age or older.

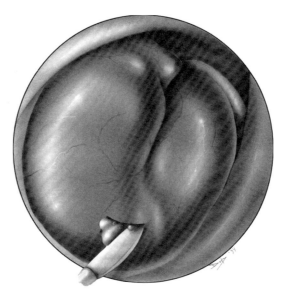

FIGURE 6.6 Myringotomy. Note the bulging appearance of the tympanic membrane. (From English GM. *Otolaryngology*. Hagerstown, MD: Harper & Row; 1976.)

In general, this approach is undertaken when a patient does not respond to medical therapy, large adenoids are present, and there is no evidence of nasal allergy. Under these conditions, it is assumed that the eustachian tube blockage causing the middle ear disease is a result of enlarged adenoids. The adenoids are removed to free the eustachian tube from the blockage.

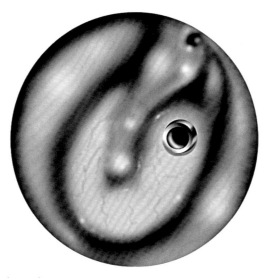

FIGURE 6.7 Ventilating tube or grommet.

A more radical surgical approach is required if chronic disease permanently impairs basic structures within the middle ear. When alteration of the middle ear structures is required, a surgical technique known as tympanoplasty is performed. Tympanoplasty may simply involve repair of a chronically perforated eardrum or may also involve reconstruction of ossicles that have been eroded away by the long-standing disease.

COCHLEAR AND RETROCOCHLEAR PATHOLOGY

Millions of Americans have sensorineural hearing loss as a consequence of cochlear pathology. For children, conductive hearing loss produced by middle ear pathology, as reviewed earlier in this chapter, is probably the most common type of hearing loss. For adults, however, sensorineural hearing loss resulting from underlying cochlear pathology is probably the most common type of hearing impairment. Recall from the previous sections of this chapter that conductive hearing loss was usually medically treatable, either through surgery, medication, or a combination of the two. With sensorineural hearing loss, however, this is usually not the case. The hearing loss is typically permanent. For those individuals with significant sensorineural hearing loss, the usual course of action is to seek assistance from amplification, often a personal wearable hearing aid. Hearing aids and other types of amplification for the hearing impaired are described in detail in Chapter 9.

The description of the hearing loss produced by cochlear pathology as "sensorineural" seems particularly appropriate. As is reviewed in Chapter 7, the presence of a sensorineural hearing loss does not tell us the exact location of the pathology along the auditory pathway; it only eliminates the outer and middle ears as possibilities. The pathology could be affecting the sensory receptors within the cochlea, the neural pathways leading from the cochlea to higher centers of the auditory system, or both the sensory and neural structures. In this context, then, "sensorineural" hearing loss is a very appropriate label.

The term sensorineural hearing loss is also an appropriate label for the hearing loss resulting from cochlear pathology for another reason. In cochlear pathology, the sensory receptors within the cochlea are destroyed. Exactly how this occurs depends on the specific cause. Research suggests that the sensory cell destruction quickly becomes sensorineural damage. Once the inner hair cells within the organ of Corti are destroyed, a phenomenon known as retrograde degeneration occurs. *Retrograde degeneration* refers to the destruction of connecting anatomic structures located more central to the structure that was destroyed. Destruction of the inner hair cells within the organ of Corti results in the eventual degeneration of some of the first-order afferent nerve fibers communicating with the damaged hair cells. Most patients with profound sensorineural hearing loss caused by cochlear pathology, therefore, most likely have underlying damage to both the sensory (cochlea) and neural (nerve fibers) portions of the auditory system.

When a sensorineural hearing loss is observed, how do the audiologist and physician determine whether it is because of cochlear pathology or a problem lying further up the ascending neural pathways (called *"retrocochlear" pathology*)? As mentioned in Chapter 7, several steps are involved in establishing the diagnosis of the hearing loss. The case history taken by the audiologist or physician can provide some important clues as to the location of the problem. The presence of other, frequently nonauditory, complaints, such as dizziness, loss of balance, and ringing in the ears (tinnitus), can aid the physician in establishing the diagnosis. A particular pattern of results from the basic audiology test battery may alert the physician to a probable underlying cause. Finally, special tests can be performed on the patient at the physician's request. These tests may be auditory, in which case they will be performed by an audiologist, or they may be nonauditory. An example of a nonauditory special test is electronystagmography, which tests the vestibular system and may also be performed by an audiologist. Other nonauditory tests, not performed by the audiologist, might involve some form of tomography or magnetic resonance imaging (MRI). Computer-assisted tomography scans and MRIs provide a visual image of the brain and brainstem structures and are increasingly commonplace for site-of-lesion testing when a retrocochlear problem is suspected. The most definitive auditory special test to evaluate retrocochlear function involves the measurement of the auditory brainstem response, or ABR. This test may also be administered by an audiologist. (The basic ABR was described briefly in Chapter 3, and clinical use of the ABR is described in more detail in Chapter 7.)

Discussion of the special tests, auditory and nonauditory, that aid the physician in establishing the diagnosis is beyond the scope of this book, although some of these fundamental tests are described briefly in Chapter 7. Suffice it to say that such tests exist and that the audiologist is frequently asked to perform some of them. Many types of cochlear and retrocochlear pathology, however, do produce distinct patterns of hearing loss and can result in breaks in the communication chain. The remainder of this chapter describes several of these more common pathologies.

Cochlear Pathology

Before describing some specific causes of cochlear pathology, some general characteristics shared by most patients with cochlear pathology are noteworthy. First, studies of human cadavers have revealed a close correspondence between the location of the damage along the length of the cochlea and the resulting pattern of hearing loss. For example, if postmortem anatomic studies of a patient's ear reveal damage in the basal high-frequency portion of the cochlea, then recent measures of hearing loss obtained before death would most likely indicate the presence of a high-frequency sensorineural hearing loss. Although there are exceptions, it is generally the case in cochlear pathology that the pattern of hearing loss or audiometric configuration provides at least a gross indication of the regions of the cochlea, from base to apex, that were damaged by the pathology. A high-frequency sensorineural hearing loss reflects damage to the basal portion of the cochlea, a low-frequency sensorineural hearing loss suggests damage to the apical region of the cochlea, and a broad hearing loss extending from low to high frequencies reflects an underlying lesion along the entire length of the cochlea. This follows directly from the mapping of sound frequency to place of maximum mechanical activity in the cochlea or tonotopic organization, noted previously in Chapter 3 (Vignette 6.5).

As noted, in sensorineural hearing loss caused by cochlear pathology, there is a close correspondence between the frequencies that demonstrate hearing loss and the region along the length of the cochlea that is damaged. There is a less certain correspondence, however, between the degree of hearing loss at a particular frequency and the degree of damage at the corresponding location in the cochlea. One popular conception is that mild or moderate degrees of sensorineural hearing loss result from destruction of the outer hair cells, to varying degrees, whereas more severe hearing loss reflects damage to both the outer and the inner hair cells of the cochlea.

There are also several perceptual consequences of sensorineural hearing loss caused by cochlear pathology. Except for those with profound impairments, patients with cochlear pathology most commonly complain that they can hear speech, but can't understand it. This may be especially true when listening against a background of noise. The reason for this common complaint in many individuals with cochlear pathology is that it is often the basal portion of the cochlea that is most severely damaged in cochlear pathology. This results in a hearing loss for high-frequency sounds. Many important consonant sounds, such as "s," "t," and "f," are low-intensity, high-frequency speech sounds. An individual who has trouble hearing high-frequency sounds will often not be able to hear these speech sounds. They will, however, be able to hear many other speech sounds, such as vowels, because these sounds have most of their energy in the lower frequencies where hearing is normal or close to normal in these individuals. When this individual is presented with a series of words such as "white, wife, wipe, wise," what is perceived may be something like "why, why, why, why" because the high-frequency consonants are too soft to be heard. As a result, the individual can tell that someone is speaking, but can't understand what was said. This, of course, can cause a breakdown in communication between the talker and the listener.

Hearing loss
demonstration

VIGNETTE 6.5 • FURTHER DISCUSSION

Illustration of the Relationship between Location of Cochlear Damage and Hearing Loss

The three figures accompanying this vignette illustrate the correspondence between the region of the cochlea that is damaged and the resultant hearing loss that is measured. The upper portion of each figure shows a "cochleogram" from three monkeys that were exposed to intense noise. A cochleogram depicts the percentage of hair cells (*HCs*) within the organ of Corti that remain at various locations along the length of the cochlea after noise exposure. The percentages are determined after careful microscopic examination of the cochlea.

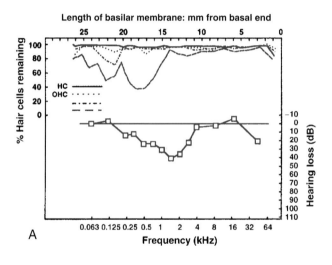

A

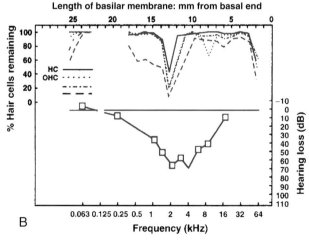

B

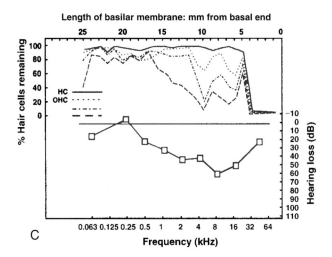

C

In Panel A, the monkey was exposed to a low-frequency noise. This resulted in destruction of outer hair cells (*OHCs*) in the region roughly 15 to 25 mm from the base of the cochlea. Before sacrificing the animal to examine the type and extent of damage produced by the noise, the audiogram in the lower portion of the panel was obtained. A sensorineural hearing loss in the low and intermediate frequencies was produced.

When another monkey was exposed to a high-frequency noise (Panel B), the cochleogram (*upper portion*) indicated that the damage appeared in the basal portion of the cochlea. Note that the audiogram obtained from the same monkey after the noise exposure and just before sacrifice (*lower portion*) revealed the presence of a high-frequency sensorineural hearing loss. As the damage to the sensory hair cells within the organ of Corti progressed from an apical (Panel A) to a basal (Panel B) region of the cochlea, the audiogram reflected the change as a shift from a low-frequency to a high-frequency sensorineural hearing loss.

Panel C shows a cochleogram and audiogram from a monkey exposed to a wideband noise. Note that the damage is much more extensive, affecting both the apical and basal portions of the cochlea. The damage, however, is most severe in the basal region. This is again reflected in the audiogram. The audiogram shows a broad hearing loss extending from low to high frequencies, more severe in the high frequencies.

Adapted from Moody DB, Stebbins WC, Hawkins JE Jr, et al. Hearing loss and cochlear pathology in the monkey [macaca] following exposure to high levels of noise. *Arch Otorhinolaryngol* 1978;220:47–72.

The patient with cochlear pathology also frequently experiences a phenomenon known as loudness recruitment (see Chapter 3 for a brief description). The hearing loss makes low-intensity sounds inaudible. Moderate-intensity sounds that are comfortably loud to a normal-hearing person may be barely audible to the person with cochlear pathology. At high intensities, however, the loudness of the sound is the same for both a normal ear and one with cochlear pathology. Let us assume, for example, that a pure tone at 2,000 Hz having a level of 110 dB SPL is uncomfortably loud for both a normal listener and a person with cochlear pathology. The person with cochlear pathology, however, has a hearing threshold at 2,000 Hz of 60 dB SPL, whereas the normal listener's threshold is 10 dB SPL. Thus, for the normal listener, the intensity of the tone has to be increased 100 dB to increase the loudness of the tone from "just audible" (threshold) to "uncomfortable." For the person with cochlear pathology, however, an increase in intensity of only 50 dB was needed to cover the same range of loudness (from "just audible" to "uncomfortable"). Loudness increases more rapidly in the ear with cochlear pathology than in the normal ear. This is known as loudness recruitment.

The presence of loudness recruitment makes it more difficult to fit a hearing aid on a person with cochlear pathology. Low-level sounds need to be amplified to be made audible to the hearing-impaired person. High-intensity sounds, however, cannot be amplified by the same amount or the hearing aid will produce sounds that are uncomfortably loud to the wearer. Possible solutions to this dilemma when fitting the patient with a hearing aid are described in more detail in Chapter 9.

Finally, the patient with cochlear hearing loss may have accompanying speech abnormalities. As noted previously, the auditory system of the talker or sender is also used to monitor the quality of the acoustic speech sounds produced by the talker. Depending on the severity, configuration, and age of onset of the hearing loss, the talker's speech may be misarticulated. In addition, if the cochlear pathology produces sensorineural hearing loss in the low and intermediate frequencies, the patient will typically use speech levels that are inappropriately loud, especially while talking without wearing a hearing aid. This is because the feedback that a speaker normally receives when talking is not available to assist in regulating the voice level.

Now that we have reviewed some features shared by most individuals with cochlear pathology, the remainder of this section will examine several types of pathology. The pathologies described here are by no means an exhaustive compilation. In keeping with the general mission of this book, the pathologies described were selected either because of their common occurrence in the general population or among children or because of their potential for severe negative impact on the communication chain.

Viral and Bacterial Diseases

Severe viral and bacterial infections can result in varying degrees and patterns of sensorineural hearing loss. Infectious disease can be transmitted to the child by the mother in utero, a condition referred to as prenatal, congenital, or sometimes perinatal disease. These terms carry slightly different meanings, yet are often used synonymously. The term *prenatal* refers to something that occurs to the fetus before birth. *Congenital* also implies before birth, but usually before the 28th week of gestation. Finally, the word *perinatal* pertains to a condition that occurs in the period shortly before or after birth (from 8 weeks before birth to 4 weeks after). A disease can also be acquired later in life, and this is usually referred to as a postnatal condition. The following discussion reviews some of the more common prenatal and postnatal infectious diseases known to cause hearing loss.

Prenatal Diseases   Many of the prenatal diseases are categorized as part of the TORCH complex, an acronym used to identify the major infections that may be contracted in utero. In the acronym TORCH, T stands for toxoplasmosis, O is for other, R is for rubella, C is for cytomegalovirus (CMV), and H is for herpes simplex. Some have used the mnemonic (S)TORCH, where S stands for syphilis. Any disease of the (S)TORCH complex is considered a high-risk factor for hearing loss, and therefore, it is important for the audiologist to have some general knowledge of these infectious conditions. Table 6.2 lists the (S)TORCH diseases. Let us now review briefly each of these conditions:

- *Syphilis* is transmitted to the child by intrauterine infection from the mother. Syphilis may manifest itself anytime from the first to the sixth decade of life. When the age of onset is early (before 10 years), the sensorineural hearing loss is profound and bilateral with sudden onset. With adult onset, the hearing loss is fluctuating and asymmetric and may appear either suddenly or gradually. Dizziness is also commonly associated with this condition.
- *Toxoplasmosis* is a disease caused by an organism (*Toxoplasma gondii*) that is transmitted to the child via the placenta. It is thought that the infection is contracted by eating uncooked meat or by making contact with feces of cats. As noted from Table 6.2, approximately 17% of infected newborns exhibit sensorineural hearing loss. The hearing loss is typically moderate and progressive.
- *Rubella* is perhaps the most well-recognized disease of the (S)TORCH complex. Rubella, sometimes referred to as German measles, infects the mother via the respiratory route. The virus is carried by the bloodstream to the placenta and to the fetus. If the mother contracts the virus during the 1st month of pregnancy, there is a 50% chance that the fetus will

be infected; in the 2nd month, there is a 22% chance; and in subsequent months, there is approximately a 6% to 10% chance. Table 6.2 lists some of the more frequently encountered symptoms. One of the symptoms is a severe-to-profound sensorineural hearing loss in both ears. The child will display a trough- or bowl-shaped pattern of hearing loss with good hearing in the middle frequencies (500 to 2,000 Hz), but poorer hearing at lower and higher frequencies.

- *Cytomegalovirus (CMV)* is easily the most common viral disease known to cause hearing loss. Approximately 33,000 infants are born each year with CMV. Ninety percent of the symptomatic children who survive (approximately 20% die) will exhibit complications. One of the common complications is sensorineural hearing loss. The hearing loss ranges from mild to profound and can be progressive. The virus is passed from the mother to the fetus via the bloodstream.
- *Herpes simplex virus (HSV)* is a sexually transmitted disease, and the acquired virus is passed on to the fetus in utero or during the birth process. Only 4% of infected infants survive without complication. Some of the complications of the disease include central nervous system involvement, psychomotor retardation, visual problems, and hearing loss. Sensorineural hearing loss occurs when HSV is contracted in utero.

Postnatal Infections   Several postnatal infections produce sensorineural hearing loss. The cochlear damage produced by these viral or bacterial infections appears to result from the infecting agent entering the inner ear through the blood supply and nerve fibers. The following is a brief review of those diseases that would be encountered most frequently.

Hearing loss is the most common consequence of acute *meningitis*. Although the pathways used by the organisms to reach the inner ear are not altogether clear, several routes have been suggested. These include the bloodstream, the auditory nerve, and the fluid supply of the inner ear and the middle ear. The prevalence of severe-to-profound sensorineural hearing loss among patients with this disorder is approximately 10%. Another 16% will exhibit transient conductive hearing loss. Interestingly, some patients with sensorineural hearing loss will exhibit partial recovery, although such a finding is rare.

Mumps is recognized as one of the more common causes of sensorineural hearing loss that affects just one ear (unilateral hearing loss). The hearing loss is usually sudden and can vary from a mild high-frequency impairment to profound loss at all frequencies. Both children and adults are affected. Because it is not uncommon for this disease to be subclinical, children with hearing loss resulting from mumps are not usually identified until they first attend school since only one ear is typically affected.

TABLE

6.2

(S)TORCH Complex of High-Risk Prenatal Infections and Clinical Manifestations

Disease	Primary Symptoms	Prevalence of Hearing Loss (%)	Type and Degree of Hearing Loss
Syphilis	Enlarged liver and spleen, snuffles, rash, hearing loss	35	Severe-to-profound bilateral SNHL; configuration and degree vary
Toxoplasmosis	Chorioretinitis, hydrocephalus, intracranial calcifications, hearing loss	17	Moderate-to-severe bilateral SNHL; may be progressive
Rubella	Heart and kidney defects, eye anomalies, mental retardation, hearing loss	20–30	Profound bilateral SNHL—cookie-bite audiogram is common; may be progressive
CMV	Mental retardation, visual defects, hearing loss	17	Mild-to-profound bilateral SNHL; may be progressive
Herpes simplex	Enlarged liver, rash, visual abnormalities, psychomotor retardation, encephalitis, hearing loss	10	Moderate-to-severe unilateral or bilateral SNHL

Measles is another cause of sensorineural hearing loss. Hearing loss affects 6% to 10% of measles patients. A typical pattern of hearing loss shows a severe-to-profound hearing loss for high frequencies and in both ears.

Ototoxic Drugs

A negative side effect of some antibiotic drugs is the production of severe high-frequency sensorineural hearing loss. A group of antibiotics known as aminoglycosides are particularly hazardous. This group, also commonly referred to as the "mycin" drugs, includes streptomycin, neomycin, kanamycin, and gentamicin. A variety of factors can determine whether hearing loss is produced in a specific patient. These factors include the drug dosage, the susceptibility of the patient, and the simultaneous or previous use of other ototoxic agents.

Ototoxic antibiotics reach the inner ear through the bloodstream. The resulting damage is greater in the base of the cochlea, and outer hair cells are typically the primary targets, with only limited damage appearing in other cochlear structures. This results in a pattern of hearing loss that is moderate to severe in the high frequencies in both ears.

Some drugs used in chemotherapy to treat cancer can produce hearing loss as a side effect. Platinum compounds, such as cisplatin, carboplatin, and oxaliplatin, are common chemotherapy agents and each can be ototoxic. In general, cisplatin is known to be particularly ototoxic, impacting the outer hair cells in the base of the cochlea first, resulting in a high-frequency sensorineural hearing loss. The hearing loss may progress to involve middle or low frequencies with high doses. Carboplatin, used in isolation, tends to be less ototoxic, but also selectively attacks the inner hair cells in the cochlea. Oxaliplatin typically results in less hearing loss than cisplatin. Laboratory research with animals has shown that this is due to much lower concentrations of oxaliplatin in the cochlea, 20% of that measured in the cochlea for cisplatin, following equivalent doses delivered intravenously.

Some ototoxic drugs cause a temporary or reversible hearing loss. Perhaps the most common such substance is aspirin. When taken in large amounts, aspirin can produce a mild-to-moderate temporary sensorineural hearing loss.

Noise-Induced Hearing Loss

Exposure to intense sounds can result in temporary or permanent hearing loss. Whether or not a hearing loss actually results from exposure to the intense sound depends on several factors. These factors include the acoustic characteristics of the sound, such as its intensity, duration, and frequency content (amplitude spectrum); the length of the exposure; and the susceptibility of the individual.

When the intense sound is a broadband noise, such as might be found in industrial settings, a characteristic pattern of hearing loss emerges after the exposure. This pattern is frequently referred to as a "4,000-Hz notch" and reflects the sharp loss of hearing that is maximum at a test frequency of 4,000 Hz. More detailed measurements of the hearing loss produced by exposure to broadband noise reveal that the sharp drop in hearing threshold is as likely to appear at 3,000 or 6,000 Hz as at 4,000 Hz. Because 3,000 and 6,000 Hz are not routinely included in audiometric testing (see Chapter 7), however, the notch is less frequently observed at these two frequencies. This same "4,000-Hz notch" configuration is observed both in temporary hearing loss after brief exposures to broadband noise and in permanent hearing loss after prolonged exposure to such noise.

Many theories attempt to explain why the region around 4,000 Hz seems to be more susceptible to the damaging effects of broadband noise. One theory is that, although the noise itself may be broadband, with roughly equal amplitude at all frequencies, the outer ear and ear canal resonances (see Chapter 3) have amplified the noise in the 2,000- to 4,000-Hz region by the time the noise reaches the inner ear. Thus, this region shows the greatest hearing loss. Other theories suggest that the region of the cochlea associated with 4,000 Hz is more vulnerable to damage because of differences in cochlear mechanics, cochlear metabolism, or cochlear blood supply. Whatever the underlying mechanism, damage is greatest in that region of the cochlea associated with frequencies of 3,000 to 6,000 Hz. The damage again seems to be more marked in the outer hair cells, although this can vary with the acoustic characteristics of the noise.

Given the permanent nature of the resulting noise-induced hearing loss, it is crucial to prevent its occurrence. Hearing conservation programs have been developed by employers to protect the hearing of their employees. At least part of the employer's motivation is the avoidance of hefty fines for noncompliance with federal standards regarding industrial noise levels. Basically, the primary components of an industrial hearing conservation program include surveys of noise levels and durations to which employees are exposed, regular (at least annual) monitoring of hearing thresholds for all employees, and the provision of hearing protection devices, such as earmuffs and earplugs. A key component of such hearing conservation programs also involves the education of employees regarding the risk of permanent hearing loss from noise exposure and instruction in the effective use of hearing protection devices.

The world in which we live, however, is increasingly noisy. Exposure to high noise levels is not confined to work environments. Many recreational sources of noise exist today, and the risk of hearing loss from prolonged exposure to high sound levels is the same whether it involves a 110-dB SPL machine-generated noise or an exposure to 110-dB SPL from loudspeakers at a rock concert (Vignette 6.6). The biggest difference in these two cases, however, is that an employee might be exposed to the high-level machine-generated noise on a daily basis for many years, whereas the audience member at a rock concert will most likely be exposed to this same high noise level much less frequently. Of course, if one considers the rock musician, including practices and performances, the differences in exposure duration, and the subsequent risk of hearing loss, might be minimal. Musicians, however, are no longer the only ones who could be exposed to high levels of music for long periods of time. For example, the nature of contemporary MP3 audio players makes long, uninterrupted periods of music listening much more feasible than previously. This is mainly due to the small size, long battery life, and expansive memory capabilities of these devices that enable uninterrupted playback of hundreds of songs. When combined with volume controls that enable outputs in the listener's ears of over 110-dB SPL, the potential risk to hearing from such devices has raised concerns among many hearing health care professionals (Vignette 6.7).

VIGNETTE 6.6 • FURTHER DISCUSSION

Recreational Sources of Noise

We live in a noise-filled society in which many recreational activities make use of devices or equipment that generates high levels of sound. In many cases, those making use of these devices may not consider the sound to be "noise," but it is nonetheless high-intensity sound. The following provides a listing of several recreational

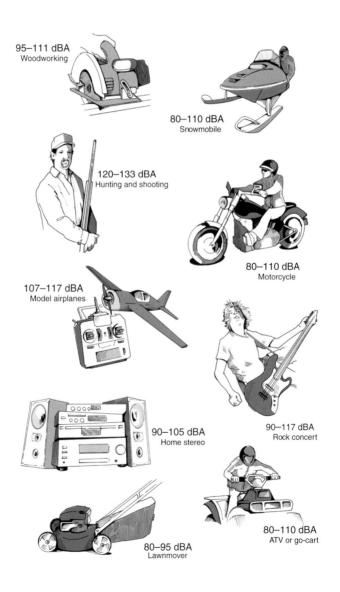

95–111 dBA
Woodworking

80–110 dBA
Snowmobile

120–133 dBA
Hunting and shooting

80–110 dBA
Motorcycle

107–117 dBA
Model airplanes

90–105 dBA
Home stereo

90–117 dBA
Rock concert

80–95 dBA
Lawnmower

80–110 dBA
ATV or go-cart

sources of noise (Adapted from Clark WW, Bohne BA. The effects of noise on hearing and the ear. *Med Times* 1984;122:17–22.). In each case, the range of maximum sound levels in dBA* reported in various studies is shown. Although not noted in the source, it is assumed that these sound levels are measured at about one meter from the source.

*Instruments used to measure noise have three weighting networks (A, B, and C) that are designed to respond differently to noise frequencies. The A network weighs (filters) the low frequencies and approximates the response characteristics of the human ear. The B network also filters the low frequencies, but not as much as the A network does. The C scale provides a fairly flat response. The federal government recommends the A network for measuring noise levels.

VIGNETTE 6.7 • FURTHER DISCUSSION

Noise-Induced Hearing Loss and "iPods"

There has been much in the news media in recent years regarding the risk of noise-induced hearing loss from Apple iPods or similar portable MP3 music-playback devices. Unpublished reports have indicated that sound levels from such devices can be as high as 100- to 115-dB SPL. Such high sound levels, however, have been documented in many published reports over the past 20 to 25 years for other personal portable music players, such as "Walkman-like" cassette and CD players. It is not clear that the sound levels produced by portable MP3 players are more hazardous than these other earlier devices.

One thing that is different, however, is that it is possible with most portable MP3 players to listen to music for much longer periods, often uninterrupted. For noise-induced hearing loss, it is the combination of the sound level and the duration of the sound exposure that is critical. For example, many national and international guidelines for hearing hazard suggest most individuals could spend a lifetime listening to sound levels below 85-dB SPL for 8 hours a day and not experience a hearing loss

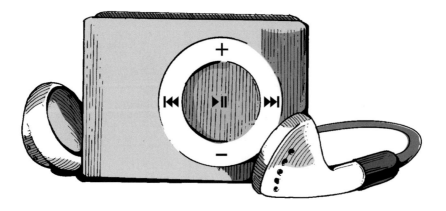

greater than that which would occur by aging alone. Many of these same national and international guidelines indicate that as the sound level increases 3 dB the safe duration of exposure must be cut in half. So, for example, most individuals could safely be exposed to sound levels of 88-dB SPL for 4 hours each day or 91-dB SPL for 2 hours per day throughout their lives without experiencing noise-induced hearing loss. Thus, the new danger with portable MP3 players, compared to earlier predecessors like portable CD players, is not necessarily in the sound levels that they produce, but in the potential for extended, uninterrupted periods of use.

Most of the research conducted on noise-induced hearing loss, however, that forms the basis for the national and international guidelines is for continuous exposures (8 hours per day, typically with brief breaks every 2 hours) to steady-state industrial noise, not fluctuating music, for periods of many years. In addition, most of these exposures occurred with open ears in sound field industrial conditions, not with sound delivered in sealed ear canals by "earbud"-style earphones. Additional research is needed to determine the impact of these and other factors on guidelines for "safe exposures." In the interim, limiting the use of high-volume control settings (e.g., less than 2/3 full-on) and length of listening each day would be the best way to minimize the risk for eventual *permanent* noise-induced hearing loss.

Presbycusis

Beyond approximately the age of 50 years, hearing sensitivity deteriorates progressively, especially in the high frequencies. The progression is somewhat more rapid for men than for women. Figure 6.8 shows the progression of hearing loss in both men and women as a function of age. The more rapid decline of hearing with age in men may not reflect differences in aging per se but may reflect their more frequent participation in noisy recreational activities such as hunting, snowmobiling, or operating power tools (e.g., lawn mowers, chain saws, and table saws).

The patterns of hearing loss associated with ototoxic antibiotics, noise-induced hearing loss, and **presbycusis** are all very similar. In all three cases, a high-frequency sensorineural hearing loss is usually observed in both ears. The underlying cochlear damage is also very similar: the basal high-frequency region of the cochlea is the main area of destruction, and the outer hair cells are primarily affected. Accompanying retrograde destruction of first-order afferent nerve fibers may also be observed, as is usually the case in cochlear pathology.

Degenerative changes associated with aging have also been observed in the brainstem and cortical areas of the ascending auditory pathway in some cases. These central changes, when present, can seriously compound the communicative impairment experienced by the elderly person with sensorineural hearing

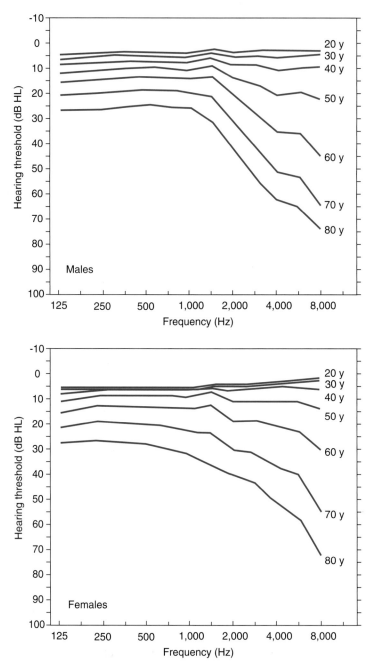

FIGURE 6.8 Hearing loss progression as a function of age in women (*top*) and men (*bottom*). (Adapted from Johansson MS, Arlinger SD. Hearing threshold levels for an otologically unscreened, non-occupationally noise-exposed population in Sweden. *Int J Audiol* 2002;41:180–194.) Perfectly normal hearing is represented in these graphs by the horizontal line at 0 dB.

loss. Approximately 5% to 15% of elderly persons may have central auditory deficits affecting their ability to communicate. Aging can also have a negative impact on some aspects of cognitive function, including memory and attention. Some of these cognitive processes are important for effective communication. In that regard, older adults may experience a "double" or "triple whammy" with regard to impairments that have a negative impact on the communication chain. They not only are likely to have some amount of high-frequency hearing loss from inner ear damage, but may also have impairments in central auditory function, cognitive function, or both.

Retrocochlear Pathology

Retrocochlear pathology refers to damage to nerve fibers along the ascending auditory pathways from the internal auditory meatus to the cortex. Most often a tumor is involved, although not always, as in the case of multiple sclerosis or cerebral vascular attacks ("strokes").

In many cases, the auditory manifestations of the retrocochlear pathology are subtle. Frequently, for example, no hearing loss is measured for pure tones. The possibility that a tumor along the auditory pathway will fail to produce measurable hearing loss for pure tones can be understood when one recalls the multiple paths by which information ascends through the brainstem within the auditory system (Chapter 3). Recall that after the first-order ascending neurons terminated in the cochlear nucleus, a variety of paths were available for the neural transmission of information to the cortex. Thus, if the tumor is located central to the cochlear nucleus, the information required for the detection of a pure tone can easily bypass the affected pathway and progress to the cortex.

For the detection of a pure tone, many of the brainstem centers along the ascending auditory pathways probably serve simple relay functions and perform little processing of the signal. For more complex signals, such as speech, however, some preprocessing probably takes place in the brainstem before complete processing by the cortex. Still, in many brainstem and cortical disorders, speech perception appears normal in quiet listening conditions. This seems to be accomplished through the use of multiple cues available in the speech signal that assist in its recognition. Some of the cues processed by a brainstem or a cortical center can be eliminated from the total information reaching the cortex by the presence of a tumor without producing a misperception of the speech signal. The patient is simply using several of the remaining cues that are not affected by the presence of the tumor. If, however, the speech signal is degraded by filtering, adding noise, temporal interruption, and so forth, the cues of the speech signal become less redundant. Every cue in the speech signal is now needed for its correct recognition. Individuals with retrocochlear pathology in the brainstem or cortex typically perform poorly on speech-recognition tests involving the recognition of degraded speech signals, such as filtered speech or speech in noise.

Again, a detailed description of retrocochlear disorders and the tests developed for their detection is beyond the scope of this book. Many special speech-recognition tests making use of degraded speech have been developed for use with this population.

Retrocochlear pathology that occurs at the first-order afferent nerve fibers, unlike that occurring at higher centers along the ascending auditory pathway, typically results in abnormal performance on the basic audiologic test battery. These tumors, referred to as vestibular schwannomas, acoustic neuromas, acoustic neurinomas, or acoustic neurilemmomas, are benign, slow-growing tumors that typically produce a high-frequency sensorineural hearing loss that is either unilateral or asymmetric between the two ears. Vestibular schwannomas affecting only one ear are fairly common, representing about 8% of all tumors inside the skull. Each year, about 1 of 100,000 people will develop a unilateral vestibular schwannoma, most commonly between the ages of 30 and 60 years. Most patients will also complain of tinnitus on the affected side, and slightly more than half of these patients complain of dizziness. The ability to understand speech for clinical tests may range from normal to extremely poor at moderate intensities, but it typically becomes poorer as speech level is increased to high intensities. Clinical measures of middle ear muscle contraction, known as acoustic reflex thresholds and decay (Chapter 7), often are also abnormal. If several of the abovementioned abnormal audiologic results are observed, the patient should be referred for additional testing. This will most likely involve measurement of the ABR, other nonauditory tests, and, depending on the results, radiologic tests, such as an MRI. Because the tumors are typically slow growing, treatment may first simply involve monitoring of hearing and the tumor (radiologically), followed by eventual treatment surgically or with radiation.

SUMMARY

The auditory system, marvelously complex and intricate, is nevertheless vulnerable to assault and damage from disease, trauma, genetic imperfection, extreme environmental conditions (i.e., noise), and aging. Many conditions affect both children and adults and can affect all levels of the auditory system, resulting in various types, degrees, and patterns of hearing loss. These problems, in turn, can have a negative impact on the development and function of the communication chain.

CHAPTER REVIEW QUESTIONS

1. If both parents have normal hearing, but carry the same genes for recessive hereditary deafness, what is the likelihood that they will have a child with impaired hearing?
2. Why is otitis media much more common among young children than adults?
3. List the prenatal infections that comprise the (S)TORCH complex. If the mother develops any of these prenatal infections during her pregnancy, does that mean that she will give birth to a child with impaired hearing?
4. What are three common forms of cochlear pathology in adults, each of which results in an inability to hear low-intensity, high-frequency sounds? What is the impact of such a hearing loss on speech communication?
5. Several viral infections that are prevalent (or have been prevalent in the past) among children can lead to severe or profound loss of hearing. Describe two of these viral infections and the most likely pattern of hearing loss that would result. For each, what do you believe would be the impact of the hearing loss on communication? Would the age at which the hearing loss developed matter? Why or why not?
6. What is meant by "retrocochlear" pathology?

REFERENCES AND SUGGESTED READINGS

Bess FH, ed. *Hearing Impairment in Children*. Parkton, MD: York Press; 1988.

Carhart R. Clinical application of bone conduction audiometry. *Arch Otolaryngol* 1950;51:798–807.

Eichwald J, Mahoney T. Apgar scores in the identification of sensorineural hearing loss. *J Am Acad Audiol* 1993;4:133–138.

English GM, ed. *Otolaryngology*. Hagerstown, MD: Harper & Row; 1976.

Fria TJ, Cantekin EI, Eichler JA. Hearing acuity of children with otitis media with effusion. *Arch Otolaryngol* 1985;111:10–16.

Gerkin KP. The high risk register for deafness. *ASHA* 1984;26:17–23.

Goodhill V, ed. *Ear Diseases, Deafness, and Dizziness*. Hagerstown, MD: Harper & Row; 1979.

Jerger J, Jerger S. *Auditory Disorders*. Boston, MA: Little Brown; 1981.

Johansson MS, Arlinger SD. Hearing threshold levels for an otologically unscreened, non-occupationally noise-exposed population in Sweden. *Int J Audiol* 2002;41:180–194.

Joint Committee on Infant Hearing. Year 2000 position statement: Principles and guidelines for early hearing detection and intervention programs. *Pediatrics* 2000;106:798–817.

Kavanaugh J, ed. *Otitis Media and Child Development*. Parkton, MD: York Press; 1986.

Lebo CP, Reddell RC. The presbycusis component in occupational hearing loss. *Laryngoscope* 1972;82:1399–1409.

Newton VE. *Paediatric Audiological Medicine*. Philadelphia, PA: Whurr Publishers; 2002.

Northern JL, ed. *Hearing Disorders*. 4th ed. Boston, MA: Little Brown; 1991.

Parving A. Congenital hearing disability epidemiology and identification: A comparison between two health authority districts. *Int J Pediatr Otorhinolaryngol* 1993;27:29–46.

Rodgers GK, Telischi FF. Ménière's disease in children. *Otolaryngol Clin North Am* 1997;30:1101–1104.

Shambaugh GE, Glasscock ME. *Surgery of the Ear*. Philadelphia, PA: WB Saunders; 1980.

Shuknecht HF: *Pathology of the Ear*. Cambridge, UK: Harvard University Press; 1974.

Seewald R, Tharpe AM, eds. *Comprehensive Handbook of Pediatric Audiology*. San Diego, CA: Plural Publishing; 2011.

Tekin M, Arnos KS, Pandya A. Advances in hereditary deafness. *Lancet* 2001;358:1082–1090.

7

Audiologic Measurement: Identifying Breaks in the Communication Chain

Chapter Objectives

- To understand how audiologists measure hearing loss for pure tones and speech;
- To be able to interpret the graphical presentation of test results on an audiogram;
- To understand how immittance measurements are performed by the audiologist and how this information is presented graphically; and
- To see how each test of the basic audiological test battery provides an important piece of the puzzle in diagnosing the hearing loss as well as understanding its impact on communication.

Key Terms and Definitions

- **Pure-tone audiometry:** The measurement of hearing thresholds for pure tones of various frequencies using standardized equipment and procedures.

- **Speech audiometry:** The measurement of speech recognition threshold (SRT) in decibels, representing the lowest sound level at which speech can be heard 50% of the time, and measures of the ability to understand speech when it is many decibels above this threshold. The latter is a speech recognition score reported as a percentage and represents the percentage of spoken words on standardized lists that were correctly perceived by the patient. When individual words are used to measure the speech recognition score, which is most often the case clinically, the score is referred to as the "word recognition score."

- **Acoustic immittance measurements:** Clinical measurement of the impedance or admittance of the flow of sound energy through the middle ear. Typically includes measurement of a tympanogram and acoustic reflex thresholds.

In the preceding chapters, the importance of an intact auditory system, from the periphery to the cortex, for the communication chain was emphasized. This system is critical for the conversion of acoustical speech sounds generated by the talker to neural signals that can be interpreted by the brain of the listener. Impairments of the auditory system, as reviewed in the preceding chapter, have the potential to disrupt or break the communication chain. Much of audiology is devoted to the detection of such impairments, their location within the auditory system, and the determination of their severity and impact on communication. This chapter reviews some of the methods and test techniques used in audiology to accomplish these tasks. Since most readers of this text are unlikely to become audiologists themselves, the approach taken here is to provide enough information so that the reader can become an "intelligent consumer" of audiological information. As a result, in this chapter, we focus on the results that are obtained by the audiologist and their interpretation, more than details about how such measurements are performed. In many cases, additional details about methods used can be found in the online supplemental material accompanying this chapter.

The nature of auditory impairment depends on such factors as the severity of the hearing loss, the age at onset, the cause of the loss, and the location of the lesion within the auditory system. The hearing evaluation plays an important role in determining some of these factors. Audiometric measurement of auditory function can (a) determine the degree of hearing loss, (b) estimate the location of the lesion within the auditory system that is producing the problem, (c) help establish the cause of the hearing problem, (d) estimate the extent of the handicap produced by the hearing loss, and (e) help to determine the client's habilitative or rehabilitative needs and the appropriate means of filling those needs. This chapter focuses on those tests used most commonly in the evaluation of auditory function. This battery of tests includes pure-tone audiometry, speech audiometry, and acoustic immittance measures.

CASE HISTORY

Before the audiologic evaluation begins, the audiologist obtains a history from the client. For adults, this history may be supplied by completing a printed form before the evaluation. The form contains pertinent identifying information for the client, such as home address and referral source. Questions regarding the nature of past and present hearing problems, including a family history of hearing loss or a history of exposure to noise, other medical problems, and prior use of amplification, are also usually included. The written responses are then followed up during an interview between the audiologist and the client before any testing.

For children, the case history form is usually more comprehensive than the adult version. In addition to questions such as the ones mentioned for adults, detailed questions about the mother's pregnancy and the child's birth are included. The development of gross and fine motor skills and the development of speech and language are also probed. The medical history of the child is also reviewed in detail, with special emphasis on childhood diseases (e.g., measles and mumps) capable of producing a hearing loss. Vignette 7.1 provides examples of common questions included on two pediatric case-history forms used by audiologists, one for children over 4 years of age and one for younger children.

VIGNETTE 7.1 • CLINICAL APPLICATIONS

Examples of Pediatric Case-History Forms Used in Audiology

CHILD OVER 4 YEARS

Date: _____

Interviewer: _____

Name: _____   DOB: _____

Nature and Onset of Problem:

Chief complaint:

Duration:

Progression/consistency:

Communication difficulties:

Medical History:

Familial history of speech/hearing/other medical problems:

Unusual prenatal conditions:

Unusual postnatal conditions:

Serious childhood diseases/conditions:

Ear infections:

Speech-Language Development:

Present speech-language behavior:

Past speech-language therapy:

Educational History:

Past educational concerns:

Present school progress:

Difficult academic subjects:

Preferential seating or extra academic help:

Special education services:

CHILD 4 YEARS AND YOUNGER

General Information: Date: _____

Name of child: _____   Age: _____

Informant: _____(relationship to child)

Who stays with the child during the day? _____

List other children in the family:

Name	Age	Grade	Speech and/or hearing problems?
_____	_____	_____	_____
_____	_____	_____	_____
_____	_____	_____	_____

Chief Concern:

_____

_____

_____

_____

How does s/he respond to various types of sounds such as speech, telephone ringing, music, whispered speech, and television? _____

_____

_____

Are there any sounds that frighten him/her? _____

_____

Any unusual responses to sounds? _____

_____

Any balance or coordination problems? _____

_____

Medical History:

Family history of speech/hearing problems? _____

_____

Unusual prenatal conditions: _____

Unusual postnatal conditions: _____

Serious childhood diseases/conditions: _____

Ear infections: _____

Developmental History (age when milestones accomplished):

Sat alone: _____

Crawled: _____

Walked alone: _____

Toilet trained: _____

Speech-Language Development:

Age at first words: _____

Current speech status: _____

_____

Current language status: _____

_____

Social Development:

Is the child easily managed at home? _____

Does s/he like to play with other children? _____

What does s/he like to do most, and how does s/he entertain him/herself? _____

_____

_____

Previous Treatment:

Please list the names and addresses of any physician or agency that has provided services for your child in the past:

Name   Address

_____   _____

_____   _____

_____   _____

_____   _____

OTOSCOPY

Once the case history has been completed, the audiologist will typically examine the patient's ear canals and eardrums with a small handheld otoscope prior to proceeding to pure-tone audiometry. A skilled audiologist will often be able to considerably narrow the list of possible auditory disorders for a particular case on the basis of the initial case history and otoscopy. The audiologist inspects the ear canal for the presence of foreign objects, excessive ear wax, signs of inflammation or irritation, and dried blood. The appearance of the eardrum is also examined closely, with special attention paid to the coloration of the eardrum, whether it is distended or bulging; the opacity of the eardrum; the visibility of fluid in the middle ear; and the presence of any scars, perforations, or tears in the eardrum. A readily visible hallmark of a healthy eardrum and middle ear is referred to the "cone of light" and results from the reflection of the otoscope's light by the malleus. The cone of light appears as a brighter strip or narrow wedge of light located in the lower front quadrant of the eardrum (typically, between 4 and 6 o'clock positions if the eardrum is visualized as the face of a clock).

PURE-TONE AUDIOMETRY

Pure-tone audiometry is the basis of a hearing evaluation. With pure-tone audiometry, hearing thresholds are measured for pure tones at different test frequencies. Hearing threshold is typically defined as the lowest (softest) sound level needed for a person to detect the presence of a signal approximately 50% of the time. Threshold information at each frequency is then plotted on a graph known as an audiogram. Before examining the audiogram, however, we shall describe the equipment used to measure hearing.

Audiometer

An audiometer is the primary instrument used by the audiologist to measure hearing threshold and by the speech-language pathologist to screen for hearing loss. Audiometers vary from the simple, inexpensive screening devices used in schools and public health programs to the more elaborate and expensive diagnostic audiometers found in hospitals and clinics. Certain basic components, however, are common to all audiometers. Figure 7.1 shows an example of one of these basic units. A frequency selector dial permits selection of different pure-tone frequencies. Ordinarily, these frequencies are available at octave intervals ranging from 125 to 8,000 Hz. An interrupter switch or presentation button allows presentation of the tone to the listener. A hearing

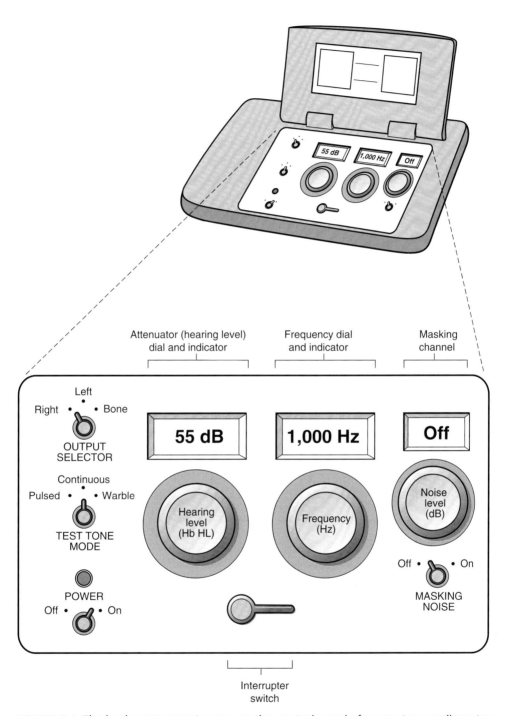

FIGURE 7.1 The basic components seen on the control panel of a pure-tone audiometer.

level (HL) dial controls the intensity of the signal. Most audiometers can deliver signals spanning a 100-dB range in 5-dB steps. An output selector determines whether the pure tone will be presented to the earphones for air-conduction testing (for either the right or the left ear) or whether the tone is to be sent to a bone vibrator for bone-conduction testing. Many audiometers also have a masking level dial, which controls the intensity of the masking noise presented to the nontest ear when masking is necessary. The more elaborate diagnostic audiometers not only can generate masking noise and pure-tone signals but also provide a means for measuring the understanding of speech signals.

Audiogram

The audiogram is a chart used to graphically record the hearing thresholds and other test results. Figure 7.2 shows an example of an audiogram and the associated symbol system recommended by the American Speech-Language-Hearing Association. The audiogram is shown in graphic form, with the signal

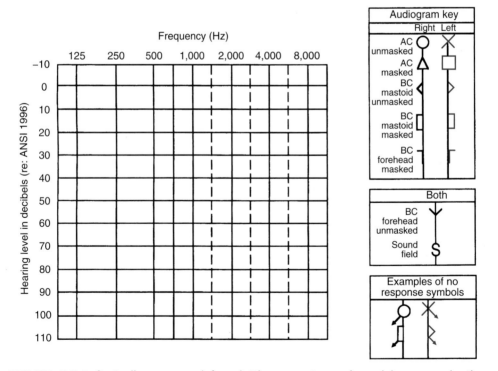

FIGURE 7.2 *Left*: Audiogram used for plotting pure-tone air and bone conduction thresholds. *Right*: The *audiogram key* displays the symbols commonly used in audiograms. *AC*, air conduction; *BC*, bone conduction.

frequencies (in hertz) displayed on the *x*-axis and the HL (in decibels) represented on the *y*-axis. The graph is designed in such a manner that the length representing one octave in frequency on the horizontal scale is equal in size to the length representing 20-dB HL on the vertical scale.

The horizontal line at 0-dB HL represents normal hearing sensitivity for the average young adult. However, as described in Chapter 3, the human ear does not perceive sound equally well at all frequencies. Recall that the ear is most sensitive to sound in the intermediate-frequency region from 1,000 to 4,000 Hz and is less sensitive at both the higher and lower frequencies. Greater sound pressure is needed to elicit a threshold response at 250 Hz than at 2,000 Hz in normal ears. The audiometer is calibrated to correct for these differences in threshold sensitivity at various frequencies. Consequently, when the HL dial is set at zero for a given frequency, the signal is automatically presented at the normal threshold sound pressure level (SPL) required for the average young adult to hear that particular frequency (Vignette 7.2).

Results plotted on the audiogram can be used to classify the extent of a hearing impairment. This information plays a valuable role in determining the habilitative or rehabilitative needs of an individual with impaired hearing. Classification schemes using the pure-tone audiogram are based on the fact that there is a strong relationship between the threshold for those frequencies known to be important for hearing speech (500, 1,000, and 2,000 Hz) and the lowest level at which speech can be recognized accurately 50% of the time. The latter measure is generally referred to as the speech recognition threshold, or SRT. Given the pure-tone thresholds at 500, 1,000, and 2,000 Hz, one can estimate the hearing loss for speech and the potential handicapping effects of the impairment. This is done by simply calculating the average (mean) loss of hearing for these three frequencies. This average is referred to as the three-frequency pure-tone average (PTA). Figure 7.3 shows an example of a typical classification system based on the PTA. This scheme, adapted from several other systems, reflects the different classifications of hearing loss as well as the likely effects of the hearing loss on an individual's ability to hear speech. The hearing loss classes, ranging from mild to profound, are based on the PTA at 500, 1,000, and 2,000 Hz. The classification of normal limits extends to 25-dB HL, and HLs within this range have typically been thought to produce essentially no problems with even faint speech. Some evidence indicates, however, that losses from 15- to 25-dB HL can have negative effects educationally on children. Children with hearing loss in this range should be considered for relatively unobtrusive ways to amplify the teacher's speech in the classroom that will also provide benefit to children with normal hearing in the same classroom (see Chapter 9 for more details).

VIGNETTE 7.2 • CONCEPTUAL DEMO

Illustration of the Relationship between Decibels SPL (dB SPL) and Decibels HL (dB HL)

The accompanying figure depicts the relationship between the dB HL scale and the dB SPL scale of sound intensity. The *circles* in the *upper panel* are the data for hearing thresholds of normal-hearing young adults. The *triangles* in the *upper panel* are hearing thresholds obtained from an individual with a high-frequency hearing loss. Note that increasing hearing loss is indicated by higher SPLs at threshold. At 4,000 Hz, for example, the average threshold for normal-hearing young adults is 10-dB SPL; the

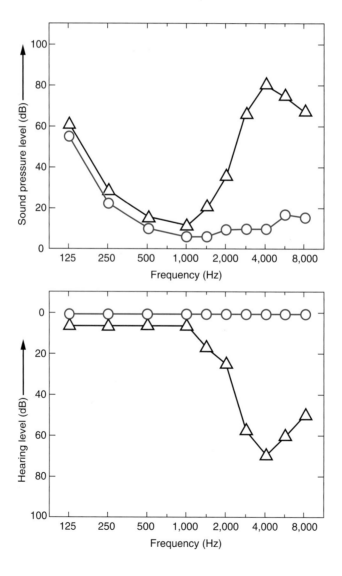

patient's threshold is 80-dB SPL, indicating a hearing loss of 70 dB. These same data have been replotted on the dB HL scale in the *lower panel*. Note now that the normal hearing threshold has been set to 0-dB HL on this scale at all frequencies. Increasing intensity is shown in a downward direction on the audiogram. Note also that the threshold for the hearing-impaired subject at 4,000 Hz is 70-dB HL. This threshold value itself then directly indicates the magnitude of hearing loss relative to normal hearing. There is no need to subtract the normal hearing threshold value from the value observed in the impaired ear, as was the case for the dB SPL scale.

Measurement of Hearing

#7

In pure-tone audiometry, thresholds are obtained by both air conduction and bone conduction. In air conduction measurement, the different pure-tone stimuli are transmitted through earphones. The signal travels through the ear canal, across the middle ear cavity via the three ossicles to the cochlea, and on to the auditory central nervous system, as reviewed in the previous chapter. Air conduction thresholds reflect the integrity of the total auditory mechanism. When a

#8

person exhibits a hearing loss by air conduction, it is not possible to determine the location of the pathology along the auditory pathway. The hearing loss

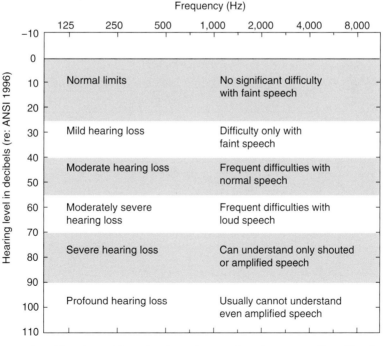

FIGURE 7.3 Classification of hearing impairment in relation to disability for speech recognition.

could be the result of (a) a problem in the outer or middle ear, (b) a difficulty at the level of the cochlea, (c) damage along the neural pathways to the brain, or (d) some combination of these. When air conduction measurements are combined with bone conduction measurements, however, it is possible to differentiate outer and middle ear problems (conductive hearing loss) from inner ear problems (sensorineural hearing loss).

In bone conduction measurement, signals are transmitted via a bone vibrator that is usually placed on the mastoid prominence of the skull (a bony prominence located behind the pinna, slightly above the level of the concha). The forehead is another position for placement of the bone vibrator. A signal transduced through the vibrator causes the skull to vibrate. The pure tone directly stimulates the cochlea, which is embedded in the skull, effectively bypassing the outer ear and middle ear systems. If an individual exhibits a reduction in hearing sensitivity when tested by air conduction yet shows normal sensitivity by bone conduction, the impairment is probably a result of an obstruction or blockage of the outer or middle ear. This condition is referred to as a conductive hearing loss. Figure 7.4 gives an audiometric example of a young child with a conductive hearing loss caused by middle ear disease. The bone conduction thresholds ([, right ear thresholds;], left ear thresholds) appear close to 0-dB HL for all test frequencies. Such a finding implies that the inner ear responds to sound at normal threshold levels. The air conduction thresholds (O-O, right ear; X-X, left ear), on the other hand, are much greater than 0-dB HL. Greater sound

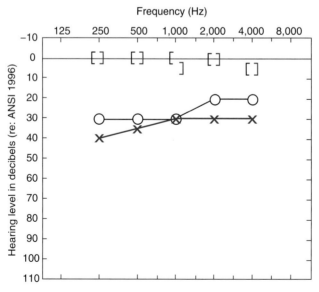

FIGURE 7.4 Pure-tone audiogram demonstrating the relation between air and bone conduction thresholds typifying mild conductive hearing impairment.

intensity is needed for this child to hear the air-conducted pure-tone signals than is required by the average normal hearer. Because the bone conduction thresholds suggest that the inner ear is normal, the loss displayed by air conduction must result from a conductive lesion affecting the outer or middle ear.

The difference between the air conduction threshold and the bone conduction threshold at a given frequency is generally referred to as the air-bone gap. In Figure 7.4, for example, at 250 Hz, there is a 30-dB air-bone gap in the right ear and a 40-dB gap in the left ear. Conductive hearing loss is especially prevalent among preschool- and young school-age children who experience repeated episodes of otitis media (middle ear infection). Other examples of pathologic conditions, known to produce conductive hearing loss, include congenital atresia (absence of ear canals), blockage or occlusion of the ear canal (possibly by cerumen or earwax), perforation or scarring of the tympanic membrane, ossicular chain disruption, and otosclerosis (bony growth fixing the stapes to the oval window).

As we noted, hearing thresholds better than a HL of 25-dB HL are considered normal. Air-bone gaps of 10 dB or more, however, represent a significant conductive hearing loss and may require medical referral, even if the air conduction thresholds are less than 25 dB at all frequencies. That is, such small air-bone gaps, although likely to have only a marginal impact on communication, may reflect an underlying medical condition that requires follow-up examination.

A sensorineural hearing loss is suggested when the air conduction thresholds *and* bone conduction thresholds are approximately the same (within 5 dB) at all test frequencies and outside the normal limits. Sensorineural hearing impairment may be either congenital or acquired. Some of the congenital causes include heredity, complications of maternal viral and bacterial infections, and birth trauma. Factors producing acquired sensorineural hearing loss include noise, aging, inflammatory diseases (e.g., measles or mumps), and ototoxic drugs (e.g., aminoglycoside antibiotics). Figure 7.5 gives three different examples of sensorineural hearing impairment. Figure 7.5A shows the audiogram of an adult with a hearing loss resulting from the use of ototoxic antibiotics. This audiogram displays a moderate bilateral sensorineural impairment with a greater hearing loss in the high-frequency region. Figure 7.5B shows the audiogram of a child whose hearing impairment resulted from maternal rubella (measles). It can be seen that the magnitude of this hearing loss falls in the profound category in the region of the most critical frequencies for hearing speech (500 to 2,000 Hz). In fact, the loss is so severe that bone conduction responses could not be obtained at the maximum output of the audiometer at all test frequencies. This is indicated by the downward-pointing arrows attached to the audiometric symbols and should not be mistaken for an

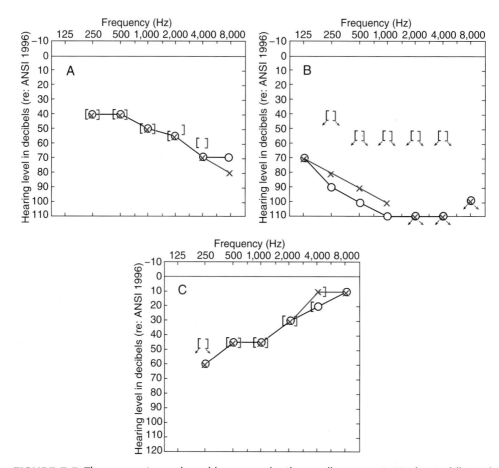

FIGURE 7.5 Three pure-tone air and bone conduction audiograms. *A*: Moderate bilateral sensorineural hearing loss. *B*: Profound bilateral sensorineural hearing loss. *C*: Low-frequency bilateral sensorineural hearing loss.

air-bone gap. Air conduction thresholds also could not be obtained at frequencies above 1,000 Hz because the hearing loss was so great.

The majority of sensorineural hearing losses are characterized by audiometric configurations that are flat, trough-shaped, or slightly to steeply sloping in the high frequencies. The latter is probably the most common configuration associated with acquired sensorineural hearing loss. Occasionally, however, patients display a sensorineural hearing loss in which the greatest hearing loss occurs at low and intermediate frequencies, with normal or near-normal hearing sensitivity at the high frequencies. Figure 7.5C shows an example of a typical low-frequency hearing loss. Low-tone hearing loss most commonly results from either some types of hereditary deafness or Ménière disease. Young children whose audiograms display low-frequency hearing impairment are difficult to identify and are sometimes the unfortunate victims of misdiagnosis. Because of their near-normal hearing sensitivity in the high frequencies, these children may respond to whispered speech and broadband stimuli at low-intensity levels. In addition, unlike children with a high-frequency hearing loss, their articulation of speech is usually good. These manifestations are not typical of sensorineural hearing loss in children, which makes them more prone to misdiagnosis.

When both air conduction thresholds and bone conduction thresholds are reduced in sensitivity, but bone conduction yields better results than air conduction, the term "mixed hearing loss" is used, meaning the patient's hearing loss is partially conductive and partially sensorineural. Figure 7.6 shows an audiogram depicting mixed hearing loss. Even though hearing loss is evident both for bone and air conduction thresholds, bone conduction sensitivity is consistently better across all test frequencies. This suggests that there has been some damage to the hair cells or nerve endings in the inner ear, causing a reduction in bone conduction thresholds, which is added to the reduction in air conduction thresholds resulting from malfunction of the outer ear or middle ear.

Vignette 7.3 provides a little more detail about the mechanisms underlying air conduction and bone conduction hearing tests. Additional explanation of the interpretation of thresholds from air conduction and bone conduction testing for the purpose of pinpointing the location of the pathology in the auditory periphery is also provided.

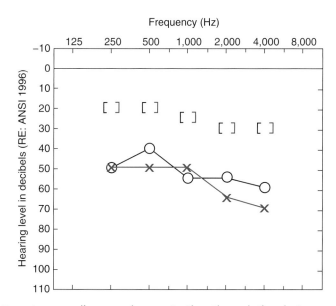

FIGURE 7.6 Pure-tone audiogram demonstrating the relation between air and bone conduction thresholds indicating a mixed (conductive and sensorineural) type of hearing loss.

VIGNETTE 7.3 • CONCEPTUAL DEMO

Mechanisms Underlying Air Conduction and Bone Conduction Thresholds

This series of panels is designed to better explain the nature of hearing thresholds obtained by air conduction and by bone conduction. Panel *A*, for example, schematically shows the sound wave and resulting mechanical energy traveling from the outer ear, through the middle ear, and mechanically stimulating the cochlea in the inner ear.

A. Air-conduction pathway

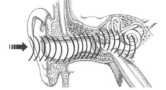

B. Bone-conduction pathway

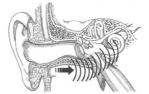

C. Outer ear damage- higher- air-conduction threshold

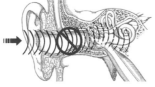

D. Outer ear damage - normal- bone-conduction threshold

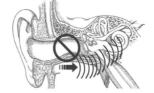

E. Middle ear damage- higher- air-conduction threshold

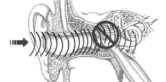

F. Middle ear damage - normal- bone-conduction threshold

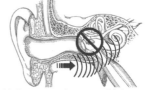

G.Inner ear damage- higher- air-conduction threshold

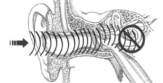

H. Inner ear damage - higher- bone-conduction threshold

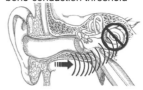

I. ME & IE damage

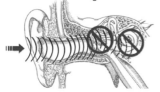

J. ME & IE damage

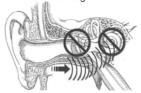

Likewise, panel *B* illustrates the mechanical vibration of the bony skull with a bone oscillator and a mechanical pathway directly stimulating the cochlea. The bone conduction pathway, for the most part, can be viewed as bypassing the outer and middle ears to directly stimulate the inner ears (Recall that *both* cochleas are stimulated through skull vibration). The symbol in the next two panels, *C* and *D*, represents the location of pathology in the outer ear (*C*) and middle ear (*D*). Clearly, the pathology in these two areas would have a negative impact on the transmission of mechanical energy through the normal air conduction pathway. To get through the blockage posed by the pathology in the outer or middle ear, the sound intensity for air conduction stimulation would have to be increased. In other words, a hearing loss would be measured for air conduction stimuli.

What about bone conduction stimulation in the case of outer or middle ear pathology? This situation is illustrated schematically in panels *E* and *F*. The mechanical bone conduction pathway is not impacted by the presence of outer ear or middle ear pathologies, and bone conduction hearing is essentially normal. Consequently, air conduction thresholds reveal elevated hearing thresholds and bone conduction thresholds do not, which results in an air-bone gap.

Now, consider the case of inner ear pathology as shown in panels *G* and *H*. Notice that the inner ear pathology occurs at the end of both the air conduction and bone conduction pathways. As a result, hearing threshold for both air and bone conduction stimulation will be impaired by the same amount. In other words, both thresholds will show the same amount of hearing loss, and, as a result, there will be no air-bone gap.

Finally, the *bottom* two panels (*I* and *J*) schematically depict the situation for a mixed hearing loss with pathology present in both the middle ear and inner ear. The air conduction pathway (*I*) is negatively impacted by both pathologies, whereas the bone conduction pathway (*J*) is only affected by the inner ear pathology. As a result, bone conduction thresholds will be higher than normal, but air conduction thresholds, having to surmount both the middle ear and inner ear pathology, will be even higher. In other words, an air-bone gap will exist and the bone conduction thresholds will indicate the presence of sensorineural (inner ear) hearing loss.

To measure hearing thresholds for pure tones, whether by air conduction or bone conduction, audiologists follow standardized procedures. That way, if an individual has a hearing test today and another test a week, month, or year later, assuming there have been no changes to the auditory system during that time period, the test results obtained at the two different times should match. Further, the use of standardized procedures ensures that someone can have a hearing test in Bloomington, Indiana, and then get retested a day later in Nashville, Tennessee, and the results once again, assuming no changes to the auditory system during this time period, should be the same.

The procedures used by audiologists to test hearing fall under a broader class of procedures known as behavioral methods. Briefly, a controlled sensory stimulus, in this case a pure tone of specified frequency, intensity, and duration, is presented to an individual, following which a response is required from the listener prior to the presentation of the next stimulus. For school-age children and adults, most frequently, the behavioral response required following the presentation of a pure tone in a hearing test is the raising of one's hand or finger to indicate that the pure tone has been heard by the listener. The audiologist usually begins the testing with a pure tone that is at a frequency and sound level easily heard and then gradually decreases the level of the pure tone watching for a change in response from the raising of the hand to no response. When this change of response occurs, the audiologist will then switch course and begin increasing the sound level of the pure tone, now watching for a change in response from no response to a raising of the hand. In this way, the "threshold," or the sound level at the boundary between "I heard it" (raised hand) and "I didn't hear it" (no response), can be established for that person at each of several pure-tone frequencies. Again, the details as to how pure-tone thresholds are measured are not necessary for the typical reader of this book. Rather, just gaining an appreciation for the general approach used by the audiologist is sufficient. For those who are interested, however, additional procedural details may be found in the online supplements accompanying this chapter.

Of course, babies, infants, and many toddlers are not able to respond to the presentation of pure tones by raising their hand or their finger. There are, however, standardized methods available for the measurement of pure-tone thresholds in these age groups too. For infants, for example, instead of presenting the pure tones via earphones, the sounds can be presented via loudspeakers, one located to the right of the infant and one to the left. At about 3 to 6 months of age, typically developing infants will learn to turn and look or "localize" the source of a sound. With training, audiologists can learn to capitalize on this natural behavioral responses by alternately and randomly presenting pure tones from either the right or left loudspeaker, changing the sound level from presentation to presentation, and using the infant's head-turn response to determine whether the sound was heard by the baby. Correct head-turn responses at higher sound levels used initially can be reinforced by visible animated toys located atop each loudspeaker. This simply reinforces and sustains the infant's head-turn response so that it can be used enough times to establish a threshold before the baby loses interest in the stimulus and the task. Again, the procedural details are not critical for the intended reader of this book. It is simply important to understand that standardized behavioral measurement procedures, considerably different from those used with older children and adults, can be used to get valid and reliable behavioral measurements of pure-tone thresholds in typically developing children as young as 3 months of age. Further procedural details are available in the online supplemental material accompanying this chapter.

Whether for a child or an adult, when hearing is assessed under earphones or with a bone vibrator, it is not always the case that the ear being tested by the clinician is the one that is stimulated. Sometimes the other ear, referred to simply as the nontest ear, will be the ear stimulated by the sound. This situation results because the two ears are not completely isolated from one another. Air-conducted sound delivered to the test ear through conventional earphones mounted in typical ear cushions is decreased or attenuated approximately 40 dB before stimulating the other ear via skull vibration. The value of 40 dB for interaural ("between-ear") attenuation is actually a minimum value. The amount of interaural attenuation for air conduction varies with the frequency of the test signal but is always more than 40 dB. The minimum interaural attenuation value for bone conduction is 0 dB. Thus, the bone oscillator placed on the mastoid process behind the left ear vibrates the entire skull such that the effective stimulation of the right ear is essentially equivalent to that of the left ear. It is impossible, therefore, when testing by bone conduction, to discern whether the right ear or the left ear is responding without some way of eliminating the participation of the nontest ear (Vignette 7.4).

Masking enables the clinician to eliminate the nontest ear from participation in the measurement of hearing thresholds for the test ear. Essentially, the audiologist introduces a sufficient amount of masking noise into the nontest ear so as to make any sound crossing the skull from the test ear inaudible.

In summary, the pure-tone audiogram provides a lot of information to the audiologist regarding the location of the impairment in the periphery (conductive, outer or middle ear; sensorineural, inner ear; mixed, both), the severity of the resulting hearing loss (mild to profound), the configuration of the hearing loss (rising, flat, or sloping), and whether one or both ears are affected. Each of these factors can contribute to a breakdown in the communication chain. The implications of the findings from pure-tone audiometry also vary with the outcome obtained. For example, in general, conductive hearing loss poses a lesser threat to the communication chain because it is typically milder in degree and is often medically treatable and, as a result, will often be of short duration. An unresolved conductive hearing loss, one that becomes long lasting, or a sensorineural hearing loss of the same degree can have much greater impact on the communication chain and its development. Thus, clearly establishing the location of a peripheral problem in the outer, middle, or inner ear is crucial. The audiologist routinely relies on more than just pure-tone audiometry to make this determination.

VIGNETTE 7.4 • CONCEPTUAL DEMO

Understanding the Need for Masking

In the drawing that accompanies this vignette, two gremlins named Lefty and Righty sit in adjacent rooms. The two rooms are separated by a wall that decreases sound intensity by 40 dB. The gremlins' job is to listen for pure tones. When they hear a sound, they are to signal by pushing a button to light a neon sign containing the words "I heard that!" Righty hears a 10-dB SPL sound coming from the loudspeaker in his room and presses the button. By using softer and louder intensities, we determine the sound intensity that Righty responds to 50% of the time and call this his threshold. Righty has a threshold of 10-dB SPL. This is the typical, or normal, threshold for most gremlins.

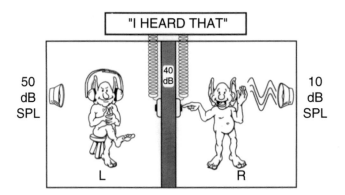

Next we measure Lefty's hearing threshold. Unbeknownst to us, Lefty has decided to wear earmuffs. (You have to be careful with gremlins.) The earmuffs reduce the sound reaching his ears by 60 dB. As we try to measure Lefty's threshold, we gradually increase the intensity of the sound coming from the loudspeaker in the left room. Finally we get a response. Approximately 50% of the time, we see the neon light flash above the rooms when the presentation level of the sound is 50-dB SPL. We conclude that Lefty's threshold is 50-dB SPL.

Is our conclusion correct? Probably not. We said that the earmuffs decrease the sound reaching Lefty's ears by 60 dB and that the typical threshold for gremlins is 10-dB SPL. If the sound level from the speaker in the left room is 50-dB SPL and the earmuffs decrease it by 60 dB, the sound level reaching Lefty's ears is -10-dB SPL. This is well below threshold for gremlins. Yet we clearly saw the neon light flash 50% of the time when the left speaker presented a sound level of 50-dB SPL. By now you have probably reasoned that it was Righty, not Lefty, responding to the sound from the left speaker. The wall decreases sound by 40 dB. A 50-dB SPL sound from the left speaker is 10-dB SPL in the right room. Righty's threshold is 10-dB SPL, and he responds accordingly by pushing the button and lighting the neon sign. Whenever the sound level presented to one room is 40 dB or more above the threshold of the gremlin in the other room, we can't be sure which gremlin is turning on the neon light.

If we used the loudspeaker in Righty's room to present a noise loud enough to make Righty's threshold higher than 10-dB SPL, we could then proceed to increase the sound from the left speaker above levels of 50-dB SPL. By introducing enough masking noise into Righty's room, we could eventually measure Lefty's real threshold of 70-dB SPL (10-dB SPL normal threshold plus 60 dB from earmuffs).

The gremlins in the drawing are like our inner ears, and the loudspeakers are like the headphones. The wall of 40 dB is the separation between the ears provided by the skull, known as the interaural (between-ear) attenuation. Masking noise is often needed to determine which ear is really responding to sound. This is true especially when testing by bone conduction, because there is no interaural attenuation between the two inner ears when the skull is vibrated. Essentially, the 40-dB wall has been removed for bone conduction testing, and the gremlin with the better hearing always responds. The hearing of the better inner ear is always measured via unmasked bone conduction testing regardless of where the bone vibrator is placed on the skull.

SPEECH AUDIOMETRY

The acoustic signals critical to communication are speech sounds, not the pure tones used in pure-tone audiometry. So, the audiologist also assesses the impact of the hearing loss on speech communication as well. This is referred to as **speech audiometry**, and additional equipment, a speech audiometer, is needed for such measurements. Typically, the audiologist makes use of a diagnostic audiometer, which includes capability for both pure-tone and speech audiometry in the same device. The speech audiometer is used to obtain two types of measurements: (a) *SRT*, which corresponds to the softest level at which speech can be recognized with 50% accuracy, and (b) *speech recognition score*, which corresponds to the percentage of speech that can be understood when presented at sound levels well above the softest that can be heard, sound levels close to the optimal level for a given hearing impairment.

Assessment of Speech Recognition Threshold

SRT is the intensity at which an individual can identify simple speech materials approximately 50% of the time. It is included in the basic hearing evaluation for two specific reasons. First, it serves as an excellent check on the validity of pure-tone thresholds. There is a strong correlation between the average of the pure-tone thresholds obtained at the frequencies known to be important for speech (i.e., 500, 1,000, and 2,000 Hz) and the SRT. Large discrepancies between the SRT and this PTA may suggest functional, or nonorganic, hearing loss. A second important reason for including the SRT in the hearing evaluation is that it provides a basis for selecting the sound level at which a patient's speech recognition abilities should be tested. Finally, besides its use in the basic hearing evaluation, the SRT is also useful in the determination of functional gain in the hearing aid evaluation process.

The most popular test materials used by audiologists to measure SRT are spondaic words. Spondaic words are two-syllable words spoken with equal stress on each syllable (e.g., baseball, hotdog, cowboy). A carrier phrase, such as "say the word," may precede each stimulus item.

Assessment of Suprathreshold Speech Recognition

Although the speech threshold provides the clinician with an index of the degree of hearing loss for speech, it does not offer any information regarding a person's ability to make distinctions among the various acoustic cues in our spoken language at conversational intensity levels. Unlike the situation with the SRT, attempts to calculate a person's ability to understand speech presented at comfortably loud levels based on data from the pure-tone audiogram have not been successful. Consequently, various suprathreshold speech recognition tests have been developed for the purpose of estimating a person's ability to understand speech. Three of the more common types of speech recognition tests are phonetically balanced (PB) lists of single-syllable words (e.g., "dog," "ball"), multiple choice tests comprised of rhyming single-syllable words (e.g., "ball," "tall," "fall," and "mall"), and sentence tests.

The most popular stimuli used to assess speech understanding are PB lists of single-syllable words, and these are the only ones reviewed here. These word lists are referred to as "phonetically balanced" because the phonetic composition of all word lists in the test is equivalent and representative of everyday English speech. All of the PB word lists use an open-set response format. This is similar to a "fill in the blank" test item in which the set of possible responses is potentially unlimited and is restricted only by the listener's vocabulary. In contrast, a closed-response format is akin to a multiple-choice test item in which the listener is presented with a set of several alternative responses for each test item, one of which is the monosyllabic word spoken by the examiner. A typical presentation includes the use of a carrier phrase, such as "Say the word...." For example, a typical sequence might be "Say the word dog" (the patient responds), "Say the word ball" (the patient responds), and so on. Typically, the instruction to the patient is simply to repeat aloud the last word heard for each test item ("dog" and "ball" in the preceding two examples).

The procedures used to obtain SRT and speech recognition scores are standardized for adults so that similar results can be obtained from clinic to clinic or from time to time for the same patient in the same clinic. There are also variations of all of these procedures, as well as for pure-tone audiometry, for use with children of various ages. The details of these adaptations are not included here. In the end, the audiologist uses a variety of age-appropriate techniques to get the best estimate of hearing for pure tones and hearing for speech from the patient and records these on the audiogram.

Pure-tone and speech audiometry, however, involve voluntary behavioral responses from the patient. As with any such measurements, there can be variability or error in the measurements, and this, in turn, can impact the certainty of the diagnosis. As a result, audiologists have developed other complementary measurements that assess the auditory system but don't require behavioral responses from the patient. These can be especially valuable in the assessment of young children who may be more variable in their behavioral responses. One set of complementary measurements has become a standard part of the basic audiologic test battery and is known as "acoustic immittance measurement."

ACOUSTIC IMMITTANCE MEASUREMENT

When an acoustic wave strikes the eardrum of the normal ear, a portion of the signal is transmitted through the middle ear to the cochlea, while the remaining part of the wave is reflected back out the external canal. The reflected energy forms a sound wave traveling in an outward direction with an amplitude and phase that depend on the opposition encountered at the tympanic membrane. The energy of the reflected wave is greatest when the middle ear system is stiff or immobile, as in such pathologic conditions as otitis media with effusion and otosclerosis. On the other hand, an ear with ossicular chain dislocation or interruption will reflect considerably less sound back into the canal because of the reduced stiffness. A greater portion of the acoustic wave will be transmitted to the middle ear under these circumstances. The reflected sound wave, therefore, carries information about the status of the middle ear system.

As noted in Chapter 2, impedance is the term used to describe the opposition to flow of acoustic (mechanical) energy through the middle ear. The reciprocal of impedance is admittance. An ear with high impedance has low admittance and vice versa. Admittance describes the relative ease with which energy flows through a system, such as the middle ear. Some commercially available devices used by the clinician measure quantities related to acoustic impedance of the middle ear, whereas others measure quantities related to acoustic admittance.

In an effort to provide a common vocabulary for results obtained with either device, professionals have decided to use the term "immittance." Immittance itself is not a physical quantity but simply a term that can be used to refer to either impedance data or admittance data.

The measurement of **acoustic immittance** at the tympanic membrane is an important component of the basic hearing evaluation. This sensitive and objective diagnostic tool has been used to identify the presence of fluid in the middle ear, to evaluate eustachian tube and facial nerve function, to predict audiometric findings, to determine the type of hearing loss, and to assist in diagnosing the site of auditory lesion. This technique is considered particularly useful in the assessment of difficult-to-test persons, including very young children.

Figure 7.7 shows how this concept may be applied to actual practice. A pliable probe tip is inserted carefully into the ear canal, and an airtight seal is obtained so that varying amounts of air pressure can be applied to the ear cavity by pumping air into the ear canal or suctioning it out. A positive amount of air pressure (usually +200 daPa) is then introduced into the airtight ear canal, forcing the tympanic membrane inward.[1] The eardrum is now stiffer than it is in its natural state because of the positive pressure created in the ear canal. A low-frequency pure tone is then introduced, and a tiny microphone measures the level of the sound reflected from the stiffened eardrum. A low-frequency tone is used because this is the frequency region most affected by changes in stiffness (see Chapter 2). Keeping the intensity of the probe tone introduced into the ear canal constant, the pressure is then reduced slowly, causing the tympanic membrane to become more compliant (less stiff). As the tympanic membrane becomes increasingly compliant, more of the acoustic signal will be passed through the middle ear, and the level of the reflected sound in the ear canal will decrease. When the air pressure in the ear canal equals the air pressure in the middle ear, the tympanic membrane will move with the greatest ease. As the pressure is reduced further, the tympanic membrane is pulled outward, and the eardrum again becomes less mobile. As before, when the eardrum becomes stiffer or less compliant, more low-frequency energy is reflected off the tympanic membrane, and the sound level within the ear canal increases.

#12

---

[1]A daPa is a measure of air pressure in units of decapascals. 1 daPa = 10 Pa = 1.02 mm H_2O. Millimeters (mm) H_2O refers to the amount of pressure to push a column of water in a special tube to a given height in millimeters. For measurements of immittance, air pressure is generally expressed relative to ambient air pressure. That is, ambient air pressure is represented as 0 daPa, and a pressure of 100 daPa above ambient pressure is represented as +100 daPa.

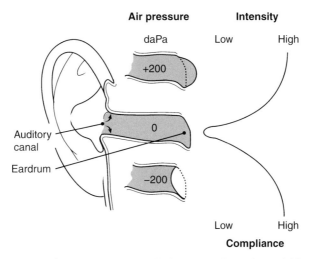

FIGURE 7.7 Concepts of immittance applied in practice. The *middle* column shows three different air pressures developed in the ear canal (+200, 0, and +200 daPa), and the *dotted line* in the drawings at the *top* and *bottom* of this column represents the resting position of the eardrum (at 0 daPa). The *right* column shows both the sound intensity of the probe tone recorded in the ear canal as the air pressure is changed from –200 daPa (*top*) to +200 daPa (*bottom*) and the corresponding changes in the compliance of the middle ear.

Figure 7.8 illustrates the basic components of most immittance instruments. The probe tip is sealed in the ear canal, providing a closed cavity. The probe contains three small ports that are connected to (a) a sound source that generates a low-frequency (usually 220 or 660 Hz) pure tone, (b) a microphone to measure the reflected sound wave, and (c) an air pump and manometer for varying the air pressure within the ear canal.

IMMITTANCE TEST BATTERY

Three basic measurements—tympanometry, static acoustic immittance, and threshold of the acoustic reflex—commonly make up the basic acoustic immittance test battery. Each of these measurements is described, in turn, below.

Tympanometry

Acoustic immittance at the tympanic membrane of a normal ear changes systematically as air pressure in the external canal is varied above and below ambient air pressure (Fig. 7.7). The normal relationship between air pressure changes and changes in immittance is frequently altered in the presence of middle ear disease.

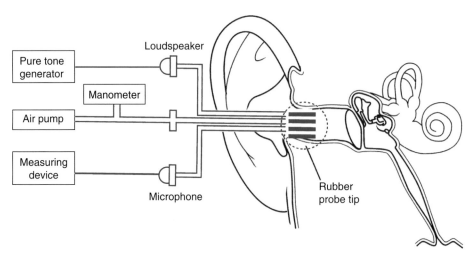

FIGURE 7.8 Components of an immittance instrument.

Tympanometry is the measurement of the mobility of the middle ear when air pressure in the external canal is varied from +200 to –400 daPa. Results from tympanometry are then plotted on a graph, with air pressure along the x-axis and immittance, or *compliance*, along the y-axis.[2] Practice surveys of audiologists have indicated that well over 90% of audiologists obtain tympanograms from their patients and the majority do so all of the time. Figure 7.9 illustrates some of the tympanograms commonly seen in normal and pathologic ears.

Various estimates have been made of the air pressure in the ear canal that results in the least amount of reflected sound energy from normal middle ears. This air pressure is routinely referred to as the peak pressure point. A normal tympanogram for an adult (Fig. 7.9A) has a peak pressure point between –100 and +40 daPa, which suggests that the middle ear functions optimally at or near ambient pressure (0 daPa). Tympanograms that peak at a point ≤ –150 daPa (Fig. 7.9B) suggest malfunction of the middle ear pressure-equalizing system. This malfunction might be a result of eustachian tube malfunction, early or resolving serous otitis media, or acute otitis media. (These and other disorders were described in detail in Chapter 6). Ears that contain fluid behind the eardrum are characterized by a flat tympanogram at a high impedance or low admittance value without a peak pressure point (Fig. 7.9C). This implies an excessively stiff system that does not allow for an increase in sound transmission through the middle ear under any pressure state. The amplitude (height)

---

[2]Throughout this text, we have assumed that immittance measurements are made with an impedance meter. With such a device, immittance values are described in arbitrary units, frequently labeled "compliance." These devices do not actually measure compliance.

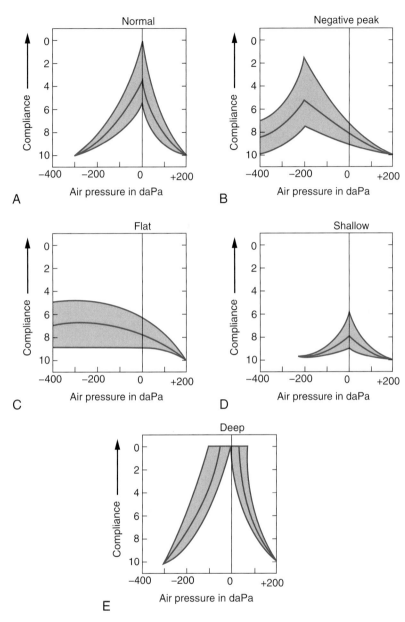

FIGURE 7.9 Tympanometric configurations for normal and pathologic ears are shown. Measured tympanograms falling in the *dotted* regions would be classified using the label at the *top* of each tympanogram (normal, negative peak, flat, etc.).

of the tympanogram also provides information about the compliance or elasticity of the system. A stiff middle ear (as in, e.g., ossicular chain fixation) is represented by a shallow amplitude, suggesting high acoustic impedance or low admittance (Fig. 7.9D). Conversely, an ear with abnormally low acoustic impedance or high admittance (as in an interrupted ossicular chain or a hyper-mobile tympanic membrane) is revealed by a tympanogram with a very high amplitude (Fig. 7.9E).

Flat tympanograms can also be observed when the probe tip of the immit-tance device is blocked (e.g., with earwax) or when there is a perforation of the eardrum. In these cases, when the shape of the tympanogram is the same (flat), the clinician relies on differences in the overall amplitude of the impedance or admittance value. A blocked probe tip, for example, will show a very high impedance (very low admittance), a perforated eardrum often shows a very low impedance (very high admittance), and a fluid-filled middle ear is somewhere in between, typically closer to the values of the blocked probe tip. Since the tympa-nograms are flat, these differences in immittance amplitude manifest themselves at the initial reading of immittance obtained with a high positive pressure (+200 daPa), a measurement often referred to as the "equivalent ear canal volume." Of course, otoscopic inspection of the ear canal and eardrum can help differen-tiate among these different causes for tympanograms having flat shape.

Tympanograms are frequently labeled as "types." Type A tympanograms (Fig. 7.9A) represent normal tympanograms (normal shape, peak-pressure point, and amplitude), Type B tympanograms are flat (Fig. 7.9C), and Type C tympa-nograms have normal shape and amplitude but a negative peak-pressure point (Fig. 7.9B). Two subtypes of "Type A" tympanograms, which are abnormal only with regard to the peak amplitude and not the shape or peak-pressure point, are Type A_s (s = "shallow"; Fig. 7.9D) and Type A_d (d = "deep"; Fig. 7.9E).

Static Acoustic Immittance

Static acoustic immittance measures the ease of flow of acoustic energy through the middle ear and is usually expressed in "equivalent volume" in cubic centimeters. To obtain this measurement, immittance is first determined under a positive pressure (+200 daPa) artificially induced in the canal. Very little sound is admitted through the middle ear under this extreme positive pressure, with much of the acoustic energy reflected back into the ear canal. Next, a similar determination is made with the eardrum in its most compliant position, thus maximizing transmission through the middle ear cavity. The arithmetic differ-ence between these two immittance values, usually recorded in cubic centimeters (cm^3) of equivalent volume, provides an estimate of immittance at the tympanic membrane. Compliance values less than or equal to 0.25 cm^3 of equivalent volume suggest low acoustic immittance (indicative of stiffening pathologies), and values greater than or equal to 2.0 cm^3 generally indicate abnormally high immittance (suggestive of ossicular discontinuity or healed tympanic membrane perforations).

Acoustic Reflex Threshold

The acoustic reflex threshold is defined as the lowest possible intensity needed to elicit a contraction of the muscles in the middle ear. Contraction of the middle ear muscles, evoked by intense sound, results in a temporary increase in the middle ear impedance. The acoustic reflex is a consensual phenomenon; acoustic stimulation to one ear will elicit a muscle contraction and subsequent impedance change in both ears. Often, the acoustic reflex is monitored in the ear canal opposite (contralateral) to the ear receiving the sound stimulus. Figure 7.10 shows how it is measured contralaterally. A headphone is placed on one ear, and the probe assembly is inserted into the contralateral (opposite) ear. When the signal transduced from the earphone reaches an intensity sufficient to evoke an acoustic reflex, the stiffness of the middle ear is increased in both ears. This results in more sound being reflected from the eardrum, and a subsequent increase in sound pressure is observed on the immittance instrument. In recording the data, it is standard procedure to consider the ear stimulated with the intense sound as the ear under test. Because the ear stimulated is contralateral to the ear in which the reflex is measured, these reflex thresholds are referred to as contralateral reflex thresholds. It is also frequently possible to present the loud reflex-activating stimulus through the probe assembly itself. In this case, the reflex is both activated and measured in the same ear. This is referred to as an ipsilateral acoustic reflex. A recent survey of audiologic practices found that more than 90% of audiologists measure acoustic reflex thresholds with more using ipsilateral measurements than contralateral.

#14

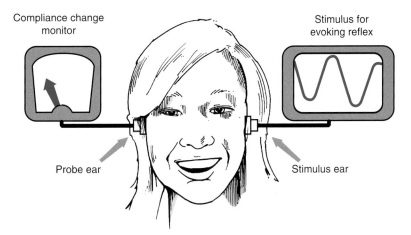

FIGURE 7.10 Example of how an acoustic reflex is obtained for contralateral stimulus presentation. Essentially, for ipsilateral measurements, the functions of the probe tip and the earphone are combined so that the reflex-eliciting stimulus and the immittance change that results from the muscle contraction can be measured in the same ear.

In the normal ear, contraction of middle ear muscles occurs with pure tones ranging from 65- to 95-dB HL. A conductive hearing loss, however, tends to either elevate or eliminate the reflex response. When acoustic reflex information is used in conjunction with tympanometry and static acoustic immittance measurements, it serves to substantiate further the existence of a middle ear disorder. With unilateral conductive hearing loss, failure to elicit the reflex depends on the size of the air-bone gap and on the ear in which the probe tip is inserted. If the stimulus is presented to the good ear and the probe tip is placed on the affected side, an air-bone gap of only 10 dB will usually abolish the reflex response. In this case, the pathology present in the "probe ear" has increased the stiffness of the middle ear so much that small increases in stiffness associated with the acoustic reflex either do not occur or cannot be measured. If, however, the stimulus is presented to the pathologic ear and the probe is in the normal ear, a gap of 25 dB is needed to abolish or significantly elevate the reflex threshold. In this case, the contralateral acoustic reflex is absent because the middle ear pathology decreases the amplitude of the reflex-activating sound reaching the cochlea to levels that are too soft to elicit the reflex.

Acoustic reflex thresholds can also be useful in differentiating whether a sensorineural hearing loss is caused by a lesion in the inner ear or to one in the auditory nerve. For hearing losses ranging from mild to severe, the acoustic reflex threshold is more likely to be elevated or absent in ears with neural pathology than in those with cochlear damage. The pattern of acoustic reflex thresholds for ipsilateral and contralateral stimulation across both ears, moreover, can aid in diagnosing brainstem lesions affecting the reflex pathways in the auditory brainstem.

Immittance can be most valuable in the assessment of young children, although it does have some diagnostic limitations. Further, although electroacoustic immittance measures are ordinarily simple and quick to obtain, special considerations and skills are required to obtain these measures successfully from infants. Variation in test stimuli, such as the use of higher frequency, might also be needed to ensure valid results. Immittance measures in young children might be confined to handheld immittance screeners that enable quick measurement of tympanograms and ipsilateral acoustic reflexes at a single high intensity (often at a single frequency too, such as 1,000 Hz).

Although immittance tests may be administered to neonates and young infants with a reasonable amount of success, tympanometry may have limited value with children younger than 7 months of age. Below this age, there is a poor correlation between tympanometry and the actual condition of the middle ear. In very young infants, a normal tympanogram does not necessarily imply that there is a normal middle ear system. However, a flat tympanogram obtained in an infant strongly suggests a diseased ear. Consequently, it is still worthwhile to administer immittance tests to this population.

Another limitation of immittance measurements is the difficulty of obtaining measurements from a hyperactive child or a child who is crying, yawning, or continually talking. A young child who exhibits excessive body movement or head turning will make it almost impossible to maintain an airtight seal with the probe tip. Vocalization produces middle ear muscle activity that, in turn, causes continual alterations in the compliance of the tympanic membrane, making immittance measurements impossible. With difficult-to-test and younger children, specialized techniques are needed to keep the child relatively calm and quiet. For young children, it is always recommended that a second person be involved in the evaluation. While the child is sitting on the parent's lap, one person can place the earphone and insert the probe tip and a second person can manipulate the controls of the equipment. With infants below 2 years of age, placing the earphones and headband on the child's head is often distracting. It may be helpful to remove the earphone from the headband, rest the band over the mother's shoulder, and insert the probe tip into the child's ear. It is also helpful to use some distractive techniques that will occupy the child's attention during the test (Vignette 7.5).

Basic Audiologic Test Battery

#23 and #24

In the measurement of auditory function, the most meaningful information can be gleaned only when the entire test battery of pure-tone and speech audiometry together with immittance measurements is used. If just one or two of these procedures are used, valuable clinical information will be lost because each of these clinical tools offers a unique and informative set of data. In particular, the reader should keep in mind the differences between pure-tone measures and electroacoustic immittance measurements. Pure-tone audiometry does not measure the immittance of the middle ear, just as immittance does not measure hearing sensitivity. Although an abnormal audiogram strongly suggests the presence of a hearing loss, abnormal immittance does not. Abnormal immittance findings in the absence of significant hearing loss, on the other hand, can be sufficient grounds for medical referral. A test-battery approach is essential. Vignettes 7.6, 7.7, and 7.8 show examples of applications of the test battery.

ADDITIONAL SPECIAL TESTS

Administration of the basic audiologic test battery determines whether the patient has any hearing loss; what affect the hearing loss, if present, has on speech understanding; and whether the nature of the hearing loss is conductive, sensorineural, or a combination of the two (mixed). Administration of the

Distractive Techniques when Obtaining Immittance Measures from Young Children

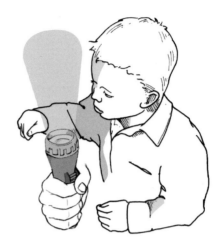

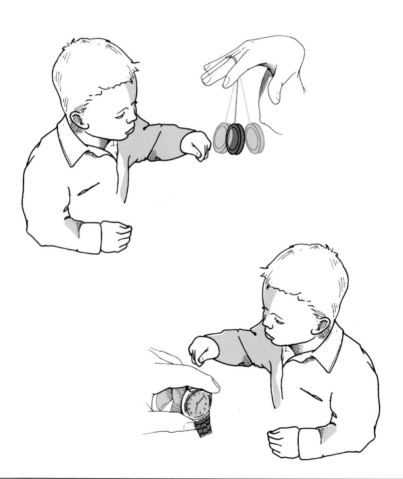

VIGNETTE 7.6 • CLINICAL APPLICATIONS

A 6-Year-Old Child with Bilateral Otitis Media

The accompanying charts show a mild-to-moderate bilateral hearing loss for air con-duction; bone conduction thresholds are normal in both ears. Such a discrepancy between air conduction and bone conduction thresholds suggests a conductive loss. The SRTs are compatible with the pure-tone data. Also, when the signal is made comfortably loud, suprathreshold speech recognition is excellent in both ears. Good speech recognition is consistent with a middle ear disorder. Immittance confirms the impression of a conductive loss. The *shaded* areas on the tympanogram and static immittance forms represent normative data. The tympanograms are flat, the static immittance is well below normal, and acoustic reflexes are absent in both ears. This general pattern is consistent with a middle ear complication and strongly sug-gests a fluid-filled middle ear, thus requiring a medical referral. If, however, there is no evidence of previous middle ear problems and the child has no complaints, a recheck should be recommended in 3 weeks. If the same results are obtained, the child should be referred to the family physician.

Educationally, such a problem can be relatively serious if medical intervention does not result in a speedy return to completely normal HLs. Such children are likely to appear listless and inattentive in the classroom, and their performance soon begins to deteriorate. Both the teacher and the parents should receive an expla-nation of these probable consequences from the audiologist. In counseling the teacher, emphasis should be placed on establishing favorable classroom seating, supplementing auditory input with visual cues, articulating clearly and forcefully,

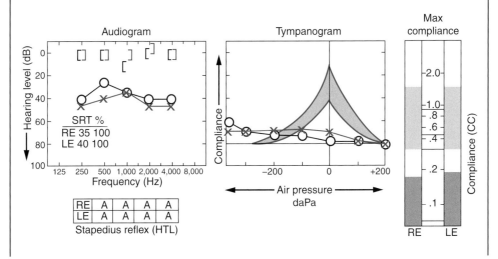

and frequently reiterating assignments. If the condition does not respond readily to medical treatment, amplification, along with other remedial measures such as speechreading instruction and training in listening skills, should not be ruled out. Above all, the child will need patient understanding while the HL is diminished and sometimes fluctuating from one day to the next.

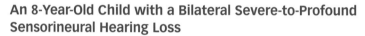

VIGNETTE 7.7 • CLINICAL APPLICATIONS

An 8-Year-Old Child with a Bilateral Severe-to-Profound Sensorineural Hearing Loss

The pure-tone results in the accompanying figure display a severe-to-profound sensorineural hearing loss. Bone conduction responses could not be obtained at the maximum output limits of the audiometer. The SRTs using selected spondees were compatible with the pure-tone data. Suprathreshold speech recognition scores could not be obtained because of the severity of the loss. Immittance results on both ears show tympanograms and static immittance values to be within the normal range. Acoustic reflexes are absent in both ears, but these usually cannot be elicited with a hearing loss in excess of 85-dB HL.

These audiologic results confirm the presence of a sensorineural hearing impairment, which is so severe that the best possible educational opportunities must be made available and, at age 8, hopefully have been in place already for several years. Periodic audiologic evaluations are highly important in the optimal educational management of such children.

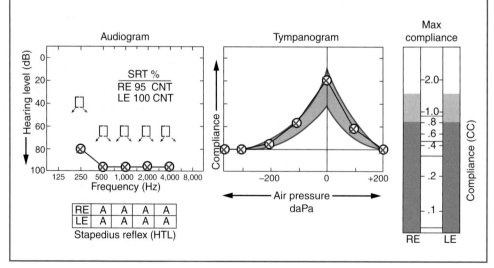

VIGNETTE 7.8 • CLINICAL APPLICATIONS

Adult with a Bilateral Mild-to-Moderate Sensorineural Hearing Loss

The pure-tone results accompanying this vignette show a bilateral sloping sensorineural hearing loss in an elderly adult. The SRTs are compatible with the pure-tone data, and suprathreshold speech recognition is only fair to good, even when the signal is made comfortably loud. Immittance results show normal tympanograms and static immittance for both ears, with acoustic reflexes present, but elevated, bilaterally.

Recommended treatment in this case would most likely be the use of two hearing aids, although there are limitations to the benefits achievable with amplification alone (see Chapter 9). It may also be necessary to provide special assistance in the form of training in auditory and visual (speechreading) communication skills.

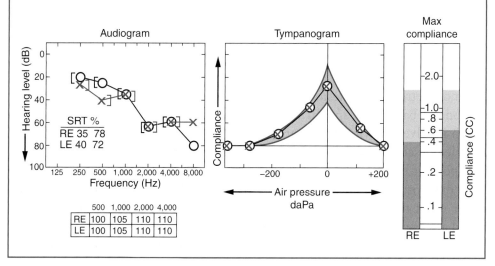

immittance battery can also evaluate middle ear function regardless of whether a measurable hearing loss is present. Thus, through interpretation of the results from the basic audiologic test battery, the clinician can determine where in the peripheral portion of the auditory system a lesion may be located.

Additional special auditory tests are needed, however, to determine whether lesions are present in more central portions of the ascending nervous system, such as the auditory nerve, brainstem, or cortex. A patient with a life-threatening tumor affecting the auditory nerve, for example, will frequently have pure-tone test results consistent with a high-frequency sensorineural hearing loss, a pattern of hearing loss most frequently associated with a variety of cochlear lesions, rather than a tumor on the auditory nerve. Other components of the basic hearing test battery, however, may provide some "warning signs" suggesting that the lesion responsible for the hearing loss is affecting the auditory nerve. For example, the hearing loss in such cases usually affects the high frequencies and is different in the two ears, often leaving one ear completely unaffected. In addition, speech recognition scores in the impaired ear are often reduced much more than would be expected on the basis of the pure-tone hearing loss. Finally, acoustic reflex thresholds for the affected ear are typically elevated above the normal range (>100-dB HL). Although these features are typical for many patients with tumors affecting the auditory nerve, many cases manifest only one or two of these features. Patients with inner ear pathology, moreover, may also manifest one or more of these features.

A battery of special auditory tests has been developed to assist in the identification of lesions occurring central to the cochlea or inner ear. These lesions are referred to as retrocochlear lesions. Historically, this test battery was based on a variety of behavioral tests that used pure tones as stimuli. After several years of test development and refinement, most of these tests were still only 60% to 70% accurate in identifying retrocochlear impairments. Many individuals with cochlear hearing loss were falsely identified as having retrocochlear lesions, and still more retrocochlear lesions were identified as cochlear.

Today's battery of special auditory tests consists of several tests, few of which involve behavioral measurements in response to pure-tone stimulation. Detailed descriptions of these procedures are beyond the scope of this book. It is important here to note only that the basic audiologic test battery is limited in its diagnostic usefulness. Additional special auditory tests can be performed in the event that any of the retrocochlear warning signs described above are found after performing the basic tests. Readers who desire to learn more about the special auditory test battery can consult the Suggested Readings at the end of this chapter.

Finally, an area that has received much attention in recent years, much of it controversial, especially in school-age children, has been the diagnosis of dysfunction in the auditory portions of the central nervous system. These problems have generally been labeled as "auditory processing disorder" or APD. The reliability and validity of many of the tests developed to identify APD, both in children and adults, are still being investigated. One of the challenges has been to demonstrate that such tests are truly measuring auditory abilities and not more general cognitive function. Until such tests are developed and norms using them established, however, the diagnosis and treatment of such disorders are likely to remain controversial. (See Vignette 7.9 on the importance of test reliability and validity.)

VIGNETTE 7.9 • FURTHER DISCUSSION

Illustration of the Importance of Test Reliability and Validity

The reliability and validity of a test represent essential information that must be known before the widespread use of that test. Unfortunately, because of the pressures of solving problems for patients today, audiologists often don't feel that they have the time to wait for the needed research to be completed before the use of a newly developed test. The testing of auditory processing disorder (APD) in children is clearly an area that exemplifies this problem. Often, tests have been pressed into use before clearly establishing their reliability or validity as tests of APD.

In general, the reliability of the test refers to its accuracy or stability. Ideally, if the same test were administered to the same individual under identical conditions on 10 successive occasions, with no memory, learning, or fatigue involved, we'd like all 10 scores to be identical. For behavioral testing of humans, especially children, however, this ideal is seldom achieved. Rather, the scores vary from test to retest because of a wide variety of factors. The greater the variation in test scores in this hypothetical scenario, the poorer the reliability of the test. Many tests of APD have been found to have unacceptable reliability. For some of the proposed APD tests, the scores can be expected to vary from test to retest such that the diagnostic disposition will likely vary from "normal" to "abnormal" (or vice versa). Clearly, such tests would be unacceptably unreliable for widespread clinical use.

Perhaps an even thornier issue, though, has to do with establishing the validity of a test. There are many kinds of test validity, but in all cases, evaluation of a test's validity attempts to determine how well the proposed test measures what it was designed to measure. In the case of APD, is the proposed test measuring "central auditory processing?" First, it must be demonstrated that poor performance on the test cannot be attributed to peripheral auditory deficits. Although this has been an infrequent problem when APD has been studied in children, it has been a very common problem when APD has been studied in the elderly. Second, it must be demonstrated that the test is sensitive to an auditory deficit and not representative of a more general cognitive problem that can affect multiple sensory modalities. Often, in this regard, clinical researchers have taken the approach that a similarity in responses implies similarity in causality. Several tests of APD, for example, make use of tasks that were validated on cases of surgically or radiologically confirmed central auditory lesions (e.g., stroke patients or patients with tumors in the central pathways). When audiologists observed similar (but usually not identical) trends in performance on proposed APD tests in individuals with no known central auditory lesions, they then concluded that the locus of the dysfunction had to be central because the response pattern was similar to that obtained from patients with known central lesions.

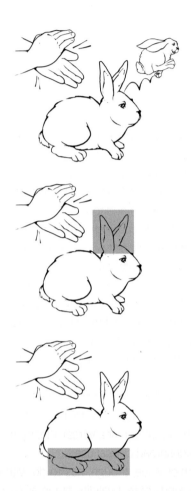

A key problem with such reasoning is shown with the fictitious "hand-clap" test of hearing illustrated here. First, the researcher establishes that normal-hearing rabbits will hop away in response to a clap of the hands (*top* panel). Next, a rabbit's ears are surgically destroyed. (Relax! This is just a hypothetical experiment.) The experimenter then demonstrates that the rabbit fails to hop away in response to a clap of the hands (*middle* panel). Thus, the test has been validated as being sensitive to the presence of a hearing impairment. Now, another rabbit's legs are surgically removed, and the experimenter again claps his or her hands. The rabbit fails to hop away and the experimenter, noting the same response from those rabbits without ears, concludes that "rabbits without legs can't hear"! Clearly, the faulty reasoning in this analogy is apparent. Similarity or even equivalence of responses does not confirm similarity (or equivalence) of the underlying causal factors.

In recent years, researchers have realized the need for reliable and valid measures of APD, in both children and adults. Several tests are under development and evaluation at present, and it is hoped that these tools will be available for widespread clinical use in the near future.

SUMMARY

We have reviewed the basic components of the test battery used in the measurement of auditory function. This includes the measurement of pure-tone threshold by air and bone conduction, speech audiometry, and immittance measurements. The results from these various approaches, when used as a battery, give the audiologist good insight into the nature and extent of the auditory disorder. The resulting diagnosis will also have implications for the development and use of the communication chain by the patient, as well as approaches to remedying any disruptions or breaks in the communication chain.

CHAPTER REVIEW QUESTIONS

1. Draw and label the axes of an audiogram. Shade in the region that is considered to be "normal hearing."
2. Using the audiogram you drew in Question 1, using the appropriate symbols, show a mild conductive hearing loss in the right ear. What disorder might be associated with this hearing loss?
3. Based on the audiogram you drew in Question 2 and the disorder that you associated with it, what immittance test results (tympanogram and ipsilateral acoustic reflex thresholds) would be expected for the right ear?
4. Now, draw a mild-to-severe sloping sensorineural hearing loss in the left ear, using the appropriate symbols. What disorder might be associated with the pattern of hearing loss you drew?
5. Based on the audiogram you drew in Question 4 and the hypothesized disorder associated with it, draw the tympanogram most likely to be measured and indicate the expected ipsilateral acoustic reflex thresholds.
6. Does tympanometry represent a measurement of hearing loss? That is, do individuals with abnormal tympanograms have hearing loss? Do individuals with hearing loss have abnormal tympanograms?

REFERENCES AND SUGGESTED READINGS

American Speech-Language-Hearing Association. Guidelines for audiometric symbols. *ASHA* 1990;32(suppl 2):25–30.

American Speech-Language-Hearing Association. Guidelines for determining threshold level for speech. *ASHA* 1988;30(3):85–90.

Bench J, Kowal A, Bamford J. The BKB (Bamford-Kowal-Bench) sentence lists for partially-hearing children. *Br J Audiol* 1979;13:108–112.

Bess FH. Clinical assessment of speech recognition. In: Konkle DF, Rintelmann WF, eds. *Principles of Speech Audiometry*. Baltimore, MD: University Park Press; 1982.

Bess FH. The minimally hearing impaired child. *Ear Hear* 1985;6:43–47.

Bess FH, Chase PA, Gravel JS, et al. Amplification for infants and children with hearing loss—1995 position statement. *Am J Audiol* 1996;5:53–68.

Bluestone CD, Beery QC, Paradise JL. Audiometry and tympanometry in relation to middle ear effusions in children. *Laryngoscope* 1963;83:594–604.

Carhart R. Future horizons in audiological diagnosis. *Ann Otol Rhinol Laryngol* 1968;77:706–716.

Carhart R, Jerger JF. Preferred method for clinical determination of pure-tone thresholds. *J Speech Hear Disord* 1959;24:330–345.

Clifton RA. Development of spatial hearing. In: Werner LA, Rubel EW, eds. *Developmental Psychoacoustics*. Washington, DC: American Psychological Association; 1992.

Cox R, Alexander G, Gilmore C, et al. Use of the Connected Speech Test (CST) with hearing-impaired listeners. *Ear Hear* 1988;9:198–207.

Diefendorf AO. Pediatric audiology. In: Lass NJ, McReynolds LV, Northern JL, et al., eds. *Handbook of Speech-Language Pathology and Audiology*. Philadelphia, PA: BC Decker; 1988.

Egan J. Articulation testing methods. *Laryngoscope* 1948;58:955–991.

Haskins HA. A phonetically balanced test of speech discrimination for children. Master's thesis. Evanston, IL: Northwestern University; 1949.

Hirsh IJ, Davis H, Silverman SR, et al. Development of materials for speech audiometry. *J Speech Hear Disord* 1952;17:321–337.

Hood JD. The principles and practice of bone-conduction audiometry: A review of the present position. *Laryngoscope* 1960;70:1211–1228.

House AS, Williams CE, Hecker MHL, et al. Articulation testing methods: Consonantal differentiation in a closed-response set. *J Acoust Soc Am* 1965;20:463–474.

Jerger S. Speech audiometry. In: Jerger J, ed. *Pediatric Audiology*. San Diego, CA: College Hill Press; 1984.

Jerger S, Lewis S, Hawkins J, et al. Pediatric speech intelligibility test I. Generation of test materials. *Int J Pediatr Otorhinolaryngol* 1980;2:217–230.

Kalikow DN, Stevens KN, Elliott, LL. Development of a test of speech intelligibility in noise using sentence materials with controlled word predictability. *J Acoust Soc Am* 1977;61:1337–1351.

Katz J. *Handbook of Clinical Audiology*. 5th ed. Baltimore, MD: Lippincott Williams & Wilkins; 2002.

Katz DR, Elliott LL. Development of a new children's speech discrimination test. Paper presented at the convention of the American Speech-Language-Hearing Association, November 18–21, Chicago, 1978.

Levitt H, Resnick SB. Speech reception by the hearing impaired: Methods of testing and the development of new tests. In: Ludvigsen C, Barfod J, eds.

Sensorineural Hearing Impaired and Hearing Aids. Scand Audiol Suppl 1978;6:107–130.

Martin FN. Minimum effective masking levels in threshold audiometry. *J Speech Hear Disord* 1974;39:280–285.

Northern JL. Acoustic impedance in the pediatric population. In: Bess FH, ed: *Childhood Deafness: Causation, Assessment, and Management.* New York, NY: Grune & Stratton; 1977.

Northern JL, Downs MP. *Hearing in Children.* 5th ed. Philadelphia, PA: Lippincott Williams & Wilkins; 2001.

Olsen WO, Matkin ND. Speech audiometry. In: Rintelmann WF, ed. *Hearing Assessment.* Baltimore, MD: University Park Press; 1979.

Owens E, Schubert ED. Development of the California consonant test. *J Speech Hear Res* 1977;20:463–474.

Ross M, Lerman J. A picture identification test for hearing impaired children. *J Speech Hear Res* 1970;13:44–53.

Sanders JW. Masking. In: Katz J, ed: *Handbook of Clinical Audiology.* 2nd ed. Baltimore, MD: Williams & Wilkins; 1978:124.

Sanders JW. Diagnostic audiology. In: Lass NJ, McReynolds NJ, Northern JL, et al., eds. *Handbook of Speech-Language Pathology and Audiology.* Philadelphia, PA: BC Decker; 1988.

Schwartz D, Josey AF, Bess FH, eds. Proceedings of meeting in honor of Professor Jay Sanders. *Ear Hear* 1987;8:4.

Shanks JE, Lilly DJ, Margolis RH, et al. Tympanometry. *J Speech Hear Disord* 1988;53:354–377.

Studebaker GA. Clinical masking in air- and bone-conducted stimuli. *J Speech Hear Disord* 1964;29:23–35.

Tharpe AM, Ashmead DH. A longitudinal investigation of infant auditory sensitivity. *Am J Audiol* 2001;10:104–112.

Tillman TW, Olsen WO. Speech audiometry. In: Jerger J, ed. *Modern Developments in Audiology.* New York, NY: Academic Press; 1973.

Tillman TW, Carhart R. *An Expanded Test for Speech Discrimination Using CNC Monosyllabic Words.* Northwestern University Auditory Test No. 6. Technical Report No. SAM-TR-66-55, USAF School of Aerospace Medicine, Brooks Air Force Base, Texas, 1966.

8

Screening for Hearing Loss and Middle Ear Status

Chapter Objectives

- To recognize the importance of screening as a tool to identify possible cases of hearing loss or middle ear pathology as the first step toward treatment;
- To understand the principles of screening, including sensitivity and specificity of screening tests;
- To carry out pure-tone hearing screening, including the procedures for performing the testing, managing the results, and seeking appropriate follow-up; and
- To carry out immittance-based screening to identify the presence of middle ear pathology, including screening procedures, management of results, and monitoring necessary follow-up testing.

Key Terms and Definitions

- **Screening:** A screening program is designed to expediently and reliably identify those likely to have a disorder within the general population. More definitive follow-up testing is typically required to confirm (or refute) the findings of the screening.
- **Test sensitivity:** The proportion of the population or sample who have the disorder or trait for which the screening is being conducted and who failed the screening test (i.e., tested positive for the disorder or trait).
- **Test specificity:** The proportion of the population or sample who do not have the disorder or trait for which the screening is being conducted and who passed the screening test (i.e., tested negative for the disorder or trait).
- **Prevalence:** The estimated proportion of the population who have a particular disorder or trait.

As reviewed in the previous chapter, the audiologist uses a variety of diagnostic tools, including pure-tone audiometry, speech audiometry, and immittance measurements, to determine whether hearing loss or middle ear dysfunction is present, the severity of the problem, and the likely location of the problem within the auditory system. These results are summarized on audiograms and tympanograms and are frequently accompanied by a brief written report. For school-age children with impaired hearing, the speech-language pathologist is often asked to interpret the results obtained by the audiologist so as to incorporate this information into the child's individualized educational plan.

Hearing problems are important to identify at any age. At a young age, the presence of an undetected hearing impairment can have negative consequences for the acquisition and development of speech and language, critical elements of the communication chain. For older adults at the other end of the age continuum, an undetected hearing impairment can impair communication with others and have negative consequences on social and psychological well-being.

For many adults, the development of a hearing loss is often readily apparent to the hearing-impaired individual, and assistance will most likely be sought out. This is often not the case, however, for older adults with mild or moderate amounts of sloping, high-frequency, sensorineural hearing loss. Such individuals often wait as long as 10 to 15 years from their (or their significant other's) first suspicion of hearing problems to their first appointment with an audiologist for a complete hearing evaluation. In a 2011 survey of 2,232 older adults, members of the American Association of Retired Persons (AARP), 47% acknowledged that their hearing was not as good as it could be or that they had hearing difficulty but had not sought out treatment. Although it is unclear exactly why this is the case, it has generally been attributed to the negative stigma associated with the use of hearing aids, including the association of hearing aid use with "old age." The physically invisible inner ear damage accompanying age-related sensorineural hearing loss is suddenly made readily visible to others via the use of a hearing aid or other assistive device. In the 2011 AARP survey, however, the majority (58%) of those with untreated hearing difficulty indicated that they did not perceive their hearing loss to be bad enough to seek treatment. The two next most frequent reasons for postponing treatment cited in the AARP study were related to the cost of hearing aids and were reported by 29% to 33% of the respondents. Thus, although there is evidence that many older adults defer treatment for hearing problems, the exact reasons for this are still being identified. Regardless of the underlying reasons, due to their reluctance to seek assistance, brief, efficient hearing screening procedures have been developed that can be administered to large numbers of older adults in an effort to identify hearing loss among this population. Once identified, solutions for the hearing loss can be explored and any breaks in the communication chain repaired.

It is very common for hearing loss, and the consequent breaks in the communication chain, to go undetected in children. The younger the child, the more likely this will be the case. Obviously, a newborn or young infant has no way to express that he or she is experiencing difficulty with hearing; they have yet to develop a communication system that would enable them to do so. Even older children, however, with developed communication systems may not realize that a hearing problem they are experiencing, especially one unaccompanied by any physical pain or discomfort, is not "normal" or "typical." For children, we rely heavily on observant parents or caregivers to identify those with hearing problems. Such problems, however, are often physically invisible to the caregiver, especially for sensorineural hearing loss.

As noted in Chapter 1, there are typical developmental milestones during the first 4 years of life for speech and language. One way parents or caregivers can identify a possible hearing problem is through observable delays in speech or language development. Table 8.1 provides some guidelines for referral of the child to a professional for a comprehensive assessment, including a hearing evaluation. Note that the referral guidelines point to ages for referral that are considerably greater than the ages for "typical" development discussed in Chapter 1. As discussed in Chapter 1, there are large individual variations in the trajectories for development of speech and language during the first years of life. The referral guidelines are designed to refer children who are considerably delayed relative to "typical" development. If a child meets any of these referral guidelines, the parent or caregiver should seek a comprehensive assessment of speech and language capabilities and the child's hearing. Meeting any one of these referral guidelines in Table 8.1 does not mean, however, that the child has a hearing loss. Hearing loss is just one of the possible causes of a delay in speech and language development. It is important, however, to rule out hearing loss as the causative factor in the initial assessment.

The referral guidelines in Table 8.1 require observant parents or caregivers, including pediatricians, and assume that the parents and caregivers are familiar with these general guidelines. Note also that these guidelines begin at 12 months of age and several pertain to children 2 years of age or older. As noted in Chapter 1, it would be advantageous to identify hearing problems earlier and *before* they begin to have a negative impact on the development of speech and language.

How does one go about detecting the presence of significant hearing loss in newborns or young children? One strategy would be to test the hearing and middle ear function of every newborn and school-age child. Although it has been estimated that there are 4,000 to 5,000 children born each year with significant hearing loss, this represents only 1 to 3 newborns out of every 1,000 live births. Clearly, it would be extremely costly and inefficient to do complete audiological evaluations on every newborn or every school-age child. What is

TABLE

8.1

Referral Guidelines for Children with "Speech" Delay

12 Months

No differentiated babbling or vocal imitation

18 Months

No use of single words

24 Months

Single-word vocabulary <10 words

30 Months

Fewer than 100 words, no evidence of two-word
combinations, unintelligible

36 Months

Fewer than 200 words, no use of telegraphic
sentences, clarity ≤50%

48 Months

Fewer than 600 words, no use of simple sentences,
clarity ≤80%

From Matkin ND. Early recognition and referral of hearing-impaired children. *Pediatr Rev* 1984;6:151–156.

needed instead is a simple, efficient, inexpensive way to screen newborns and young children and identify those who are *likely* to have a significant hearing loss. This represents the basic purpose of hearing screening programs for any age group: identify those individuals *at risk* for hearing loss so that those individuals can have more thorough and comprehensive audiological evaluations to confirm (or refute) the presence of a hearing loss. Again, once such cases have been identified and confirmed through follow-up testing, efforts can be made to repair the break in the communication chain.

Screening is designed to separate persons who are likely to have an auditory disorder from those who are unlikely to have an auditory disorder and to do so in a simple, safe, rapid, and cost-effective manner. Screening programs are intended to be preventive measures that focus on early identification and subsequent intervention. The objective is to minimize the consequences of hearing loss or middle ear disease as early as possible so that the disorder will not produce a disabling condition.

The purpose of this chapter is to present information on screening for hearing loss and middle ear disease. The review will cover the general principles of screening, discuss screening procedures for hearing loss and otitis media used with different age groups, and recommend follow-up protocols for those identified as having an auditory disorder. The focus in this section is on the screening of children from birth through 18 years of age, but screening procedures for adults are discussed at the end of this chapter.

UNDERSTANDING THE PRINCIPLES OF SCREENING

Factors that Determine Whether to Screen

How does one know whether to screen for the presence of a particular disorder? Several criteria are used in establishing the value of screening for a specific disorder. First, a disorder should be important. If left unidentified, the disorder will likely diminish an individual's functional status. It is also essential that the program be capable of reaching those who could benefit. Another important criterion is the prevalence of the disorder or how frequently it occurs within a given population. There should be acceptable criteria for diagnosis. Specific symptoms of a disease must occur with sufficient regularity that it can be determined with assurance which persons have the disorder and which do not. Once detected, the disease should be treatable. Diagnostic and treatment resources must also be available so that adequate medical and educational follow-up can be implemented. Finally, the health system must be able to cope with the program, and the program must be cost-effective. It is generally believed by most, but not all, that hearing loss in people of all ages and middle ear disease in children satisfy many of these criteria and that screening for auditory disorders is justifiable.

What is an Acceptable Screening Test?

A screening test must be selected that will most effectively detect the conditions to be identified. A good screening tool should be acceptable, reliable, valid, safe, and cost-effective. An acceptable test is simple, easy to administer, readily interpretable, and generally well received by the public. A reliable test should be consistent, providing results that do not differ significantly from one test to the next for the same individual. It does little good, for example, to have a screening test that the same healthy individual passes five times and fails five times when the test is administered 10 times in succession. Furthermore, the test should allow examiners to be consistent in the evaluation of a response. Two different examiners testing the same person should obtain the same results.

Validity may best be defined by asking, "Are we measuring what we think we are measuring?" The emphasis in this question is on what is being measured. For example, a clinician who wants to identify middle ear disease has selected a screening test that involves the measurement of hearing by air conduction. Such a test would not be valid because, although it might reliably measure a child's hearing loss, it cannot indicate the presence or absence of otitis media. (Recall from the last chapter that a child with a fluid-filled middle ear from otitis media may not have air-conduction thresholds outside the normal range, even though a significant air-bone gap might exist.) Validity of screening tests consists of two components: **sensitivity** and **specificity**. Sensitivity refers to the ability of a screening test to identify accurately an ear that is abnormal (whether from hearing loss or from otitis media); specificity denotes the ability of a screening tool to identify normal ears. Thus, a valid test is one that identifies a normal condition as normal (high specificity) and an abnormal one as abnormal (high sensitivity).

Finally, a good screening test is one that is safe and cost-effective in relation to the expected benefits. Because the instruments designed to screen for hearing loss and middle ear disease are considered safe and reasonable in cost, the greatest direct expense is usually the salary for personnel. Other factors should be taken into consideration when estimating the expense of a screening program. These include the time required to administer the test, the cost of supplies, the number of individuals to be screened and rescreened, and the cost of training and supervising screeners.

Calculation of the costs of any screening program should also consider indirect costs, such as the cost of the comprehensive audiologic assessment, monitoring, and intervention that would occur as a result of the screening. A special concern is the cost associated with "false-positive" tests, those individuals who fail the screen but who have normal hearing. For children, such costs might include a parent's lost time from work, transportation to health care facilities, administration of unnecessary follow-up tests, and, possibly, unnecessary treatment, as well as the more human cost of the anxiety of parents or caring others, the potential of misunderstanding, and the disturbance of family function. Finally, the possible cost savings resulting from a screening program must be entered into the equation. For example, educational costs might be reduced as a consequence of early identification and subsequent intervention.

PRINCIPLES OF EVALUATING A SCREENING TEST

In this section, we will cover some of the basic principles of how to assess the usefulness of a screening test. Figure 8.1 sets the stage for understanding this process. Our primary goal is to distinguish within the population at large those individuals who exhibit an auditory disorder ($A + C$) from those who do not ($B + D$). Within the group with an auditory disorder, subgroup A represents those

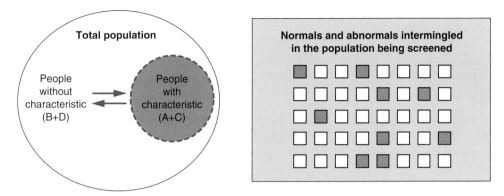

FIGURE 8.1 Illustration of the general notion of screening. On the left, a Venn diagram is used to illustrate that the individuals with a particular disorder represent a subset of the general population and the key is to be able to reliably identify this subset of the population. This is also illustrated on the right where the total set of *squares, blue* and *white*, represent the general population; those with the disorder represented by the *blue squares* and those without the disorder represented by the *white squares*.

people with the disorder who test positive (true positives); subgroup C represents those with the disorder who test negative (false negatives). Within the group without an auditory disorder, subgroup B represents those persons without the disorder who test positive (false positives); subgroup D is comprised of all those persons without the disorder who test negative (true negatives).

Any screening test must be evaluated against an independent standard, often referred to as a "gold standard." The results of the gold standard test are universally accepted as proof that the disease or disorder is either present or absent. In the case of hearing loss, pure-tone audiometry typically serves as the gold standard for any screening tool, whereas for middle ear disease, the gold standard is usually pneumatic otoscopy or electroacoustic immittance.

Figure 8.2 illustrates how the characteristics of a screening test can be evaluated against the gold standard. Toward this end, several terms and definitions need to be understood. First is sensitivity [$100A/(A + C)$]. (The factor 100 is introduced to convert the result to a percentage.) We have already learned that sensitivity refers to the proportion of individuals with the characteristic correctly identified by the test. If 100 subjects have a hearing loss and the test correctly identifies 75 of them, the sensitivity of the test would be 75%. Sensitivity is typically affected by the severity or duration of the characteristic or disease. This is only logical in that the milder an impairment is, the closer it is to a normal condition and the more difficult it is to distinguish from normal. However, the measure is not affected by how prevalent the disease is in the general population. Another important measure is specificity, [$100D/(B + D)$], which refers to the proportion of individuals without the characteristic correctly identified by the test. If, in a group of 100 normal subjects, the test identifies 70 as normal

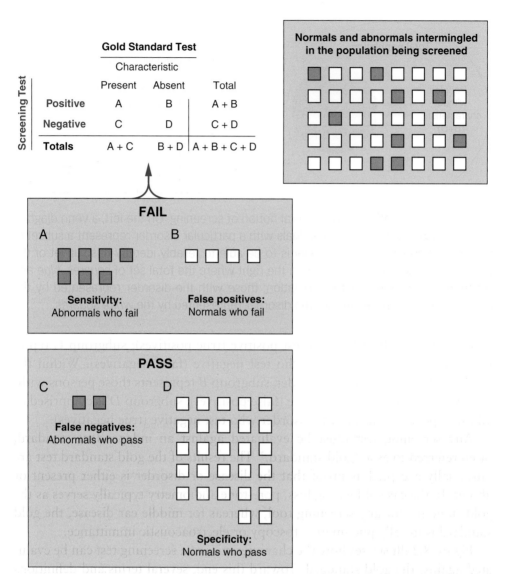

FIGURE 8.2 Schematic illustration of the "sorting" of the general population (*all squares*) into those who have the disorder ("fail") and those who do not ("pass"), according to the screening test used, compared to their true grouping (*blue or white squares*). Ideally, the individuals represented by *blue squares*, those who truly have the disorder, would be the only ones who fail the screening and those represented by the *white squares*, who do not have the disorder, would be the only ones who pass. Errors of both types, passing those who have the disorder (group C) and failing those who don't (group B), are almost always made. The table at the left illustrates the four subgroups, A through D, in tabular format, together with various column and row sums used in the evaluation of a screening test.

and 30 as abnormal, the specificity would be 70%. Like sensitivity, specificity is not affected by the prevalence of the disorder. The best screening tool will be one that provides the highest degree of both sensitivity and specificity.

It is possible to vary the accuracy of a screening test by altering the pass/fail criteria. A cutoff on a hearing screening test, for example, might be 15-dB HL or 40-dB HL. A 15-dB HL cutoff will provide high sensitivity but lower specificity. This is because the 15-dB HL criterion will result in a larger portion of normal or near-normal individuals being classified as hearing impaired. If a 40-dB HL cutoff is used, however, sensitivity will decrease, but specificity will increase. The 40-dB HL cutoff will miss some of the mildly impaired individuals but will avoid misclassifying most of those with normal hearing.

An important concept in any screening program is the prevalence of the disorder that is to be screened. **Prevalence** (derived from the word *prevail*) refers to the proportion of individuals in the population who demonstrate the characteristic $[100(A + C)/(A + B + C + D)]$. An important use of prevalence data is as a pretest indicator of the probability of the disorder being present. To illustrate how the prevalence of a disorder may be important to a screening program, consider the following two extremes. If 99% of the population has the disorder, it is easier to simply assume that everyone has it and treat it accordingly. In this case, we would only be mistreating 1% of the population. If one in a million people have the disorder (prevalence = 0.0001%), then it may be safer and more efficient to assume that no one has it. Failure to screen for such a disorder would miss 0.0001% of the population.

Additional test characteristics of key importance in screening for a disorder are positive predictive value (the probability of an individual having the disorder when the test is positive) and negative predictive value (the probability of not having the disorder when the test is negative). Unlike sensitivity and specificity, predictive values are very dependent on the prevalence of the disorder in the population being tested. For a disorder of very low prevalence, even a highly specific test is likely to have a low positive predictive value. For example, a test that has a sensitivity of 90% and a specificity of 90% in detecting a disorder will have a positive predictive value of 79.4%, and thus a false-positive rate of 20.6%, if the prevalence of the disorder is 30%. However, the positive predictive value decreases to 50% if the prevalence is only 10% and to 8.3% if the prevalence is only 1%.

In most hearing clinic settings, especially when screening for hearing loss, we need tests that yield maximum accuracy. The ideal test would be one that always gave positive results in anyone with a hearing loss and negative results in anyone without a hearing loss. Unfortunately, no such test exists. As a rule, one attempts to maximize the sensitivity and specificity of a screening test. This is done by evaluating different pass/fail criteria and test protocols in comparison to the gold standard. Vignettes 8.1 and 8.2 give examples of how to apply these general principles to actual screening data.

VIGNETTE 8.1 • CONCEPTUAL DEMO

Guidelines for Calculating the Operating Characteristics of a Screening Tool

Let us go through the step-by-step procedures for calculating the characteristics of a screening tool. To assist in this process, some screening data are presented. The gold standard was pure-tone audiometry. In this example, 99 patients were screened and then tested using pure-tone audiometry. Of the 47 patients who failed the screening test, 27 actually had a hearing loss and 20 did not. On the other hand, 52 patients passed the screening. Of these, the gold standard showed that three had a hearing loss and 49 did not. The prevalence of hearing loss in the population screened $[100/(A + C) (A + B + C + D)]$ is 100(30/99) or about 30%.

First, the sensitivity, or the percentage of valid positive test results, is calculated from the data. The formula for computing sensitivity is $100A/(A + C)$. When applied to our data, this gives 100(27/30) = 90%. This is excellent.

Next, compute specificity, or the percentage of valid negative test results, using the formula $100D/(B + D)$. This results in 100(49/69) = 71%. This is adequate but not excellent.

In this example, we see that the screening test appears to be a valid tool for the identification of a hearing loss, offering acceptable sensitivity and specificity values. Now, on your own, calculate the operating characteristics of a screening tool for the example in Vignette 8.2.

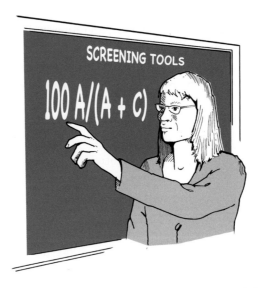

VIGNETTE 8.2 • EXPERIMENT

Computing the Characteristics of a Screening Tool Using Hypothetical Screening Data

Now compute the characteristics of a screening tool for the example. For this example, compute prevalence, sensitivity, and specificity.

Example:

GOLD STANDARD TEST

Hearing Impairment Characteristic

Screening Test		Present	Absent	Total
	Fail	160	20	180
	Pass	40	180	220
	Total	200	200	400

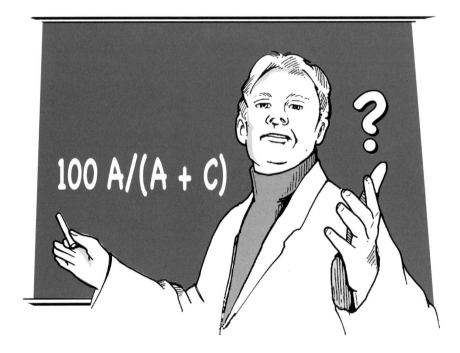

How did you do? You can find the answers in the back of the chapter.

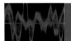

STATUS OF IDENTIFICATION PROGRAMS IN THE UNITED STATES

Screening: A Common Health Care Practice

No single procedure in health care is more popular than that of screening. Tests are performed for a variety of conditions including blood pressure, cholesterol, genetics, diabetes, breast cancer, colorectal cancer, other types of cancer, and, of course, hearing and middle ear status. New screening tests are developed each year, and legislation is always being introduced to mandate a given screening protocol. It is important to recognize that screening tests usually lead to additional procedures, which, in turn, constitute a large part of today's health care practice. It is one of the factors that contribute to the high costs of health care. For example, the billions of dollars expended for just three of the widely recognized screening programs (cervical cancer, prostate cancer, and high blood levels of cholesterol) are sufficient to fund a basic health care system for all of the poor and uninsured. Today's health care system actively encourages us to obtain screenings for a variety of conditions. Vignette 8.3 highlights a typical screening advertisement published in a local newspaper and illustrates how such screening advertisements can sometimes mislead the consumer.

VIGNETTE 8.3 • FURTHER DISCUSSION

Screening: A Popular Procedure in Today's Health Care Environment

Screening is one of the most popular procedures in health care, and health care facilities aggressively promote the need to be screened for a variety of conditions. The accompanying figure illustrates a typical advertisement in a local community newspaper. The advertisement states, "One out of every 11 men will develop prostate cancer, with the risk rising dramatically after the age of 40." The message is clear, the risk is high, and we'd better get screened for this condition right away. Unfortunately, the information presented in this advertisement does not tell the whole story. That is, the digital rectal examination used for screening prostate cancer is not very accurate. Studies illustrate that when we screen asymptomatic males, the examination detects only about 33% of those with cancer; the test misses most cases.

Moreover, the test produces many false positives. Fewer than one-third of the positive tests actually turn out to be cancer, whereas two-thirds or more of the failures are false positives. This means that the test suggests probable cancer in a large group of individuals who are normal. Hence, many individuals who fail the test but do not have cancer will be referred for additional tests, which adds to the costs of the screening program, not to mention the cost of fear, anxiety, confusion, and misunderstanding. Finally, there is no evidence to suggest that the digital rectal screening is worthwhile. No one has shown that individuals who are screened for this problem are any better off than those who are not screened. This lack of evidence has caused some national groups to recommend against screening for prostate cancer. The lesson—just because a screening procedure is popular and we are encouraged to be screened by health care facilities—does not necessarily mean that the screening is beneficial. To determine whether a screening procedure is beneficial, we must first consider the principles of screening discussed earlier in this chapter and apply these principles to the available evidence.

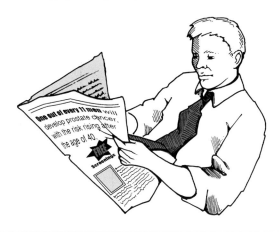

Hearing and Immittance Screening Programs for Children

Identification programs for hearing loss in children have been implemented in the United States for various age groups including the neonate, the infant, the preschooler, and the school-age child. Despite the importance of early identification, most screening has occurred at the school-age level. It has only been within the past decade that newborn hearing screening has become widespread; in fact, because of the undaunted efforts of Marion Downs (see Vignette 8.4) and others, as of February 2012, 36 states and 4 US territories legally mandate universal newborn screening and all 50 states and US territories have implemented Early Hearing Detection and Intervention (EHDI) programs to identify and treat hearing loss in young children.

Interestingly, although hearing screening is endorsed by the American Academy of Pediatrics, many practicing pediatricians do not recognize the importance of screening very young infants for hearing loss. It has been estimated, for example, that only 3% of children from 6 months to 11 years of age receive a screening test at their primary health care source. Although it is true that more reliable responses can be obtained from infants and young children than from neonates, there is the

VIGNETTE 8.4 • HISTORICAL NOTE

Marion P. Downs (1914–): Advocate for Early Identification of Hearing Loss in Infants

Throughout her professional career, Marion Downs championed the early identification of hearing loss in very young infants. Having recognized the value of early auditory stimulation, while teaching at the University of Denver in the early 1950s, she introduced the concept of early identification. After entering the faculty of the University of Colorado Medical School in 1959, she was able to implement the concept by developing a comprehensive early identification program for all newborns in the Denver area and screened more than 10,000 babies using the arousal test, which was later judged to be impractical. Consequently, Downs proposed to the ASHA the formation of the national JCIH and chaired the committee in its first few years. The committee continues to be instrumental in promoting the concept of universal newborn hearing screening.

Downs served as an advocate for early identification and habilitation throughout the world as a consultant to foreign governments and by presenting workshops and lectures in some 18 countries. In 1997, Downs was honored by having a national center on hearing and infants named after her. The center promotes her lifelong dream of achieving early intervention for newborns not only in Colorado but throughout the country. Now over 90, Downs continues to advance her long ideal of newborn hearing screening and early intervention.

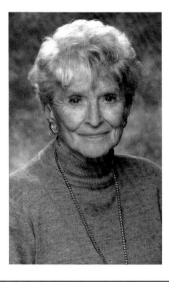

problem of locating all of the older groups of youngsters for the hearing test. Once newborns leave the hospital, it is not until age 5 years, at the kindergarten level, that these children are available for testing at one common location. Those few screening programs that do exist are conducted in daycare centers, well-baby clinics, and Head Start programs. These programs, however, attract only a specific segment of children, primarily those from lower socioeconomic levels. Even if a massive national effort were made to screen all preschoolers at these various centers, a large percentage of children would still be missed. Yet screening the preschool child has some advantages over the screening of newborns. First, children become easier to test as age increases and yield more reliable and valid results. Second, children with a progressive hearing loss and those whose hearing loss was not detected at the newborn screening stand a good chance of being identified.

Under our present system, children whose hearing loss was not detected at the newborn identification program or who moved into a community at preschool age are not identified until screening occurs in kindergarten. There is a critical need for a national effort directed at infant and preschool hearing screening programs in every state.

Hearing screening programs using pure-tone audiometry are most often conducted in the school system because it affords easy access to the children. However, the availability, accessibility, comprehensiveness, and quality of school screening programs vary significantly from one state to the next. A major problem and source of frustration for audiologists involved in school screening programs is the lack of appropriate follow-up services offered to children who fail the screen.

The incorporation of immittance screening programs is not as universal. It is estimated that about one-half of the states incorporate immittance (tympanometry) as part of their screening procedures. Some of the problems associated with mass immittance screening are discussed later in this chapter.

Figure 8.3 shows the percentage of school programs that conducted pure-tone and immittance screening in 1999. The trends apparent in these data are still believed to provide an accurate reflection of screening practices in the schools today. It is seen that the emphasis for pure-tone and immittance screening in the schools is at the elementary level and that few programs conduct screening in the secondary grades. Moreover, a much larger percentage of school programs use pure-tone screening than immittance screening.

Screening the Neonate

The advantages of detecting sensorineural hearing loss as early as possible in young children are important enough to encourage the implementation of newborn screening programs. It has now been demonstrated that children who receive intervention from the age of 3 years or younger show significantly better

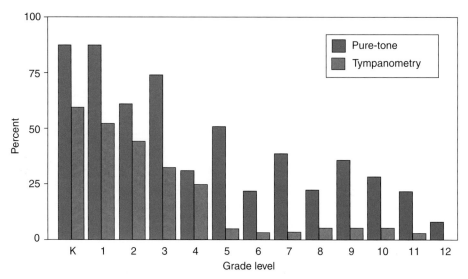

FIGURE 8.3 Percent of school-age children receiving either air-conduction pure-tone hearing screening or tympanometric screening as a function of grade level. (Sources: Roush J. Screening school-age children. In: Bess FH, Hall JW, eds. *Screening Children for Auditory Function*. Nashville, TN: Bill Wilkerson Center Press; 1992; Pure-tone data from Penn T. A summary: School-based hearing screening in the United States. *Audiol Today* 1999;11:20–21.)

speech and language outcomes later in life. Early identification and intervention (the word *intervene* means "to come in and modify") also result in substantial cost savings. For example, a deaf infant who receives educational and audiologic management during the first years of life has a better than 50% chance of becoming "mainstreamed" into a regular classroom.

Historically, the screening procedures advocated for the newborn nursery have been controversial. Audiologists have not agreed on the most effective and appropriate techniques. The national Joint Committee on Infant Hearing (JCIH, a committee of representatives from the American Academy of Otolaryngology, the American Academy of Pediatrics, the American Academy of Audiology, the American Speech-Language-Hearing Association (ASHA), the Council on Education of the Deaf, and the Directors of Speech and Hearing Programs in State and Welfare Agencies) endorsed universal newborn screening. In the 2007 JCIH Position Statement, the committee stated that the goal of EHDI programs was "…to maximize linguistic and communicative competence and literacy development for children who are deaf or hard of hearing." The 2007 Position Statement, an update of an earlier 2000 statement, established the following goals for EHDI programs: (a) all infants should have their hearing screened with a physiologic measure, such as auditory brainstem response (ABR) or evoked otoacoustic emissions (OAEs), before 1 month of age; (b) all infants who fail such a hearing screening, and rescreening, should have follow-up audiologic and medical evaluations to confirm the presence of hearing loss before 3 months of age; and (c) all infants with confirmed permanent hearing loss (e.g., not conductive loss due to acute otitis media) should receive intervention services by 6 months of age. These goals are often referred to as the 1-3-6 goals: identify by 1 month, confirm by 3 months, and intervene by 6 months of age.

Despite the past controversies and challenges, universal newborn hearing screening in the United States today is considered a great success. The number of newborns screened in the United States has grown steadily over the past decade—in the year 2000, approximately 40% of newborns were screened for hearing loss; in 2010, 98% of newborns were screened. Moreover, the success of screening programs in the United States has led to an impressive reduction in the age at which children with hearing loss are identified, from an average age of 24 to 30 months to 2 to 4 months of age. One of the greatest challenges that remain for newborn screening programs is the large numbers of infants who fail the newborn screen but are then lost to follow-up. According to the CDC (CDC, 2010), of those infants referred for follow-up after a newborn screening, more than 30% failed to receive a follow-up audiologic evaluation. The problem of lost to follow-up is an issue associated with other screening programs—not just newborn hearing screening (see Vignette 8.5 for more details).

If universal hearing screening was not available, which the above-mentioned committee acknowledged was unlikely today (see Vignette 8.5), the committee

VIGNETTE 8.5 • FURTHER DISCUSSION

A Review of the Data on the Performance of Early Hearing Detection and Intervention (EHDI) Programs in the United States for 2009

In January of 2012, the Center for Disease Control and Prevention (CDC) of the US government published the most recent national statistics on the performance of EHDI programs in the United States. Data were available from slightly more than 4 million births in the United States in 2009. Of these 4 million births, 97.4% received a hearing screening in 2009. This represents excellent compliance with the JCIH goal for screening of hearing before 1 month of age. The performance with regard to the other two targets of the "1-3-6" objective of the JCIH guidelines, however, was unacceptably poor.

For those not passing the screening ($N = 62,501$), 45.1% either were not followed up or were followed up, but there was no documentation to support follow-up. Of those who were followed up, 8.9% had a confirmed hearing loss at follow-up, and, in about 2/3 of the cases, the follow-up evaluation had been completed by the targeted age of 3 months. Thus, there is considerable improvement needed in the follow-up to the newborn screening programs. Too many screening failures are not being followed up at all, and, of those who are, too many are not being followed up in a timely fashion (by 3 months of age).

Finally, with regard to the final recommended step of the EHDI program, intervention by 6 months of age, for 24.5% of those who had a hearing loss confirmed by follow-up evaluation, either no intervention services had been provided or there was no documentation of such services having been provided. Of those 75.5% with confirmed hearing loss who did receive intervention services, two-thirds received the services by the targeted age of 6 months. Again, these data suggest considerable room for improvement with regard to the final intervention stage of the EHDI program.

In summary, these data from 2009 indicate that there has been tremendous progress in a fairly short period of time in the screening of newborn hearing. However, this initial step in the "1-3-6" EHDI program is just that, an initial step. Ultimately, it is of little value without the follow-up confirmation of hearing loss, which is extremely important because these data indicate that only 8.9% subsequently had confirmed hearing loss, as well as early intervention for those who have confirmed hearing loss. Hopefully, with further refinement, the EHDI program in the United States will become more successful in complying with the recommended "1-3-6" benchmarks.

recommended, at a minimum, screening infants who were considered at high risk for hearing loss. Table 8.2 lists the Joint Committee's neonatal intensive care criteria (risk indicators) for both newborns and infants. Infants who previously passed a newborn screen, but possess risk factors for hearing loss or speech-language delay, should receive periodic audiologic monitoring, medical surveillance, and ongoing observation of communication development, especially if the risk indicators are associated with progressive forms of hearing impairment. Unfortunately, studies have demonstrated that, although the use of such a high-risk register can identify some infants with hearing loss, many children with hearing impairment do not manifest any of the risk factors listed in the register.

Auditory Brainstem Response

The ABR (see Chapter 3 and, for more details, see the online supplement for Chapter 7) has been suggested as a reliable indicator of hearing sensitivity in infancy. The advantages of the ABR for newborn screening include (a) the use of less intense, near-threshold stimuli, making it possible to detect milder forms of hearing impairment; (b) the ability to detect both unilateral and bilateral hearing losses; and (c) the use of a physiologic measurement that depends entirely on a

TABLE

8.2

JCIH 2007 Risk Indicators Associated with Permanent Congenital, Delayed-Onset, or Progressive Hearing Loss in Childhood

1. Caregiver concern[a] regarding hearing, speech, language, or developmental delay
2. Family history[a] of permanent childhood hearing loss
3. Neonatal intensive care of >5 days or any of the following regardless of length of stay: extracorporeal membrane oxygenation (ECMO)[a] assisted ventilation, exposure to ototoxic medications (gentamicin and tobramycin) or loop diuretics (furosemide/lasix), and hyperbilirubinemia requiring exchange transfusion
4. In utero infections, such as CMV,[a] herpes, rubella, syphilis, and toxoplasmosis
5. Craniofacial anomalies, including those involving the pinna, ear canal, ear tags, ear pits, and temporal bone anomalies
6. Physical findings, such as white forelock, associated with a syndrome known to include a sensorineural or permanent conductive hearing loss
7. Syndromes associated with hearing loss or progressive or late-onset hearing loss,[a] such as neurofibromatosis, osteopetrosis, and Usher syndrome. Other frequently identified syndromes include Waardenburg, Alport, Pendred, and Jervell and Lange-Nielsen
8. Neurodegenerative disorders,[a] such as Hunter syndrome, or sensory motor neuropathies, such as Friedreich ataxia and Charcot-Marie-Tooth syndrome
9. Culture-positive postnatal infections associated with sensorineural hearing loss,[a] including confirmed bacterial and viral (especially herpes viruses and varicella) meningitis
10. Head trauma, especially basal skull/temporal bone fracture[a] requiring hospitalization
11. Chemotherapy[a]

[a]Risk indicators that are marked with an asterisk are of greater concern for delayed-onset hearing loss.

sensory response. Limitations to the technique include the cost and sophisticated nature of the instrumentation, the use of an acoustic click that makes the ABR primarily sensitive to only high-frequency hearing loss, and the fact that the ABR is not a conscious response at the level of the cortex (presence of an ABR does not mean the individual can hear). Nevertheless, the measure is thought to provide a good estimate of hearing status when used carefully, especially when one considers the limitations of the alternative procedures. A child who fails an ABR screening in the intensive care nursery must be retested later under more favorable conditions.

Several ABR-based screening systems with automated response collection and evaluation have been designed for use with neonates. These devices are portable, automatic, and microprocessor based. Their primary function is to screen for handicapping hearing loss in newborn infants. These simplified and cost-effective systems use various automated algorithms to determine whether an infant passes or fails. These devices are generally preferred for screening because they do not require test interpretation, they reduce the possible influence of tester bias, and they insure test consistency.

Otoacoustic Emissions

As noted in Chapter 3 (and in an online supplement for Chapter 7), OAEs have been used as a screening tool to identify hearing loss in neonates. Although there is some disagreement as to the details of such a screening protocol, including which type of OAE to use and the appropriate stimulus parameters to optimize screening efficiency, the scientific and clinical communities have recommended that OAEs become an integral part of a universal neonatal hearing screening program for the United States. It has generally been recommended that either OAEs or ABR be used for the initial screening, with all screening failures retested with the alternative measure. Many of the advantages and disadvantages described for the use of ABR as a screening tool also apply to the use of OAEs as a screening measure. One limitation to OAE measurement is that the test will not identify individuals with neural complications.

Screening the Infant and Preschool-Age Child

Identification Tests and Procedures

Selection of screening techniques will depend on the age, maturity, and cooperation of the child. Generally speaking, a test using sound localization in the sound field will be required for those children between the ages of 4 months and 2 years. Conventional audiometric screening using earphones can usually be used with children 3 years of age or older. Children between the ages of 2 and 3 years make up the most difficult group for which to select an appropriate test. Some of these children can be conditioned for traditional screening techniques with earphones, whereas others will require the test based on sound localization.

Infant and Pre–Nursery Child (4 Months to 3 Years)

Certainly, OAEs or ABR may be used to screen this population for hearing loss. Too often, however, these devices are not available in settings where infants and preschool-age children are typically screened.

The use of calibrated acoustic stimuli (e.g., narrow-band noise) is often suggested for eliciting a localization (head-turn) response in a sound field setting. The child is placed on the parent's lap, and the acoustic stimulus is presented about 2 feet from either ear. If the child fails to localize the signal, a rescreening is recommended. A second failure results in a third test 1 week later. If the child again fails the test, a complete diagnostic examination is conducted. Unfortunately, this technique does not offer ear-specific information, and a child with unilateral hearing loss will probably be missed.

Sometimes, delays in speech-language development are the most sensitive and valid indicators of hearing impairment among preschool children. It has been suggested that primary care physicians and other allied health personnel screen young children for hearing loss simply by asking the parent three basic questions: (a) How many different words do you estimate your child uses? Is it 100 words, 500 words, or what? (b) What is the length of a typical sentence that your child uses? Is it single words, two words, full sentences, or what? (c) How clear is your child's speech to a friend or neighbor? Would they understand 10%, 50%, 90%, or what? These questions are framed around the referral guidelines shown previously in Table 8.1.

#21

Preschooler (3 to 6 Years)

When the child reaches 3 years of age, the more traditional hearing test with earphones can be used for screening. By means of a portable pure-tone audiometer, signals may be presented at various frequencies at a fixed intensity level. The child merely indicates to the examiner, usually by raising a hand, if a tone was perceived. The ASHA and the AAA have both recommended that 1,000, 2,000, and 4,000 Hz be used as test frequencies. If immittance testing is not part of the program, the ASHA guidelines recommend that the frequency 500 Hz should also be tested (assuming that background noise levels in the test area are acceptable). The AAA guidelines indicate that tympanometry should be used in conjunction with pure-tone screening for children in this age range. The ASHA and AAA guidelines further recommend a screening level of 20-dB HL for all frequencies tested. A lack of response at any frequency in either ear, following two to four presentations per stimulus, constitutes a test failure. Children who fail should be rescreened, preferably within the same test session, but no later than 1 week after the original test. The practice of rescreening can significantly reduce the overall number of test failures. The value of rescreening is illustrated in Figure 8.4, which shows that the total number of failures has been significantly reduced via rescreening. Children who also fail the rescreening should be referred for a complete audiologic evaluation.

Procedural Considerations for Preschool-Age Children   In developing a screening program at the preschool level, special attention should be directed toward the groundwork and orientation process that occurs before the screening. The success of any screening program depends, to a large extent, on the cooperation of the teachers, the children, and the parents. All three of these parties must be familiarized with the screening process that is to take place.

First, a letter should go to the teacher outlining the need for and the purpose of the screening program. The letter should also review the teacher's responsibilities in preparing the children for the screening. Prescreening instructional activities can be used by the teacher to orient the children to the listening task. Such activities performed before the identification program can help avoid

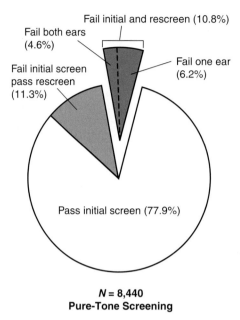

FIGURE 8.4 Illustration of the value of rescreening. Note that the number of children failing the screening has decreased considerably following immediate rescreening. (Data from Wilson WR, Walton WK. Public school audiometry. In: Martin FN, ed. *Pediatric Audiology*. Englewood Cliffs, NJ: Prentice-Hall; 1978.)

wasted time during the actual screening. It is also most helpful to provide the teacher with a list of the screening responsibilities of those individuals who will be conducting the screening, as well as of those who will be receiving the screening. This list will serve as an excellent guide and provide the teacher and/or administrator with a better understanding of the entire screening process from start to finish. Finally, a letter to the parents of each child should be included in the packet of materials, as well as a parental consent form. The letter should explain the screening program so that the parents will understand the value of screening and support the screening process.

The person who will be responsible for conducting the screening program should visit the facility and meet with the teacher(s) and administrator(s). Together they should review carefully the sequence of the screening program and discuss any concerns they might have. This is also an excellent opportunity to review with the program officials the sites available for the screening. Needless to say, a quiet room is essential. Other considerations in selecting a testing site have been identified by others. The site should (a) have appropriate electrical outlets (only grounded three-prong outlets should be used) and lighting; (b) be located away from railroad tracks, playgrounds, heavy traffic, public toilets, or cafeterias; (c) be relatively free of visual distractions; (d) have carpet and curtains to help reduce the room noise; (e) have nearby bathroom facilities to accommodate the needs of the children and screeners; and (f) have chairs and tables appropriate for small children.

Some other suggestions and hints for screening preschool children include the following. One person should be individually responsible for ensuring that the children move through the screening process smoothly and that all children receive the test. Arrangements should be made for the children to have name tags showing their legal names and nicknames. All forms should be accurately completed before the screening date. Each child should have his or her own individual preschool record form. When screening children between the ages of 3 and 6 years, it is wise to alternate age groups during the screening day, for example, 3-year-olds should be followed by 5-year-olds. Three-year-olds are much harder to test and take more time. Another factor to keep in mind is that the younger children tire more easily than older children and need to be screened earlier in the day.

Screening the School-Age Child

The practice of screening school-age children is over 50 years old, and all states conduct some form of hearing screening in the schools. The Joint Committee on Health Problems in Education (consisting of members of the National Education Association and the American Medical Association) has described the following primary responsibilities to be met by a hearing-screening program: an awareness of the importance of early recognition of suspected hearing loss, especially in the primary grades; intelligent observation of pupils for signs of hearing difficulty; organization and conduction of an audiometric screening survey; and a counseling and follow-up program to help children with hearing difficulties obtain diagnostic examinations, needed treatment, and such adaptations of their school program as their hearing condition dictates.

Who is Responsible for the Audiometric Screening Program?

Health and education departments are the agents primarily responsible for coordinating audiometric screening programs. Ideally, the state department of education should coordinate the periodic screening of all school children as well as provide for the necessary educational, audiologic, and rehabilitative follow-up. The state department of health, on the other hand, should coordinate the activities of identification audiometry, threshold measurement, and medical follow-up for students who fail the screening tests.

Personnel

The personnel designated to conduct the screening tests have been nurses, audiologists, speech-language pathologists, graduate students in speech and hearing, and even volunteers and secretaries. To assure quality programs, only professionals trained in audiology should be used to coordinate and supervise hearing screening programs. Volunteers and lay groups can best be used for support, such as in the promotion of screening programs. Certified audiologists or speech-language pathologists should oversee screening programs and use trained assistants or technicians to perform the screening. Public health nurses may serve as organizers and supervisors but can be of most value in the follow-up phase of the program. A nurse's responsibilities might include (a) counseling parents and children about the child's needs for medical diagnosis and treatment, (b) using all available facilities for diagnosis and treatment, and (c) coordinating information about the child and family with specialists in the health and education field.

Who Should Be Screened?

It is not economically feasible to mass screen all children in the schools. A target population must be identified. Most programs have concentrated their annual screening efforts on children of nursery school age through grade 3. In fact, all of these grades are recommended for screening by the ASHA guidelines, and the AAA guidelines recommend preschool, kindergarten, first grade, and third grade. After grade 3, children may be screened at 3- to 4-year intervals, according to the ASHA guidelines, whereas the AAA makes explicit recommendations for screening grade 5 and either grade 7 or 9. By concentrating the screening efforts on the first 3 or 4 years of school, it is still possible to carefully observe other special groups of school children. Several groups of children require more attention than is provided by routine screening. Included among these groups are children with preexisting hearing loss, multiple handicaps, frequent colds or ear infections, delayed language, or defective speech. In addition, children returning to school after a serious illness, enrolled in special education programs, who experience school failure or who exhibit a sudden change in academic performance, who are referred by the classroom teacher, or who are new to the school also require more attention to their hearing than provided by routinely scheduled screenings. The 2011 AAA hearing screening guidelines also make provision for the use of OAEs for the screening of "...preschool and school age children for whom pure-tone screening is not developmentally appropriate (ability levels <3 years)."

Equipment, Calibration, and the Test Environment

An important component of any identification program is the audiometric equipment used in the screening. The equipment needed for individual pure-tone screening should be simple, sturdy, and portable. Most screening audiometers are portable and weigh as little as 2 or 3 pounds. The performance characteristics of these instruments must remain stable over time. An audiometer that does not perform adequately could result in a higher-than-normal false-positive or false-negative rate. Care should be taken to ensure that all of the equipment used in screening satisfies the national performance standards. Unfortunately, this is not always done. Audiometers used in the schools often fail to meet calibration standards. School audiometers should receive weekly intensity checks with a sound level meter, as well as daily listening performance checks. All aspects of the audiometer should be thoroughly calibrated each year. It is also suggested that spare audiometers be available in case a malfunction occurs during a screening identification program.

Older audiometers will be most subject to instability and malfunction and should receive careful surveillance. Clinical audiologists who use these instruments for threshold measurement (after a screen failure) should know that the masking stimuli generated by many of these portable audiometers are often inadequate.

Once again, screening must be conducted in a quiet environment to ensure accurate measurements. Although some modern schools have sound-treated rooms or mobile units with testing facilities, most do not. Screening programs must be conducted in a relatively quiet room designed for some other purpose. Some helpful guidelines for selecting an appropriate room for screening have been outlined in the section on preschool screening.

Screening Procedures

The ASHA guidelines for pure-tone air-conduction hearing screening are the most widely used in the schools. The more recent AAA guidelines are very similar to the ASHA guidelines, and noteworthy differences between the two will be pointed out (as they have in the preceding paragraphs as well). Both procedures recognized that sound-treated environments were not readily available in the schools and focus only on middle and higher frequencies. In particular, screening is conducted at 20-dB HL at 1,000, 2,000, and 4,000 Hz in each ear. Failure to detect any one of these pure tones, following two to four immediate presentations of the stimuli, results in the failure of the screening. It is recommended that all failures be rescreened at a later date prior to referral for a complete audiological evaluation.

Why do these specific values for hearing level (20-dB HL) and these three frequencies (1,000, 2,000, and 4,000 Hz) form the basis of screening guidelines for school-age children by ASHA and AAA? As described in Chapter 7, for example, the normal limits for hearing threshold are generally considered to be 0 to 25-dB HL at each frequency. Why not screen at 25-dB HL? Briefly, because of the potential negative impact of even very mild hearing loss on the educational development of children, the maximum amount of hearing loss tolerable in school-age children is considered to be 20-dB HL instead of 25-dB HL.

What about other test frequencies? Aren't we concerned about hearing loss at frequencies of 250 or 500 Hz in addition to that from 1,000 through

4,000 Hz? Yes, we are concerned about hearing loss at all of these frequencies. However, because most test environments in which the screening is conducted have high noise levels at the lower frequencies, it is often not possible to get valid results for pure-tone screening at these lower frequencies. Inclusion of these lower frequencies would result in many more children failing the screening and requiring follow-up testing, but not necessarily due to the presence of hearing loss. Rather, they may fail simply because the background noise at the time of testing was too great at the lower frequencies and made it impossible to hear sounds softer than 20-dB HL, even while wearing earphones. The severity of hearing loss at 1,000 Hz is related in most cases to the severity of hearing loss at 500 Hz. In that sense, inclusion of 1,000 Hz in the screening protocol provides indirect information about the child's hearing status at 500 Hz.

Finally, it cannot be overemphasized that screening is designed to identify those "at risk" for hearing loss, not to confirm the presence of hearing loss. Thus, failure of the hearing screening does not mean that the person has a hearing loss. It simply means that the child "probably" has a hearing loss. Only through a complete follow-up audiological evaluation can the presence of hearing loss be confirmed.

IDENTIFICATION OF MIDDLE EAR DISEASE IN CHILDREN

Electroacoustic Immittance

There is considerable interest in using electroacoustic immittance measures to identify middle ear disease among children. Several factors have contributed to the interest in using immittance as a screening tool. Some factors relate to immittance in particular, and others relate to screening for middle ear disease in general. These factors include the ease and rapidity with which immittance measurement can obtain accurate information, the relative ineffectiveness of pure-tone audiometry in detecting a middle ear disorder, the high prevalence of otitis media, and the growing awareness of the medical, psychological, and educational consequences that may result from middle ear disease. Today this popular technique is used routinely, not only in audiology centers but also in public health facilities, pediatricians' and otologists' offices, and schools. The AAA screening guidelines recommend the use of tympanometry as a second-stage screening following failure of either the pure-tone or OAE screen in the first stage for children 3 years of age and older and as a "targeted" or desired screening procedure for all children between the ages of 3 to 6 years.

A problem with immittance screening has been the difficulty of developing appropriate pass/fail criteria. The pass/fail criteria developed have often resulted in unacceptably high referral rates (32% to 36%). The screening criteria known as the Hirtshal program seem to produce a better result. The program uses only tympanometry and does not include the acoustic reflex. At the first screen, all children with normal tympanograms are cleared. The remaining children receive a second screen in 4 to 6 weeks, and all cases with flat tympanograms are referred. Those children still remaining receive a third screen 4 to 6 weeks later. Children with normal tympanograms or tympanograms having peaks greater than (more positive) 200 daPa are cleared. Children with flat tympanograms (and equivalent ear canal volume outside the normal range) or tympanograms with peaks less than or equal to –200 daPa at the third screen are referred. With the Hirtshal screening approach, sensitivity and specificity values are 80% and 95%, respectively. Moreover, the program yields an acceptable referral rate of only 9%.

The ASHA developed a new guideline for screening children that involves the use of case history, visual inspection of the ear canal and eardrum, and tympanometry with a low-frequency (220 or 226 Hz) probe tone. The ASHA recommended that children be screened as needed or if an at-risk condition existed. Children 7 months of age to 6 years should be screened if they present with any of the following conditions: (a) first episode of acute otitis media before 6 months of age; (b) were bottle-fed; (c) have craniofacial anomalies, stigmata, or other syndromic conditions; (d) are members of ethnic populations known to have a higher prevalence of middle ear disease (Native Americans and Eskimo populations); (e) have a family history of middle ear disease with effusion; (f) reside in daycare or in crowded conditions; (g) have been exposed frequently to cigarette smoke; or (h) have been diagnosed with sensorineural hearing loss, learning disabilities, or other developmental complications.

Typically, the first scheduled screening program should occur in the fall in conjunction with screening for hearing loss. A second scheduled screening is recommended for those who failed or were missed in the fall.

For case history, the protocol simply considers recent evidence of otalgia (earache) or otorrhea (discharge from the ear). Visual inspection via otoscopy is performed to identify gross abnormalities; the use of a lighted otoscope or video otoscope is recommended. A child is referred for medical observation and/or audiologic evaluation if (a) ear drainage is observed, (b) structural defects or ear canal abnormalities are seen in the ear, (c) tympanometry reveals a flat tympanogram and equivalent ear canal volume outside normal range, and (d) tympanometric rescreen results are outside test criteria. It should be noted that data pertaining to the performance of this protocol are limited.

Handheld Tympanometers

Small portable handheld immittance screening tympanometers are also sometimes used in screening programs. These handheld otoscope-like units typically run on rechargeable batteries and incorporate a small printer to record a hard copy of the data. The tip of the tympanometer is placed into the ear, and when a pneumatic seal is obtained, a microcomputer initiates the miniature pump that varies pressure to the ear canal from +200 daPa to –300 daPa with a 226-Hz probe tone at 85-dB SPL. These handheld screening instruments record data recommended by screening guidelines.

FOLLOW-UP PROGRAMS FOR CHILDREN

Screening is of little value if follow-up is not provided for the appropriate management of children who fail the screen. This aspect of the program takes as much planning and effort as any other phase of the screening program. Noncompliance has been one of the principal problems of existing hearing screening programs for newborns. In some studies, 25% to 80% of infants who failed newborn screening have been lost to follow-up despite aggressive recruiting efforts and the offering of cost-saving incentives to parents. In other studies, after early identification of hearing loss, lag times of 8 to 9 months have transpired before infants returned for intervention services. Vignette 8.5 provides the most recent data available (from 2009) regarding the performance of neonatal screening programs and the follow-up intervention. Presently, there are no data on compliance in hearing screening programs for infants beyond the newborn period.

For preschool- and school-age programs, the screening coordinator will be responsible for the follow-up under most circumstances. A child who fails the rescreen should receive a comprehensive audiologic test at the screening site as soon as possible. Within a few days after the screening, those steps essential to appropriate follow-up should begin. Letters should be sent to parents indicating whether their child passed or failed the screening test. For those children who failed the screening, the letter should also recommend that the child be referred for medical evaluation. Approximately 6 weeks after the screening, the parents should be asked whether the recommendations were followed.

Frequently, the public health nurse handles this phase of the follow-up program. In some states, audiologists, speech-language pathologists, and educators coordinate this activity. After the medical examination, the child is referred to an audiologic facility for comprehensive testing and counseling. Parent counseling is an important aspect of the follow-up process and too often is overlooked by the supervisors of screening programs. Parents must receive special assistance and guidance to understand and cope with the prospect of having a hearing-impaired child. They must receive help before they can help their child.

Finally, the child will need to be referred to educational services that will be used for planning and placement. The follow-up is a lengthy and ongoing process requiring close coordination among all persons involved.

HEARING SCREENING PROGRAMS FOR ADULTS

There are almost no formalized hearing screening programs in the United States for adult populations. In this regard, the United States lags behind many European nations. The Netherlands, for example, pioneered the development of a valid and reliable screening protocol that was based on the hearing of digit triplets (e.g., "8 5 9") in noise for stimuli delivered either over the telephone or via the Internet. Today, it is available in several languages as a national hearing screening test for adults in several European countries (http://hearcom.eu/prof/DiagnosingHearingLoss/SelfScreenTests/ThreeDigitTest_en.html), but no comparable "national hearing screening test" has been developed for the United States. Screenings do occur, however, in the armed forces, and most communities conduct health fairs where individuals can have their hearing tested. Adult hearing screening programs are also known to take place at community health centers, retirement communities, and nursing homes. Interestingly, evidence suggests that the primary care physician typically does not screen for hearing even if the patient complains of a hearing loss. There is a critical need for audiologists to educate both consumers and health care professionals about the importance of hearing health care, including early identification and intervention.

Audiologists and other health professionals have failed to sensitize both the lay public and the educational and medical communities to the effects of auditory impairment on total development and quality of life. The importance of early detection of hearing loss and the effectiveness of the screening methods available are two concepts that have not been presented well to the educational or medical community. Until we begin to educate these other professional groups, we cannot hope to improve our present identification programs.

With the increased awareness of hearing loss in the elderly population, we have witnessed an increased interest in the hearing screening of adult populations. Unfortunately, in primary care medical practices wherein most older adults are seen regularly, we find that they are seldom screened and referred for audiologic evaluation. There seem to be several reasons for this.

First, the elderly accept their hearing loss as part of getting older and believe that there is simply no recourse for improvement. Second, it is found that primary care physicians often fail to recognize a hearing loss. Even when hearing loss is suspected or is reported to the physician, more than half of the patients are not referred for follow-up audiologic services.

It seems that the primary care physician looks upon hearing loss in the elderly in the same way that our society at large does. Deafness is viewed as a common by-product of aging, and little value is seen in rehabilitating the individuals affected by it. Those physicians who do screen for hearing loss rely on such techniques as the case history, or whisper or watch-tick tests, approaches whose validity or reliability has not been tested. Studies have shown, however, that primary care practitioners will, indeed, screen for hearing loss if provided with appropriately validated screening tools and if they are convinced that hearing loss is important to the life quality of their patient. Again, just as with preschoolers, the task confronting the audiologist is one of educating and informing the public and the health care community.

Pure-Tone Screening

There is no accepted standard or guideline for the identification of hearing loss in the adult population. Some clinicians have suggested that a pure-tone screening level of 20- or 25-dB HL be used for frequencies of 1,000 and 2,000 Hz and that 40-dB HL be used for 4,000 Hz. ASHA recommends that a 25-dB HL level should also be used for all frequencies including 4,000 Hz. Unfortunately, there are limited data to support the validity of a 20- or 25-dB HL criterion at any frequencies for screening adults. We do not know with certainty the sensitivity, specificity, and test accuracy of pure-tone screening when using 20- or 25-dB HL as the cutoff point. Some have suggested that hearing screening in the aged should be done at the test frequencies 1,000 and 2,000 Hz, with a level of 40-dB HL serving as the pass/fail criterion. Failure for two test conditions (one frequency in each ear or both frequencies in one ear) constitutes a test failure. Data using this guideline are presented later in this section. Regardless of the test protocol, it is advisable to rescreen test failures. The recommendations related to environment, calibration, personnel, and procedural setup that were discussed above regarding the screening of children can be followed with some modifications for screening the adult population.

Alternatives to the conventional pure-tone screening, such as the digit-triplet test in noise noted previously, have also been explored in recent years. These tests are designed to gain access to the millions of older adults who feel that they may be having difficulty hearing but are reluctant to seek treatment at a clinic or other facility. Instead, they can receive a reliable and valid screen of their hearing for no or minimal cost and do so at their convenience and in the comfort of their home. Unfortunately, to date, the results are mixed regarding follow-up for those who fail the screen with many screen failures not seeking treatment. Research on these alternative approaches to screening continues, however, with a key emphasis on the ultimate impact of such mass screening services on the improvement of hearing health care for adults.

Follow-Up Programs for Adult Populations

If a person fails the screening protocol, he or she should receive an otologic examination and a comprehensive audiologic evaluation. Needless to say, the hearing evaluation will provide information about the extent and nature of the hearing loss, as well as determine whether the patient could benefit from amplification. If amplification is warranted, the individual should be referred for hearing aid selection and evaluation.

Several tools have been advocated for screening the older adult population. One of these is the Welch-Allyn AudioScope, a handheld otoscope with a built-in audiometer that delivers a tone at 20-, 25-, or 40-dB HL for 500, 1,000, 2,000, and 4,000 Hz (Fig. 8.5). To use the AudioScope, the clinician selects the largest ear speculum needed to achieve a seal within the ear canal. A tonal sequence is then initiated, with the subject indicating the tone was heard by raising a finger. The AudioScope is found to perform very well against the gold standard of pure-tone audiometry when using the 40-dB HL signal at 1,000 and 2,000 Hz. The sensitivity of the AudioScope has been reported to be 94%, and its specificity is between 72% and 90% for identifying a hearing loss. In addition, the test has been found to have excellent test-retest reliability.

Communication Scales

Communication scales are another type of screening tool that can be used efficiently with the older adult population. A popular scale at present is the Hearing

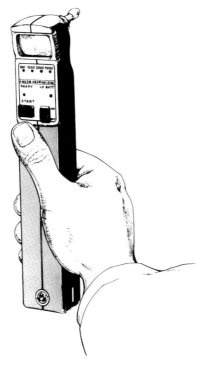

FIGURE 8.5 An AudioScope. (From Lichtenstein MJ, Bess FH, Logan SA. Validation of screening tools for identifying hearing impaired elderly in primary care. *JAMA* 1988;259:2875–2878.)

Handicap Inventory for the Elderly—Screening Version (HHIE-S). This screener is a self-report test that contains 10 items, five dealing with the social-situational aspects and five with the emotional aspects of hearing loss. Figure 8.6 lists the test questions and the instructions for scoring. The test has been reported to

Enter 4 for a "yes" answer, 2 for a "sometimes" answer, 0 for a "no" answer.	
1. Does a hearing problem cause you to feel embarrassed when you meet new people?	
2. Does a hearing problem cause you to feel frustrated when talking to members of your family?	
3. Do you have difficulty hearing when someone speaks in a whisper?	
4. Do you feel handicapped by a hearing problem?	
5. Does a hearing problem cause you difficulty when visiting friends, relatives, or neighbors?	
6. Does a hearing problem cause you to attend religious services less often than you would like?	
7. Does a hearing problem cause you to have arguments with family members?	
8. Does a hearing problem cause you to have difficulty when listening to television or radio?	
9. Do you feel that any difficulty with your hearing limits/hampers your personal or social life?	
10. Does a hearing problem cause you difficulty when in a restaurant with relatives or friends?	

TOTAL _____

HHIE-S scores may be interpreted as shown below. (Hearing loss is defined as [a] the inability to hear a 40-dB HL tone at 1,000 Hz or 2,000 Hz in each ear or [b] the inability to hear both frequencies in one ear.)

HHIE-S score	Probability of hearing loss (%)
0–8	13
10–24	50
26–40	84

FIGURE 8.6 The Hearing Handicap Inventory for the Elderly—Screening Version (HHIE-S). (Adapted from Ventry IM, Weinstein BE. Identification of elderly people with hearing problems. *ASHA* 1983;25:37–42; from Lichtenstein MJ, Bess FH, Logan SA. Validation of screening tools for identifying hearing-impaired elderly in primary care. *JAMA* 1988;259:2875–2878.)

identify the vast majority of elderly persons with high-frequency hearing losses exceeding 40-dB HL in the better ear. Again, this tool yields acceptable sensitivity and specificity values. Using a cutoff score of 8, one finds a sensitivity value of 72% and a test specificity of 77%. Although these values are not as high as those reported for the AudioScope, they do represent acceptable values for a screening tool. The pencil-and-paper format and the low number of test items are additional advantages of the HHIE-S.

Even though the AudioScope and the HHIE-S provide acceptable sensitivity and specificity values, the best test result is obtained when these two tools are used in combination. Table 8.3 lists the screening characteristics of the AudioScope and the HHIE-S when used in combination. This table shows the sensitivity and specificity for each of the screeners alone and for the two instruments used in combination. Two specific pass/fail criteria seem to afford the most favorable outcome. These criteria are (a) AudioScope fail and HHIE-S score greater than 8 and (b) AudioScope pass and HHIE-S score greater than 24. When these criteria are used, it is seen that the sensitivity is 75%, whereas the specificity is 86%. Although there is some loss of sensitivity compared with that seen when either of the screeners is used alone, there is considerable improvement in specificity. This reduces the potential for overreferrals—an important factor when one is screening on a large-scale basis. Once again, as with most screening protocols, it is recommended that one retest before referral is made.

TABLE

8.3

Sensitivity and Specificity of Screening Tests for Hearing Loss in the Hearing-Impaired Elderly

Screening Test	Sensitivity (%)	Specificity (%)
AudioScope	94	72
HHIE-S score		
>8	72	77
>24	41	92
Combined scores: Audio-Scope fail and HHIE > 8 or AudioScope pass and HHIE > 24	75	86

Name _____	Date _____
Raw Score ___ X 2 = ___ –20 = ___ X 1.25 ___%	

Please select the appropriate number ranging from 1 to 5 for the following questions. Circle only one number for each question. If you have a hearing aid, please fill out the form according to how you communicate when the hearing aid <u>is not</u> in use.

Various Communication Situations

1. Do you experience communication difficulties when speaking with one other person (for example, at home, at work, in a social situation, with a waitress, a store clerk, with a spouse, boss)?

 1) almost never 2) occasionally 3) about half 4) frequently 5) practically always
 (or never) (about ¼ of the time) of the time (¾ of the time) (or always)

2. Do you experience communication difficulties when conversing with a small group of several persons (for example, with friends or family, co-workers, in meetings or casual conversations, over dinner or while playing cards)?

 1) almost never 2) occasionally 3) about half 4) frequently 5) practically always
 (or never) (about ¼ of the time) of the time (¾ of the time) (or always)

3. Do you experience communication difficulties while listening to someone speak to a large group (for example, at a church or in a civic meeting, in a fraternal or women's club, at an educational lecture)?

 1) almost never 2) occasionally 3) about half 4) frequently 5) practically always
 (or never) (about ¼ of the time) of the time (¾ of the time) (or always)

4. Do you experience communication difficulties while participating in various types of entertainment (for example, movies, TV, radio, plays, night clubs, musical entertainment)?

 1) almost never 2) occasionally 3) about half 4) frequently 5) practically always
 (or never) (about ¼ of the time) of the time (¾ of the time) (or always)

5. Do you experience communication difficulties when you are in an unfavorable listening environment (for example, at a noisy party, where there is background music, when riding in an auto or bus, when someone whispers or talks from across the room)?

 1) almost never 2) occasionally 3) about half 4) frequently 5) practically always
 (or never) (about ¼ of the time) of the time (¾ of the time) (or always)

6. Do you experience communication difficulties when using or listening to various communication devices (for example, telephone, telephone ring, doorbell, public address system, warning signals, alarms)?

 1) almost never 2) occasionally 3) about half 4) frequently 5) practically always
 (or never) (about ¼ of the time) of the time (¾ of the time) (or always)

Feelings About Communication

7. Do you feel that any difficulty with your hearing limits or hampers your personal or social life?

 1) almost never 2) occasionally 3) about half 4) frequently 5) practically always
 (or never) (about ¼ of the time) of the time (¾ of the time) (or always)

8. Does any problem or difficulty with your hearing upset you?

 1) almost never 2) occasionally 3) about half 4) frequently 5) practically always
 (or never) (about ¼ of the time) of the time (¾ of the time) (or always)

Other People

9. Do others suggest that you have a hearing problem?

 1) almost never 2) occasionally 3) about half 4) frequently 5) practically always
 (or never) (about ¼ of the time) of the time (¾ of the time) (or always)

10. Do others leave you out of conversations or become annoyed because of your hearing?

 1) almost never 2) occasionally 3) about half 4) frequently 5) practically always
 (or never) (about ¼ of the time) of the time (¾ of the time) (or always)

FIGURE 8.7 The Self-Assessment of Communication. (Adapted from Schow RL, Nerbonne MA. Communication screening profile; use with elderly clients. *Ear Hear* 1982;3:135–147.)

Another commonly used self-report communication scale is the Self-Assessment of Communication (SAC). Similar to the HHIE-S, the SAC is a 10-item questionnaire that queries an individual regarding his or her perceptions of communication problems resulting from hearing loss. The SAC was standardized on a sample of adults over the age of 18 years; the posttest probabilities of hearing loss are similar to that of the HHIE-S. Figure 8.7 lists the test questions for the SAC.

SUMMARY

Often, it is more important to efficiently determine in a large group of children if there are breaks in any child's communication chain, rather than pinpoint the exact nature and severity of the break. Screening programs have been designed and developed for just this purpose. We have defined and justified screening and discussed important considerations and techniques of identification programs. Identification is an important first step in the overall hearing conservation program. The early identification of hearing loss and middle ear disease is the key to effective and appropriate management. There is still much to be learned about our screening programs for the identification of both hearing loss and middle ear disease. In particular, we need to learn more about the feasibility of universal screening of healthy newborns. Currently, there is widespread implementation of newborn hearing screening programs but less than desirable follow-up at this stage. Other critical issues, such as performance of screening tools, accessibility and availability of follow-up services, compliance, and costs, need to be further explored. There is also a need for more research on screening with immittance for middle ear disease in children and alternatives to conventional pure-tone screening for older adults.

CHAPTER REVIEW QUESTIONS

1. What is the basic purpose of any screening program?
2. What are some of the desirable features of screening tests?
3. What do sensitivity and specificity of a screening test indicate? What are ideal values for each? What are typical values for screening for hearing loss in newborns?
4. If 1 in 100 million Americans suffered from a serious life-threatening disease, would it be appropriate to screen all Americans for this disorder? Why or why not? What other factors might need to be considered?
5. If 99.9 million of every 100 million Americans suffered from a serious disease, would it be appropriate to screen all Americans for this disorder? Why or why not? What other factors might need to be considered?

REFERENCES AND SUGGESTED READINGS

Anderson KL, et al. *American Academy of Audiology: Childhood Hearing Screening Guidelines.* American Academy of Audiology; 2011.

American Academy of Pediatrics: Newborn and infant hearing loss: Detection and intervention. Taskforce on newborn and infant hearing. *Pediatrics* 1999;103:527–530.

American National Standards Institute. *American National Standards Specifications for Audiometers.* ANSI S3.6-1989. New York, NY: American National Standards Institute; 1989.

American Speech-Language-Hearing Association. *Guidelines for Audiologic Screening.* ASHA Desk Reference, Rockville, MD: ASHA; 1997.

American Speech-Language-Hearing Association. Considerations in screening adults/older persons for handicapping hearing impairments. *ASHA* 1992;34:81–87.

Bess FH. *Children with Hearing Impairment: Contemporary Trends.* Nashville, TN: Vanderbilt Bill Wilkerson Center Press; 1998.

Bess FH, Hall JW. *Screening Children for Auditory Function.* Nashville, TN: Bill Wilkerson Center Press; 1992.

Bess FH, Penn TO. Issues and concerns associated with universal newborn hearing screening programs. *J Speech Lang Pathol Audiol* 2001;24:113–123.

Center for Disease Control and Prevention. *Summary of 2009 National CDC EHDI Data.* Atlanta, GA: CDC; 2012.

Downs M: Early identification of hearing loss: Where are we? Where do we go from here? In: Mencher GT, ed. *Early Identification of Hearing Loss.* Basel, Switzerland: S Karger; 1976.

Harford ER, Bess FH, Bluestone CD, et al., eds. *Impedance Screening for Middle Ear Disease in Children.* New York, NY: Grune & Stratton; 1978.

Hayes D. State programs for universal newborn hearing screening. *Pediatr Clin North Am* 1999;46:89–94.

Joint Committee on Infant Hearing. *2000 Position Statement: Principles and Guidelines for Early Hearing Detection and Intervention Programs.* American Speech-Language-Hearing Association; 2000.

Joint Committee on Infant Hearing. *Year 2007 Position Statement: Principles and Guidelines for Early Hearing Detection and Intervention.* Available from www.asha.org/policy; 2007.

Kileny PR. ALGO-1 automated infant hearing screener: Preliminary results. In: Gerkin KP, Amochaev A, eds. *Hearing in Infants: Proceedings from the National Symposium. Seminars in Hearing.* New York, NY: Thieme-Stratton; 1987.

Lous J. Screening for secretory otitis media: Evaluation of some impedance programs for long-lasting secretory otitis media in 7-year-old children. *Int J Pediatr Otorhinolaryngol* 1987;13:85–97.

Matkin ND. Early recognition and referral of hearing-impaired children. *Pediatr Rev* 1984;6:151–156.

Northern JL, Downs MP. *Hearing in Children*. 5th ed. Baltimore, MD: Lippincott Williams & Wilkins; 2002.

Nozza RJ, Bluestone CD, Kardatzke D, et al. Towards the validation of aural acoustic immittance measures for diagnosis of middle ear effusion in children. *Ear Hear* 1992;13:442–453.

Nozza RJ, Bluestone CD, Kardatzke D, et al. Identification of middle ear effusion by aural acoustic admittance and otoscopy. *Ear Hear* 15:310–323, 1994.

Roush J, Bryant K, Mundy M, et al. Developmental changes in static admittance and tympanometric width in infants and toddlers. *J Am Acad Audiol* 1995;6:334–338.

Roush J. Screening school-age children. In: Bess FH, Hall JW, eds. *Screening Children for Auditory Function*. Nashville, TN: Bill Wilkerson Center Press; 1992.

Sackett DL, Haynes RB, Guyatt, GH, et al. *Clinical Epidemiology: A Basic Science for Clinical Medicine*. 2nd ed. Boston, MA: Little Brown; 1991.

Smits C, Kapteyn TS, Houtgast T. Development and validation of an automatic speech-in-noise screening test by telephone. *Int J Audiol* 2004;43:15–28.

Smits C, Houtgast T. Results from the Dutch speech-in-noise screening test by telephone. *Ear Hear* 2005;26:89–95.

Stevens JC, Parker G. Screening and surveillance. In: Newton VE, ed. *Paediatric Audiological Medicine*. London, UK: Whurr Publishing; 2002.

US Preventive Services Task Force. Universal screening for hearing loss in newborns: US Preventive Services Task Force Recommendation Statement. *Pediatrics* 2008;122:143–148.

Walton WK, Williams PS. Stability of routinely serviced portable audiometers. *Lang Speech Hear Serv Sch* 1972;3:36–43.

Weber BA. Screening of high-risk infants using auditory brainstem response audiometry. In: Bess FH, ed. *Hearing Impairment in Children*. Parkton, MD: York Press; 1988.

Welsh R, Slater S. The state of infant hearing impairment identification programs. *ASHA* 1993;35:49–52.

White KR. Universal infant hearing screening: Successes and continuing challenges. In: Seewald R. *A Sound Foundation Through Early Amplification*. Chicago, IL: Phonak; 2011.

Wilson WR, Walton WK. Public school audiometry. In: Martin FN, ed. *Pediatric Audiology*. Englewood Cliffs, NJ: Prentice-Hall; 1978.

ANSWERS TO PROBLEM IN VIGNETTE 8.2

Prevalence = 50%; Sensitivity = 80%; Specificity = 90%

"Repairing" Breaks in the Communication Chain

9

Auditory Prosthetic Devices for People with Impaired Hearing

Chapter Objectives

- To understand the function of various auditory prosthetic devices, such as hearing aids, classroom amplification systems, and cochlear implants: devices that are designed to restore auditory perception to those individuals with impaired hearing;

- To recognize the differences between hearing aids, classroom amplification systems, assistive listening devices, and cochlear implants;

- To appreciate that the selection and fitting of the appropriate device is just the initial step in the process of aural rehabilitation; and

- To realize that, especially for school-age children, maintenance of the auditory prosthetic device to ensure its function is critical to the successful use of the device.

Key Terms and Definitions

- **Hearing aid:** A personal electroacoustic device, typically worn in or on the ear of persons with impaired hearing, which primarily serves to amplify sound arriving at the wearer's ear so as to compensate for hearing loss.

- **Classroom amplification system:** An electroacoustic system typically making use of a detached microphone worn by the teacher with the microphone's output sent to personal amplification units worn by members of the class who have impaired hearing.

- **Assistive listening devices:** A wide assortment of electronic devices designed as either alternatives to or supplements of other auditory prosthetic devices. Depending on the severity of the hearing loss, common assistive listening devices include wireless systems designed for use while watching television, systems to use with the telephone, and the use of visual stimulation (e.g., flashing lights) for doorbells, alarm clocks, or other alerting devices.

■ **Cochlear implant:** An electronic device that is surgically implanted under the skin behind the ear with electrodes (wires) extending through the middle ear and inserting into the fluid-filled cochlea. The normal transducer function of the inner ear is bypassed, and the nerve fibers exiting the cochlea are stimulated directly by electrical current. These devices currently are reserved for use by individuals with severe or profound amounts of hearing loss who demonstrate little benefit from conventional hearing aids.

Hearing loss can result in a break in the communication chain negatively impacting the listener's or the receiver's ability to communicate. Ideally, this break in the chain would be repaired to restore normal communication. In the case of conductive pathology, the repair is often medical or surgical intervention to eliminate the pathology or disease causing the communication break. For individuals with sensorineural hearing loss from cochlear pathology, however, such medical repair is not possible. Instead, prosthetic devices are used to restore function to be as close to normal as possible. Everyday examples of prosthetic devices used to restore function in other parts of the body include eyeglasses or contact lenses to correct visual problems and artificial limbs to compensate for the loss of a limb. In our case, however, we are specifically interested in prosthetic devices designed to compensate for hearing loss. Some of these devices, such as **hearing aids** or other amplification systems, primarily increase the intensity of sounds at the frequencies for which the person has hearing loss. These devices deliver more intense sounds to the outer ear and make use of the normal air-conduction transmission/transduction path from the middle ear to the inner ear. Alternatively, some devices are designed to bypass entirely the damaged portion of the normal auditory transmission/transduction path. A **cochlear implant**, for example, skips the outer ear, middle ear, and much of the inner ear by stimulating the auditory nerve fibers in the cochlea directly with electrical energy.

The reader should keep in mind that auditory prosthetic devices, such as hearing aids and cochlear implants, are typically used for persons with sensorineural hearing loss resulting from inner ear pathology. Although eyeglasses were mentioned as another common prosthetic device, this analogy often leads individuals to think that hearing is restored to "20/20" as soon as the hearing aid or cochlear implant has been fitted. This is often not the case in hearing, however, even following prolonged use of the devices, because the nature of the problem being treated in vision and in hearing is entirely different. To explain, in vision, the problems typically treated with eyeglasses (nearsightedness or farsightedness) are equivalent to *conductive* problems in hearing. Hearing aids work wonderfully with conductive impairments and can restore hearing to normal, but they are rarely used in such cases, as noted frequently in earlier chapters, because these hearing losses can be remedied medically or surgically. In fact, optometrists and ophthalmologists are turning increasingly to surgical corrections of near-sightedness and farsightedness, through procedures such as laser-assisted in-situ keratomileusis (i.e., lasik surgery), as alternatives to use of prosthetic devices for these vision problems. The overwhelming majority of persons using hearing aids or cochlear implants, however, do not have conductive hearing loss; rather, the problem lies in the auditory sensory receptors in the cochlea (the inner and outer hair cells). The visual analog to sensorineural hearing loss would be vision disorders that impact the sensory cells for vision, the rods and cones in the retina. When retinal damage is the source of the visual problem, as in vision disorders associated with macular degeneration, then prosthetic devices such as eyeglasses are generally incapable of restoring vision to "20/20."

Thus, although eyeglasses and hearing aids both represent prosthetic devices designed to assist individuals who have lost sensory function, the problems being treated with these devices are usually quite different and the expectations regarding benefits should be tempered accordingly. Sometimes, just making the hearing-impaired adult aware of the differences between eyeglasses and hearing aids, both in terms of the nature of the problem being treated by each and the expected benefits provided by each, can help the individual set realistic expectations and increase the odds for successful rehabilitation.

Given the foregoing, it is extremely rare for an individual with impaired hearing to receive maximum benefit as soon as the device is fitted. Instead, a period of adjustment, training, and rehabilitation is required. As a result, before we describe various prosthetic devices used by individuals with hearing impairment in detail, a broad overview of the aural rehabilitation process will put the use of these prosthetic devices in the proper context. The main point is that the intervention phase of rehabilitation, described briefly below, *begins*, rather than ends, with the fitting of the prosthetic device.

AN OVERVIEW OF THE AURAL REHABILITATION/ HABILITATION PROCESS

The aural rehabilitation process involves at least two phases. The first phase is the identification of the problem. Before an intervention strategy can be developed, one must know about the type and degree of hearing loss as well as the impact of the impairment on communicative, educational, social, or cognitive function. For the adult with hearing impairment, the measurement of the patient's audiogram, the administration of speech recognition tests, and the use of self-report surveys or questionnaires can provide much of this information. Pure-tone and speech audiometry have already been discussed (see Chapter 7). Self-report surveys are often used to assess in detail the social, psychological, and communicative difficulties experienced by the hearing impaired. For the child with hearing impairment, additional assessment considerations might include the extent of parental support and the evaluation of skills in language, speech, auditory training, and speechreading (lip reading).

After the problem has been identified, the next phase of the rehabilitation process is intervention. For the hearing impaired, the nature of the intervention package is determined, in large part, by the identification phase. Consider, for example, just the degree and type of hearing loss, ignoring other factors such as age and social or emotional difficulties. First, regarding type of hearing loss, the most appropriate candidates for amplification are those with sensorineural hearing loss. Occasionally, individuals with chronic conductive hearing loss not amenable to medical or surgical intervention will be fitted with a hearing aid. For these individuals, a bone-anchored hearing aid that delivers sound to the inner ear via bone conduction is a viable option. Most often, though, the individual with sensorineural hearing loss as a result of cochlear pathology is the type of patient fitted with a rehabilitative device, such as a hearing aid.

Generally, as the degree of sensorineural hearing loss increases, speech-understanding difficulties increase. The need for intervention increases in proportion to the degree of speech-understanding difficulty. Thus, those with mild hearing loss (pure-tone average [PTA] of 20- to 30-dB HL) generally have less need for intervention than do those with profound hearing loss (PTA > 85-dB HL). Conventional hearing aids provide the greatest benefit to those hearing-impaired persons whose average hearing loss is between 40- and 85-dB HL. For milder amounts of hearing loss, the difficulties experienced and the need for intervention often are not great enough for full-time use of a conventional hearing aid. Part-time use of a hearing aid, or another type of device known as an assistive listening device, is usually recommended for these patients. For the profoundly impaired, on the other hand, the difficulties in communicating and the need for intervention are great. Unfortunately, the conventional hearing aid is of limited benefit in such cases. For patients with profound impairments, alternative devices, such as cochlear implants, are explored. For patients with profound impairments fit with either high-powered hearing aids or cochlear implants, the fitting of the device is usually accompanied by extensive training in several areas, including speechreading (lipreading), auditory training, and/or manual communication (finger spelling and sign language).

Consider also the time of onset of the hearing loss. Of course, the intervention approach will be much different for a congenitally hearing-impaired child than for someone who acquired the hearing loss later in life (after communication has developed). With a congenital onset, the emphasis will focus on such critical issues as early intervention, parental guidance, and a comprehensive habilitation package designed to facilitate communication development.

In summary, the intervention phase of aural rehabilitation/habilitation typically begins with the selection and fitting of an appropriate rehabilitative device, such as a hearing aid or cochlear implant. This is followed by extensive training with the device in communicative situations.

Many of the procedures used in the identification phase of the rehabilitation process have been reviewed in earlier chapters. This chapter focuses on the devices available to hearing-impaired adults and children during the intervention phase, with emphasis on the conventional hearing aid and the cochlear implant. Chapter 10 focuses on the training methods and philosophies for rehabilitation/habilitation of children and adults once a device has been selected and fitted.

AMPLIFICATION FOR INDIVIDUALS WITH HEARING LOSS

Classification of Conventional Amplification

Today, the following six types of hearing aids are available: (1) body aid, (2) eyeglass aid, (3) behind-the-ear (BTE) aid, (4) in-the-ear (ITE) aid, (5) in-the-canal (ITC) aid, and (6) completely-in-the-canal (CIC) aid. Figure 9.1 shows five of the six types of hearing aid (1 through 5), whereas the CIC hearing aid type is illustrated in Vignette 9.1. When electroacoustic hearing aids were first developed several decades ago, the body aid was the only type available. In the ensuing years, the other types of instruments were developed. In 1960, eyeglass hearing aids were the most popular, accounting for 44% of all hearing aids sold, with the remaining 56% divided evenly between body and BTE instruments. As indicated in Figure 9.2, BTE hearing aids became the most common type of hearing aid sold in the two-decade period from 1962 through 1982. From 1983 to 2003, however, the trend had been for ITE aids to capture an increasingly larger portion of the hearing aid market. In particular, from 1987 to 2003, approximately 80% of the hearing aids sold in the United States were ITE instruments; the bulk of the remaining 20% of instruments sold had been of the BTE type. Since 2003, however, there has been a considerable upturn in the percentage of BTE hearing aids sold in the United States, increasing to about 70% in 2011, owing to new innovations in these devices and the resulting decrease in their visibility (see Vignette 9.2).

The sales percentages for ITEs shown in Figure 9.2 actually represent the combination of all types of ITE hearing aids, including the ITE, ITC, and CIC types. From 1995 through 2000, approximately 43% of the aids sold were custom ITE aids, most of which were full-concha devices like the type shown as no. 3 in Figure 9.1; 22.5% were the ITC type, shown as no. 4 in this figure; and 14.5% were the CIC type. Since 2000, the sales percentages for ITC and

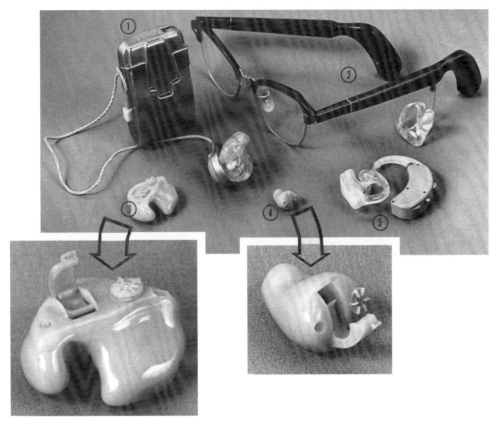

FIGURE 9.1 The different types of hearing aids. *1*, body aid; *2*, eyeglass; *3*, ITE aid; *4*, ITC aid; and *5*, BTE aid.

VIGNETTE 9.1 • CLINICAL APPLICATIONS

The Completely-in-the-Canal Hearing Aid

The drawing below depicts the size and position of a CIC hearing aid in the ear canal of an adult hearing aid wearer. The CIC hearing aid is the smallest commercially available hearing aid. As a result, it is the least conspicuous visually. Its small size, though, presents some special challenges to the audiologist, the wearer, and the manufacturer. First, for the manufacturer, the circuitry had to be miniaturized so as to have all components fit within this small space. In addition, given its small size and deep insertion, it is not possible to adjust controls on the hearing aid manually, as in other hearing aids. In most cases, manufacturers produce their CIC instruments with an electronic feature known as automatic volume control (AVC). The AVC circuit monitors the input level and gradually adjusts the gain to maintain a constant output level, much like the wearer would do with a manual volume control wheel. For the audiologist, two of the major challenges with such devices are the need for deep earmold impressions, because the device is designed to fit deeper within the ear canal than most other hearing aids, and the verification of a good fit with real-ear measurements. Finally, for the user, the primary adjustment is centered on the small size of the device. It is inserted and removed with a semi-rigid extraction string that is very small itself. Because the majority of hearing aid users are elderly adults, many of whom have diminished manual dexterity, the insertion and removal of these tiny devices, as well as battery replacement and hearing aid cleaning, can be challenging tasks for the user.

Since 1994, the average price of the CIC hearing aid has been approximately twice that of the BTE and full-shell ITE hearing aid and approximately 50% higher than the ITC hearing aid for the same electronic circuitry. In 2000, the percentage of hearing aids returned to the manufacturer for credit (i.e., the wearer returned the hearing aids to the dispenser within the 30-day money-back trial period) was highest for the CIC type at 23%. The return rate for ITC hearing aids was 19% in 2000, whereas the return rate for full-shell ITE hearing aids was 15.3%. Return rates have remained fairly stable since 2000.

Incidentally, at one time, the industry apparently considered naming these hearing aids "totally-in-the-canal" devices, or TIC. However, it was probably considered inadvisable to tell people that they had just paid a fair amount of money for "a TIC in their ear"—the industry wisely opted for CIC instead.

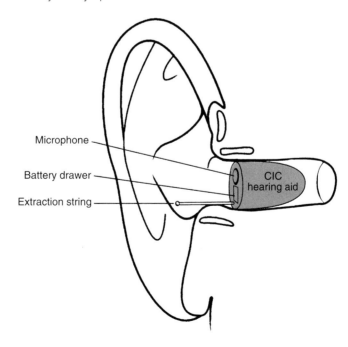

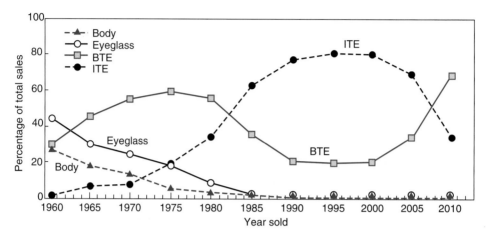

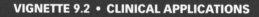

FIGURE 9.2 Sales trends for various hearing aid types since 1960. *BTE*, behind-the-ear; *ITE*, in-the-ear.

VIGNETTE 9.2 • CLINICAL APPLICATIONS

Open-Fit Mini-BTE Hearing Aids

As demonstrated previously in Figure 9.2, there has been a rapid upturn in the sales of BTE-style hearing aids in recent years. About 70% of the hearing aids sold in 2011 in the United States were BTE-style devices, and the vast majority of these devices were "mini-BTE" hearing aids connected to the ear canal of the wearer with a thin tube and open earmold or earpiece. The top photo below shows several representative mini-BTE devices. The bottom drawing below from WebMD shows the mini-BTE device itself and as worn by an adult male in the middle panel and compares this to conventional BTE (left panel) and full-concha ITE (right panel) devices. The "mini" size of the BTE, together with the use of very thin tubing, make the mini-BTE much less visible than either of the other options shown in the bottom drawing. In addition, because the microphone is on the top and behind the outer ear, any amplified sound leaving the ear canal through the open-fit earpiece has a longer way to travel to reach the microphone and cause the whistling sound associated with feedback. This results in superior electroacoustic performance than when the microphone and loudspeaker (receiver) of the hearing aid are close together in other cosmetically appealing options, such as the CIC style (see the previous Vignette 9.1). As noted, one of the engineering developments that made such open-fit mini-BTE devices feasible was improved feedback cancellation with digital hearing aids. Allowing the ear canal to remain open, rather than plugged (occluded), results in a much more comfortable listening experience for the wearer, especially when the wearer is talking, chewing, drinking, etc. Thus, there are a number of reasons, cosmetic, electroacoustic, and comfort based, that the open-fit mini-BTE devices have led to the resurgence in the popularity of BTE hearing aids.

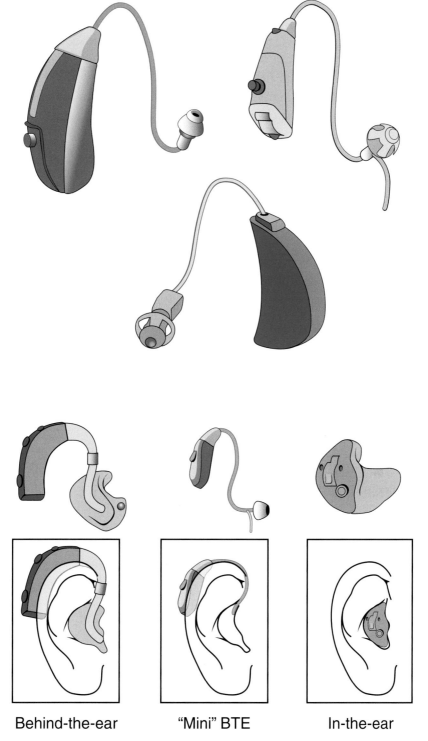

Behind-the-ear   "Mini" BTE   In-the-ear

From Kochkin S. MarkeTrak VII: Mini-BTEs tap new market, users more satisfied. *Hearing J* 2011;64(3):17–24.)

CIC types have remained about the same, but full-concha ITE hearing aids have decreased by 15% to 20% (to about 25% of ITEs since 2005), about the same as the increase in BTE hearing aid sales over this same period. The increasing popularity of the less visible BTE and the sustained popularity of the ITC and CIC hearing aids are results of both consumer pressures to improve the cosmetic appeal of the devices and rapid developments in the field of electronics. High-fidelity electronic components and the batteries to power them have been drastically reduced in size, making the smaller BTE and ITE devices possible.

Operation of Amplification Systems

Components and Function

Although the outer physical characteristics of the types of hearing aids shown in Figure 9.1 differ, the internal features are very similar. The hearing aid, for example, is referred to as an electroacoustic device. It converts the acoustic signal, such as a speech sound, into an electrical signal. The device then manipulates the electrical signal in some way, converts the electrical signal back to an acoustic one, and then delivers it to the ear canal of the wearer. A microphone is used to convert the acoustic signal into an electrical signal. The electrical signal is usually amplified or made larger within the hearing aid. It may also be filtered to eliminate high or low frequencies from the signal. A tiny loudspeaker, usually referred to as a receiver, converts the amplified electrical signal back into a sound wave. Up to this point, the hearing aid could be thought of as a miniature public-address (PA) system with a microphone, amplifier, and loudspeaker. Unlike a PA system, though, the hearing aid is designed to help a single person, the hearing aid wearer, receive the amplified speech. The microphone is positioned somewhere on the hearing aid wearer, and the amplified sound from the receiver is routed directly to the wearer's ear. For ITE and ITC hearing aids, the sound wave is routed from the receiver to the ear canal by a small piece of tubing within the plastic shell of the instrument. For the other types of hearing aids, an earmold is needed. The earmold (or shell for the ITE and ITC hearing aids) is made of a synthetic plastic or rubber-like material from an impression made of the outer ear and ear canal. The earmold is custom made for the patient's ear and allows the output of the hearing aid to be coupled to the patient's ear canal. As a result, only the patient receives the louder sound and not a group of people, as with a PA system (see Vignette 9.3).

Nearly all of the hearing aids sold in the United States since 2005 have been digital devices; only a decade earlier, the only hearing aids available were analog devices with tiny amplifiers inside. The amplifier referred to previously has basically been replaced by a small computer in contemporary digital devices. The computer can process the sound input received from the microphone prior

VIGNETTE 9.3 • FURTHER DISCUSSION

Basic Components of an Electronic Hearing Aid

The top part of the schematic drawing shows the basic components of an analog electronic hearing aid. As illustrated here, the hearing aid is like a miniature PA system, with a microphone, amplifier, and loudspeaker (or receiver). The microphone and receiver are transducers: their primary job is to convert waveforms from one form of energy to another. The microphone converts sound waves to electrical voltage waveforms. The amplifier makes this incoming electrical waveform larger, and the receiver converts it back to a sound wave. The amplifier necessitates a portable power supply, and this is supplied by a battery. There may be other controls for the patient to adjust, such as a manual volume control (not shown). A volume control allows the user to adjust the loudness so that sound is comfortably loud in different environments. In 2005, however, only about 50% of the hearing aids sold included an adjustable volume control. Since most hearing aids sold in 2005 were digital, this illustrates an additional potential advantage of digital hearing aids; the ability to incorporate a suitable AVC in the digital processor eliminates the need for manual adjustment.

The bottom portion of the drawing shows the basic components of a digital hearing aid. The overall structure of the analog and digital hearing aids is very similar, each type including a microphone, receiver, and battery. The primary difference is that the analog amplifier is replaced by the digital signal processor (DSP). Although this can seem like a minor difference, swapping one red box for another, it is a very significant change in hearing aid technology. The move to digital circuitry provides manufacturers and clinicians with almost unlimited flexibility to have the signal processed or modified for the patient's benefit. The real challenge now is in determining how best to do that.

In the DSP in the bottom drawing are three main modules or components: (a) an analog-to-digital converter (A/D), (b) a DSP, and (c) a digital-to-analog converter (D/A). The function of the A/D and D/A is described in more detail in Vignette 9.4. The DSP is the computer in the hearing aid, and it is this component that gets programmed by the audiologist with the manufacturer's software so that the digital hearing aid will have the appropriate gain, frequency response, compression characteristics, output limiting, and so on. The manufacturer's software is installed on the audiologist's personal computer, and a special cable is used to make an electrical connection between the personal computer and the hearing aid to enable programming of the hearing aid. This also reflects one of the great advantages of digital hearing aids: flexible programming. The same hearing aid can be programmed to fit a wide range of patients, rather than requiring the production of numerous analog models to do this.

In addition, for the same patient, the hearing aid can be reprogrammed over time to accommodate changes in hearing loss or wearer preferences without requiring purchase of a new device.

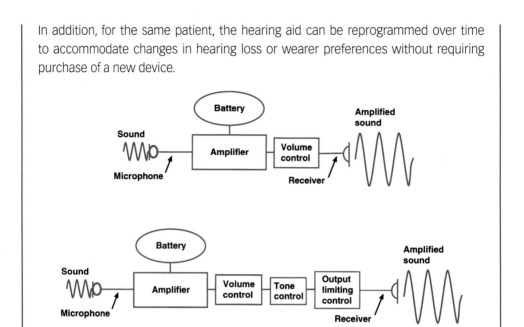

to sending it to the loudspeaker or receiver. This change to digital circuitry has greatly expanded the options available to hearing aid manufacturers, audiologists, and patients. The basic concept behind the hearing aid is the same, and one of the primary purposes served by the digital processor is the amplification of sound, but the way in which this can be accomplished has been enhanced considerably.

If the fundamental function of the components in analog and digital hearing aids is so similar, as suggested in Vignette 9.3, why did hearing aid manufacturers change from analog-to-digital technology? There were several reasons for this significant move in the industry. Among these are (a) a move in the broader consumer electronics markets to digital technologies, which had positive impacts on the availability of less expensive microchips needed for digital processing and improvements in battery technology to support such circuits; (b) more reliable mass production of the circuitry comprising digital hearing aids; (c) enhanced flexibility of the devices with the capability of the same hardware performing substantially different functions through changes to the programming software; and (d) capability to perform certain signal-processing strategies that could only be realized practically in digital form.

Regarding the latter potential advantage of digital circuitry, one point of emphasis has included reduction of the acoustic feedback that can occur in hearing aids. Feedback is typically a "whistling sound" that is generated by the hearing aid when the amplified sound coming out of the hearing aid inadvertently feeds back into the microphone, gets amplified again, feeds back into the microphone again, gets amplified again, and so on. (Keeping with our PA system analogy, the reader has probably experienced the squeal of feedback in a PA system when the speaker or performer wearing a microphone moves into the sound path of the loudspeaker presenting the amplified signal, the loud squeal making everyone in the audience cringe.) In the past, the solution has often been to reduce the gain or volume of the hearing aid, but this also decreases the amplification for sounds of the same frequency that *should* be amplified for the hearing aid wearer, such as speech sounds. Digital signal processing has enabled the development of more sophisticated approaches to feedback cancellation that are directed primarily at the unwanted feedback sound and not other similar sounds of interest to the wearer. It is really this single change more than any other that led to the possibility of practical open-fit BTE hearing aids (Vignette 9.2), devices capable of delivering sufficient amplification without feedback while keeping the ear canal unoccluded, that have driven the upswing in BTE hearing aid sales over the past decade.

Many of the other potential advantages of digital hearing aid circuitry differ in detail but share a common objective: decrease the level of the background noise amplified by the hearing aid. The hearing aid microphone transduces all sounds entering it, not just the wanted sounds. Speech communication, for example, often takes place in a background of other competing sounds, such as traffic, music, or other people talking. About two-thirds of the hearing aids sold in the United States are sold to individuals 65 years of age or older. It has been demonstrated repeatedly that older adults not only require amplification of soft and moderate level sounds due to their age-related sensorineural hearing loss (see Chapter 6) but must also have the background noise decreased to achieve sufficient benefit from hearing aids. Digital hearing aids have held great promise for reduction of the background noise level, although clear benefits to speech communication in older adults have not yet been substantiated. Although numerous approaches have been and are being pursued to use digital signal processing to reduce background noise levels, the two general areas receiving the most attention to date have been various directional microphone technologies and noise reduction strategies. Of these two general approaches to reducing background noise levels, various implementations of directional microphone technologies have been the most promising. As noted previously, the ability to better implement directional microphone technologies in larger BTE hearing aids has also been one of the reasons for the recent surge in sales of this type of hearing aid. In 2005, according to the Hearing Industries Association, 35% of the hearing aids sold used directional technology and about half of all BTEs sold in 2005 included directional technology. Basically, directional microphones are more sensitive to sounds coming from a specific direction and less sensitive to sounds coming from other directions. In general, in hearing aids, they are designed to be more sensitive to sounds coming from the front and less sensitive to sounds coming from behind the wearer. Thus, if the wearer faces the sound source and is able to position competing background sounds to the rear, directional microphones will selectively decrease the background noise. Directional microphones have been around, even in hearing aids, for decades, but it is the pairing of directional technologies with digital signal processing that holds great promise for the future in terms of noise reduction. At present, however, although large reductions in background noise can be demonstrated for select laboratory listening conditions when using some hearing aids with directional microphones, benefits to hearing aid wearers in typical, everyday listening conditions have been found to be much more modest. Further research is needed in the areas of directional technologies and noise reduction approaches to demonstrate a clear benefit of digital hearing aids in everyday speech communication. Nonetheless, as enumerated previously, there are many other advantages to digital technology in hearing aids, and, because of these factors alone, hearing aid manufacturers have almost universally moved to the use of digital circuitry in their products. Consequently, digital circuitry appears to be the circuitry of choice in hearing aids for the foreseeable future, and it is important to understand some of the fundamental concepts of digital processing. These are reviewed in Vignette 9.4.

Electroacoustic Characteristics of Hearing Aids

The primary purpose of the hearing aid is to make speech that is inaudible to the hearing-impaired person audible without causing discomfort. Modern-day conventional hearing aids have several electroacoustic characteristics that are used to describe the hearing aid's performance. Probably the two most important of these characteristics are the amount of amplification provided, referred to as the gain of the instrument, and the maximum possible sound pressure level (SPL) that can be produced, referred to as the maximum output. Currently, these characteristics can be measured in several ways. For instance, there is a standard issued by the American National Standards Institute, ANSI S3.22, which describes a set of measurements that must be made on all hearing aids sold in the United States. It is not necessary in an introductory text such as this, however, to review the ANSI standard in detail. Rather, the concepts underlying gain and maximum output and their importance in fitting the hearing aid to the patient are critical.

Gain, for example, is simply the difference, in decibels, between the input level and the output level at a particular frequency. Consider the following example. A 500-Hz pure tone is generated from a loudspeaker so that the sound level at the hearing aid's microphone is 60-dB SPL. The output produced by the

VIGNETTE 9.4 • CONCEPTUAL DEMO

Basics of Digital Signal Processing

It seems everything is digital these days, and hearing aids are no exception. What exactly is digital signal processing? Entire textbooks have been devoted to this topic, and it is impossible to cover all the details in much depth. However, some fundamental concepts of digital signal processing can be explained without going into too much detail or assuming too much background in engineering.

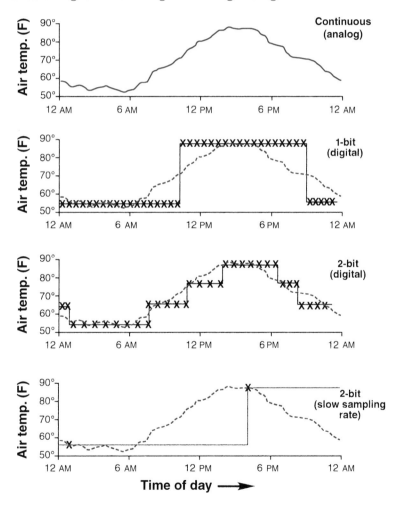

To explain these fundamental concepts, we'll make use of temperature variations during a 24-hour period, as shown in the *top panel*. The temperature in this particular location and on this particular day was around 50°F to 60°F in the early morning and gradually increased to a peak of around 87°F by midafternoon before cooling again in the evening. In this *top panel,* temperature is plotted as a continuous function of the time of day. There is a temperature indicated for every moment in time in the 24-hour span. This continuous function can be considered an analog representation of the daily temperature variations. Is it necessary to have a continuous function to capture all of the important information about daily temperature variation? Can we sample the temperature at intervals and get the same amount of information? Yes, the temperature can be measured and quantified at discrete points during the day without losing important information about the temperature changes. In fact, a mathematically derived frequency, the Nyquist frequency, indicates the lowest rate at which temperature readings could be obtained without loss of information. For this example, let's assume that by sampling the temperature at half-hour intervals, we can safely capture the information in the waveform. (For audio signals, the sampling rate or frequency should be at least twice the highest frequency of interest in the signal. Generally, this means sampling frequencies of at least 10,000 Hz but preferably >20,000 Hz.)

In the digital world, numeric values that are sampled at each point are represented as bits of information. The word *bits* is derived from ***b****inary dig****its***. Most digits with which we are familiar are from the base 10, or decimal, number system. In grade school, we learned that the decimal system organized numbers into the 1's column, the 10's column, the 100's column, and so on. Thus, in the decimal system, 752 is known to mean 7 hundreds plus 5 tens plus 2 ones. The possible numbers in each column for the decimal or base 10 system range from 0 through 9 (you can't represent a 10 *in a single column* for base 10 numbers). A more formal way of expressing this example is that 752 equals $7 \times 10^2 + 5 \times 10^1 + 2 \times 10^0$.

The binary number system, on the other hand, is a base 2 system. In this case, there is a 1's (2^0) column, a 2's (2^1) column, a 4's (2^2) column, an 8's (2^3) column, and so on. In addition, the only two digits available for use are 0 and 1 (you can't have a 2 in a base 2 system). In a system that uses only one binary digit or one bit, only two possible values exist: 1 and 0.

If we chose to code the temperatures sampled each half hour with a one-bit system, the resulting digital representation of the temperature variations would resemble that in the second panel. Essentially, we would have only two temperature values to work with, in this case with 0 corresponding to 55°F and 1 corresponding to 85°F. Clearly, one bit of information is not enough to code the temperature variations. Too many temperatures between 55°F and 85°F are lost in this 1-bit code. If the coding is doubled to 2 bits, four values are available to quantify the temperature variation: 00, 01, 10, and 11 (or 0, 1, 2, and 3 in the decimal system). The third panel shows that the accuracy of our quantification of daily temperature variation has improved considerably with 2-bit resolution. The bottom panel illustrates the case of a sampling rate that is too low. Even though enough amplitude values (4) are available, information is lost because the temperature is not sampled often enough.

Imagine that instead of temperature variations during a 24-hour period, the waveform of interest is a sound wave transduced by a hearing aid microphone. For most audio applications, including hearing aids, 8-bit coding of amplitude variations in the sound wave is adequate, but 12- or 16-bit resolution is preferred. The device that converts the continuously varying analog waveform into a discrete series of binary numbers is called an analog-to-digital (A/D) converter. Once converted to a string of 1's and 0's, the sampled signal is in the same digital language as that used by computers to process information. The computer can be programmed to adjust the gain characteristics of the hearing aid with great precision, to enhance the speech signal, or to cancel out some of the background noise. Once processed by the computer, the string of 1's and 0's representing the sound wave is reconverted to an analog signal using a digital-to-analog (D/A) converter and transduced by the hearing aid receiver (loudspeaker).

hearing aid under these conditions is 90-dB SPL. The acoustic gain provided by the hearing aid is 30 dB. The gain is simply the difference between the 60-dB SPL input and the 90-dB SPL output. The gain of the hearing aid can be measured at several frequencies. Most hearing aids provide some amplification or gain over the frequency range 200 Hz to at least 5,000 Hz. When the gain is measured across this whole frequency range by changing the frequency of the input signal and holding the input level constant, a frequency response for the hearing aid is obtained. The frequency response displays how the output or gain varies as a function of frequency. The concepts of gain and frequency response are illustrated in Figure 9.3. Because the gain is seldom constant at all frequencies, an average gain value is frequently calculated and reported. In the

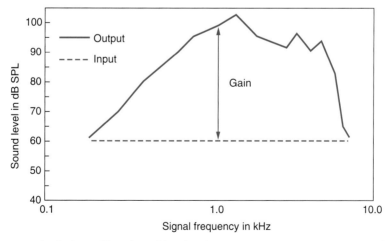

FIGURE 9.3 Calculation of hearing aid gain. The *output curve* represents the frequency response of the hearing aid for a constant 60-dB *input*.

current ANSI standard, the gain is measured at three frequencies, 1,000, 1,600, and 2,500 Hz, and the values are averaged. These frequencies are used because of their importance to speech understanding and because the hearing aid usually has its greatest output in this frequency region.

A feature shared by many hearing aids is a volume control wheel that adjusts the gain of the hearing aid under manual control by the user. In many contemporary digital hearing aids, the adjustment of the volume is accomplished automatically by the digital processor. The frequency response of the hearing aid can be measured while the position of the volume control is varied, either manually or electronically. Usually, at least two sets of measurements are obtained: one with the volume control in the full-on position and one designed to approximate a typical or "as worn" volume setting. The volume control is designed to provide about a 30-dB variation in gain. It is typically assumed that a hearing aid wearer will select a volume setting somewhere in the middle of this 30-dB range, that is, approximately 15 dB below the full-on position. If the frequency response is measured with the volume control of the hearing aid in the full-on position, the gain is referred to as "full-on" gain. When the volume control is in the middle of the usable range, the gain approximates "use" gain or "as worn" gain.

As mentioned, a second fundamental electroacoustic characteristic of the hearing aid is the maximum output. Maximum output is measured to determine the maximum possible acoustic output of the hearing aid. Consequently, a high-level input signal is used (90-dB SPL), and the volume control is set to the full-on position. Under these conditions, the hearing aid is likely to be at maximum output. The maximum output should be adjusted carefully by the audiologist to optimize the amount of gain available to the wearer while simultaneously minimizing the amount of time the hearing aid is in saturation during use.

The gain and maximum output of a hearing aid are interrelated, as illustrated in Figure 9.4. The function shown in this figure is known as an input-output

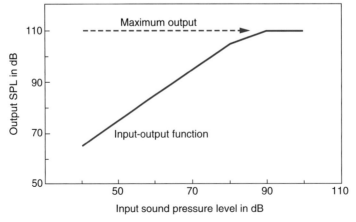

FIGURE 9.4 Input-output function for a hearing aid.

function because it displays the output along the y-axis as a function of the input level along the x-axis. For this hypothetical input-output function, the volume control is assumed to be in the full-on position. Note that low input levels (50- to 60-dB SPL) reveal output values that exceed the input by 25 dB. The gain (output minus input) is 25 dB at low input levels. At high input levels (90- to 100-dB SPL), on the other hand, the output remains constant at 110-dB SPL. This is the maximum output of the hearing aid. The instrument set so that it cannot produce an output higher than 110-dB SPL. Because the hearing aid is at maximum output, the gain at these higher input levels is lower. The gain for the 90- and 100-dB inputs is 20 and 10 dB, respectively. Because of this interaction between gain and maximum output, gain is usually measured for lower input levels (e.g., 50-dB SPL), levels that also approximate those of conversational speech, the input signal of greatest interest.

Over most of the range of input sound levels in Figure 9.4, every time the input was increased 10 dB, the output demonstrated a corresponding increase of 10 dB. This was true until the maximum output or saturation level of the hearing aid was reached. Such a circuit is generally referred to as a linear circuit. Many hearing aids dispensed today have intentionally nonlinear amplification circuits, often referred to as compression circuits, which are designed to obtain a better match between the wide range of sound levels in the environment and the narrower range of listening available in the hearing-impaired person.

Along with a wider range of possible settings and processing options associated with digital hearing aids, these devices often have multiple memories that can hold different combinations of settings. This allows the hearing aid wearer to adjust the various settings of the hearing aid easily and quickly for specific listening situations, such as listening to the television alone at home or conversing with an acquaintance at a bustling restaurant.

Candidacy for Amplification

How does one know whether an individual is a good candidate for amplification? We have already indicated that the typical candidate for amplification is one who displays a sensorineural hearing loss. Many audiologists use the degree of hearing loss as a "rule of thumb" for determining hearing aid candidacy. Figure 9.5 shows a general guideline based on the average (500 to 2,000 Hz) pure-tone hearing loss in the better ear. As hearing loss increases, the need for assistance increases, reaching a maximum for moderate amounts of hearing loss. Potential benefit from amplification, however, is lowest at the two extremes, mild and profound impairment. Those individuals with the mildest hearing losses and those with the most profound hearing deficits are usually the candidates who will benefit the least from a hearing aid. There are many

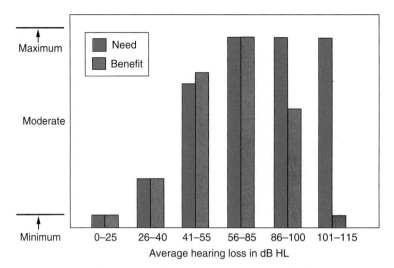

FIGURE 9.5 Illustration of the need for and potential benefit from amplification as a function of degree of hearing loss.

exceptions to this "rule of thumb" that is based simply on pure-tone thresholds. Because of this, there is now a tendency to move away from these pure-tone guidelines and to consider anyone with a communicative difficulty caused by hearing impairment as a candidate for amplification.

There are other considerations in determining hearing aid candidacy. Some of these factors are the patient's motivation for seeking assistance, the patient's acceptance of the hearing loss, and the patient's cosmetic concerns. Even if a significant hearing loss is present, some older adults put off seeking assistance for several years. The reasons for this delay are not altogether clear, although the cost of the hearing aid and the failure of the primary care physician to refer for a hearing aid are considered contributing factors. Factors that influence individuals to pursue amplification include communication problems at home, communication problems in noisy situations or in social settings, communication problems at work, and encouragement from a spouse or other loved one.

Acceptance of a hearing loss is another consideration in determining hearing aid candidacy. Some individuals simply deny that a hearing problem exists. This is particularly true for persons with very mild losses, those who fear loss of employment, and those who have suffered gradual onset of hearing loss.

Finally, one cannot overlook cosmetic concerns when considering a patient's candidacy for amplification. Amplification is still considered stigmatic. Although the acceptance of hearing aids is improving, many hearing-impaired individuals are concerned about the stigma associated with readily visible amplification devices. (This is discussed in more detail later in Vignette 10.1.)

Hearing Aid Selection, Fitting, Verification, and Evaluation

#17

Once it has been established that an individual can benefit from amplification, an appointment for hearing aid selection and evaluation is usually scheduled. In the selection phase, some important clinical decisions must be made. For example, what type of hearing aid would be most appropriate for a given hearing-impaired person? Recall from Figure 9.1 that a number of different types of hearing aids are available. The audiologist and patient need to decide whether the patient will benefit most from a body-type hearing aid, a BTE instrument, or one of the ITE systems (ITE, ITC, or CIC). As noted earlier, most hearing aids sold today are BTE, ITE, ITC, or CIC units. BTE hearing aids have several distinct advantages over body aids, the most important of which are cosmetic appeal, improved sound localization, and better speech understanding in noise when two aids are worn. Importantly, very few young children wear ITE, ITC, or CIC systems because of the frequent need to recast the earpiece because of a growing ear canal. Currently, approximately 75% of hearing aids selected for children are BTE systems.

Another important clinical decision that must be made in the selection phase is whether to recommend one hearing aid (monaural amplification) or two hearing aids (binaural amplification). Decades ago, there had been considerable controversy over the true benefits of binaural amplification, but this is no longer the case. For the past decade or longer, 75% to 80% of hearing aids dispensed in the United States have been binaural fittings. The primary reason that binaural amplification is not even more widespread is undoubtedly the added cost to the patient of buying two hearing aids rather than one. Nonetheless, there is mounting clinical evidence that failure to fit hearing aids on both ears of patients with bilateral hearing loss can result in temporary, and perhaps permanent, decreases in auditory function in the unaided ear. The deterioration over time of auditory perceptual function in the hearing-impaired ear left unaided has been referred to as an "auditory deprivation" effect.

In addition to avoiding these possible deprivation or adaptation effects, some of the reported advantages to binaural amplification include better sound localization, binaural summation (a sound is easier to hear with two ears than with one and the user can make use of lower volume settings as a result), and improvement in speech recognition in noise. Experienced hearing aid users often favor binaural amplification and report that two aids offer more balanced hearing, better overall hearing, improved speech clarity in noise, improved sound localization skills, and more natural and less stressful listening. Accordingly, binaural amplification is being recommended with increasing regularity. Some clinical research indicates that the benefits of binaural fittings over monaural ones increase as the amount of hearing loss increases. Monaural fittings may be appropriate for many persons with mild hearing impairment.

Several other factors must be considered in the selection process but are beyond the scope of an introductory text. Briefly, the audiologist must consider the type of microphone (directional versus omnidirectional), earmold material (soft silastic versus hard acrylic), and type of earmold or shell (e.g., open versus vented versus unvented). For children, an additional consideration is the adaptability of the instrument to various classroom amplification systems.

Modern-day hearing aids provide a wide range of electroacoustic characteristics that can be tailored to the patient's individual needs. The process of selecting a hearing aid with the appropriate electroacoustic characteristics for a particular patient is referred to as hearing aid selection. This process has undergone major changes in recent years. Today, most audiologists use a prescriptive approach to hearing aid selection. Using information obtained from the patient, such as the pure-tone thresholds, the appropriate gain can be prescribed according to some underlying theoretical principles. From the mid-1970s through the mid-1980s, at least a dozen different prescriptive hearing aid selection methods were developed. Although they differ in detail, these methods have the same general feature that more gain is prescribed at those frequencies for which the hearing loss is greatest. As an example, one of the simplest approaches makes use of the so-called half gain rule. One simply measures the hearing threshold at several frequencies and multiplies the hearing loss at each frequency by a factor of one-half. Thus, for a patient with a flat 50-dB hearing loss from 250 through 8,000 Hz, the appropriate gain would be 25 dB (0.5 × 50 dB) at each frequency. A person having a sloping hearing loss with a 40-dB HL hearing threshold at 1,000 Hz and an 80-dB HL threshold at 4,000 Hz would require gains of 20 and 40 dB, respectively, using this simple one-half gain rule. Regardless of the prescriptive method used, once the prescription is made, the audiologist searches among existing hearing aids capable of producing the desired gain and maximum output at each frequency and then programs the digital processor accordingly.

Maximum output can also be prescribed for the patient. Usually, additional information is required from the patient. One common approach is to measure the loudness discomfort level (LDL) of the patient for tones or narrow bands of noise. The LDL is a measure of the maximum sound level that the patient can tolerate at each frequency. When it is not possible to measure LDLs at several frequencies in each ear, as with most young children, LDLs can be estimated from pure-tone thresholds. It would not be desirable for the hearing aid's acoustic output to exceed the maximum tolerable level of the patient because this might cause the patient to reject the hearing aid. The maximum output of the hearing aid is frequently adjusted to a value slightly lower than the LDL. In this way, the audiologist can be assured that the acoustic output of the hearing aid will not exceed the maximum tolerance level of the patient. As noted, many modern hearing aids have intentionally nonlinear input-output functions so that the gain available steadily decreases as the input level increases. Although these hearing aids require different prescription procedures than linear hearing aids, the basic process is very similar regardless of the type of hearing aid circuit.

#18

Once the appropriate prescription has been made and the hearing aid has been selected, the next process, the hearing aid fitting, is conducted. In this process, the hearing aid is inserted into the patient's ear, and its acoustic performance on the wearer is verified. This is most commonly accomplished using real-ear measurements of the SPL generated in the ear canal, in close proximity to the eardrum, with and without the hearing aid in place. This is made possible by using a tiny microphone connected to a long, thin tube made of flexible plastic. The tube can be safely inserted into the ear canal, yet it is strong enough to resist being squeezed shut when the hearing aid is inserted into the ear canal over the thin tube. When SPL measurements are made at several frequencies in the patient's ear canal with and without the hearing aid, the difference between these two measurements provides a measure of the real-ear insertion gain (REIG) of the hearing aid (see Vignette 9.5). The measured insertion gain is compared with the target gain generated by the particular prescriptive method chosen by the audiologist (e.g., half gain rule), and the hearing aid's settings are adjusted until a reasonable match is observed. Similar adjustments should also be made in the maximum output of the hearing aid to assure that real-ear SPLs measured in the aided conditions for high-level input signals (90-dB SPL) do not exceed the LDL. Today, in many cases, rather than expressing targets in relative gain measured in the ear canal of the hearing aid wearer, prescriptive procedures will specify the SPLs that should be met for speech-like sounds when measured in the ear canal.

After fine-tuning the gain and maximum output of the hearing aid to match the targeted values, the hearing aid is evaluated. Again, there are several hearing aid evaluation procedures from which the audiologist can choose. These alternatives, however, have a common goal: evaluation of the benefit provided by the hearing aid when it is worn by the hearing-impaired patient. Because the primary benefit to be derived from use of the hearing aid is improved understanding of speech, the hearing aid evaluation usually involves the measurement of the patient's speech recognition performance with and without the hearing aid. The patient is typically presented with a sample of continuous speech or speech-shaped noise at a level approximating conversational levels (65- or 70-dB SPL). While listening to this stimulus, the patient adjusts the volume control on the hearing aid to a comfortable setting. Next, speech recognition testing is conducted, with the materials being presented at the same overall level (65- to 70-dB SPL). Speech recognition testing is often performed both in quiet and in a background of noise to permit evaluation of the benefit provided

VIGNETTE 9.5 • CONCEPTUAL DEMO

Measurement of Real-Ear Insertion Gain

As noted in the text, the measurement of REIG is a common first step in the verification of the fit of the hearing aid. The drawing below illustrates the basic arrangement of equipment needed for this measurement. Basically, a small loudspeaker is located at ear level about 1 m from the patient (either straight ahead or at a slight angle). A long, very narrow, flexible tube, referred to as the probe tube, is inserted into the ear canal. The closed end of the probe tube terminates at a microphone, and the microphone is connected to the real-ear measurement device. This device sends stimuli to the

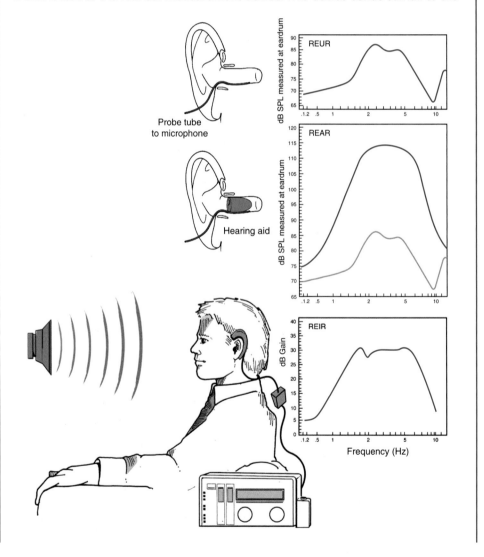

loudspeaker and records the measurements made with the microphone at the end of the probe tube. (Often, another microphone is attached to the side of the patient's head to monitor and regulate the output level of the loudspeaker at the patient's ear.)

The top panel above illustrates the position of the probe tube in the ear canal for the initial unaided measurements. When the sound is presented from the loudspeaker as a series of 60-dB SPL pure tones increasing in frequency from 100 to 10,000 Hz and measured in the open ear canal with the probe tube, a frequency response like that shown in the top panel is obtained. This is referred to as the real-ear unaided response or REUR. It shows the 15- to 20-dB resonant boost provided by the ear canal and pinna (see Chapter 3). The middle panel above shows the next measurement made with the hearing aid inserted and adjusted to the appropriate settings. Sound is again presented from the loudspeaker as a series of 60-dB SPL pure tones increasing in frequency from 100 to 10,000 Hz. The sound levels recorded with the probe-tube microphone in the aided condition are referred to as the real-ear aided response or REAR.

The lower panel shows the difference between the REAR and REUR curves and is referred to as the real-ear insertion response or REIR. Essentially, this curve shows how much REIG was provided, in dB, at each frequency from 100 to 10,000 Hz as a result of hearing aid insertion. If the REIR was flat at 0 dB, for example, this would imply that there was no gain provided by the hearing aid. The audiologist compares the REIR to target values generated by various prescription procedures and fine-tunes the hearing aid until the REIR demonstrates a close match to the target values. The REIR is a reliable measure, can be obtained in a matter of minutes, provides a very detailed picture of the hearing aid's response on that particular patient, and requires no active participation on the part of the hearing aid wearer. It has become a very common and powerful tool for the verification of a hearing aid's performance on an individual wearer.

by the hearing aid for a range of conditions representative of those in which the hearing aid is to be worn. The speech recognition measures are also often obtained from the patient in quiet and in noise under identical stimulus conditions without the hearing aid. The difference in performance between the aided and unaided measures provides a general indication of the benefit provided by the hearing aid under various listening conditions. These direct measures of the effects of the hearing aid on speech recognition performance have sometimes been referred to as "objective" measures of benefit.

In addition to these objective measures of hearing aid benefit, the hearing aid evaluation should also include some "subjective" measures of performance and benefit. Most commonly, self-assessment surveys or inventories of hearing handicap and hearing aid performance have been used with adults. Self-report measures of hearing aid benefit, satisfaction, and usage should also be obtained at a follow-up visit about 4 to 6 weeks following the hearing aid fitting.

Hearing Aid Orientation

Hearing aids are typically sold in the United States on a 30-day trial basis; dissatisfied patients are given a refund at the end of that trial period. During the trial period, the patient is encouraged to visit the audiologist two or three times for a series of hearing aid orientations. During the hearing aid orientations, the patient is instructed in the use and care of the hearing aid, counseled about its limitations, given strategies to maximize its benefit, and given an opportunity to voice any complaints about its function. Frequently, modification of the earmold or the earpiece (shell) of the aid is needed to make the hearing aid fit more comfortably in the patient's ear. The hearing aid may require some electronic adjustments as well. After the 30-day trial period, the hearing aid user is encouraged to return for further evaluation in a year or sooner if he or she experiences difficulty.

ALTERNATIVE PROSTHETIC DEVICES

Assistive Listening Devices

As mentioned previously, full-time use of a hearing aid is not necessary or beneficial for many hearing-impaired individuals. A number of adults with mild hearing loss require only part-time use of a hearing aid or alternative device. For many of these individuals, a practical alternative is a class of devices known as **assistive listening devices**. These devices are typically electroacoustic devices designed with a much more limited purpose in mind than that of the conventional hearing aid. Two of the most common purposes for which these devices were developed include use of the telephone and listening to the television. Several telephone handsets have been developed, for instance, that can amplify the telephone signal by 15 to 30 dB. These devices are effective for adults with mild hearing loss who have difficulty communicating over the telephone.

Many of the assistive listening devices physically separate the microphone from the rest of the device so that the microphone can be placed closer to the source of the desired sound. Recall that the microphone converts an acoustic signal into an electrical one so that it can be amplified by the device. If the microphone on the assistive listening device is separated by a great distance from the rest of the device, then the electrical signal from the microphone must somehow be sent to the amplifier. This is accomplished in various ways, with some devices simply running a wire, several feet in length, directly from the microphone to the amplifier. Other devices convert the electrical signal from the microphone into radio waves (FM) or invisible light waves (infrared) and send the signal to a receiver adjacent to the amplifier and worn by the individual. The receiver converts the FM or infrared signal back to an electrical signal and sends it to the amplifier to be amplified.

The FM and infrared systems are frequently referred to as wireless systems because they eliminate the long wire running directly from the microphone to the amplifier. The wireless feature of these assistive listening devices makes them more versatile and easier to use, but it also makes them more expensive. These assistive listening devices overcome the primary disadvantage of the conventional hearing aid; they improve the speech-to-noise ratio. By separating the microphone from the rest of the device and positioning it closer to the sound source (e.g., the talker's mouth or the loudspeaker of the television set), the primary signal of interest is amplified more than the surrounding background noise. On a conventional hearing aid, the ear-level microphone amplifies both the speech and the surrounding noise equally well; therefore, the speech-to-noise ratio is not improved, and all sound at the position of the microphone is simply made louder by the conventional hearing aid (see Vignette 9.6).

Separating the microphone from the rest of the device, however, has its drawbacks. It is only a reasonable alternative when the sound source is fairly stable over time. If the microphone is positioned near the loudspeaker of the television, for example, the voice of a talker seated next to the impaired person will not be amplified. The impaired individual is forced to listen to the sound source closest to the microphone. For assistive listening devices, this is not a serious drawback because they have a limited purpose.

Selection and evaluation of assistive listening devices are not as formalized as it is for hearing aids. Most hearing clinics today have a room designated as the "assistive listening device area." This room or area is set up to simulate the conditions under which the devices are to be used. Typically, the room takes on the atmosphere of a living room or family room, with television, stereo, and telephones available. After the patient's needs have been assessed through a written or oral questionnaire, several assistive devices are tried by the patient under controlled conditions in the simulated environment. If the patient finds the device beneficial, it is dispensed by the audiologist, or the patient is referred to an appropriate source for its purchase.

Assistive devices of various types also benefit the severely or profoundly impaired. In addition to those devices mentioned above, some nonauditory devices have been developed. Devices have been produced that flash lights in response to various acoustic signals occurring in the home, such as the ringing of the doorbell or the telephone. Other special telephone devices enable text to be sent over phone lines (in printed form) so that a profoundly impaired person can carry on a telephone conversation by sending and receiving text messages. Special keyboard-like devices are needed at both ends of the phone line to enable such communication.

In addition to the preceding assistive listening devices, some of the alternative amplification systems described below in the section on "Classroom

VIGNETTE 9.6 • FURTHER DISCUSSION

Effects of a Hearing Aid on Speech Understanding in Quiet and in Noise

The *left-hand panel* in the figure a high-frequency sensorineural hearing loss, not unlike that found in many elderly individuals, has been superimposed on the speech audiogram. Notice that many of the high-frequency, low-intensity consonants are no longer heard by the individual with this hearing loss, although many low- and mid-frequency speech sounds (such as vowels and nasal sounds) remain audible. As noted previously, a frequent complaint of individuals with this very common type of hearing loss is that they can hear speech but they can't understand it.

In the *right-hand panel*, the speech sounds have been amplified by a well-fit hearing aid. In this case, a well-fit hearing aid would amplify the high frequencies to make the high-frequency consonants audible to the patient while not amplifying the low frequencies, where hearing is essentially normal. With the audibility of all of the speech sounds in conversational speech restored by the hearing aid as shown in this panel, the hearing aid wearer will regain the ability to understand speech as well as a normal-hearing listener. Depending, in part, on how long they have become accustomed to hearing speech through their hearing loss, the time required to perform normally will vary from patient to patient.

In noise, however, the microphone of the hearing aid amplifies the noise as much as the speech; thus, the speech-to-noise ratio is not improved by the conventional hearing aid. If the conversational speech of the person in front of the listener is 6 dB greater at the input to the hearing aid (microphone) than the background of babble produced by the other attendees at a cocktail party, then this 6-dB speech-to-noise ratio will remain at the output from the hearing aid. The speech will be made audible by the hearing aid but so will the noise. Consequently, conventional hearing aids are generally not considered to work as well in noise as in quiet.

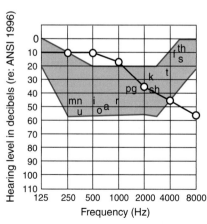

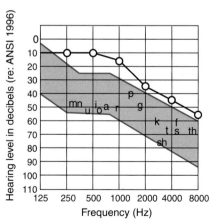

Amplification" are also available to adults in other public meeting places aside from school classrooms. Auditoriums, theaters, churches, synagogues, and other gathering places make frequent use of the FM and infrared systems described below. One alternative that used to be more commonplace in school classrooms, but has now come to the forefront for other public meeting places, such as those noted above, as well as airports and train stations, is the induction loop system. Basically, a microphone or other audio input is directed to an amplifier connected to a loop of wire that runs under the flooring or carpet in a public space (or in a suspended ceiling). There are a wide variety of ways the wire loop may be arranged under the flooring or above the ceiling, and the particular pattern selected varies widely with room size and purpose. Regardless of the loop pattern used, the method underlying this approach is the same. As the electrical signal from the audio input runs through the wire under the flooring, a magnetic field is generated. This is a natural by-product of electric current running through wire. The magnetic field, however, radiates several feet through the space around the wire. Hearing aid wearers and cochlear implant wearers simply switch their devices from microphone input to telecoil input (an option included in just about all devices), and the telecoil receives (transduces) the magnetic field, converting it into an electrical signal within the hearing aid or cochlear implant. For the reasons noted below when describing classroom amplification systems, the desired signal, such as the speech of a talker, is picked up clearly and any background noise is reduced. There have been various initiatives taking place around the world to install such induction loops in all public gathering spaces with "Let's Loop America!" being a representative initiative in the United States (http://www.hearingloop.org//loopAmerica.htm).

Classroom Amplification

A discussion of hearing aids would not be complete without a review of the special amplification systems designed for education. Classroom amplification is a term used to describe a hearing aid device that provides amplified sound to a group of children while in the classroom. Classroom amplification gained added importance with the advent of IDEA, a federal mandate regarding the education of all handicapped children. The law required that schools provide hearing-impaired children with adequate services and funding. This included habilitative/rehabilitative services, such as selection and evaluation of personal hearing aids and group systems, auditory training, speech training, speechreading, and any other services deemed necessary for the child's educational development.

Why should a child need a special educational amplification system? A primary concern is the acoustic environment that children are exposed to in the classroom. Children are continually bombarded with excessively high noise levels that interfere with their ability to understand the teacher and other children in the classroom. These noise levels originate from sources outside the school building (aircraft or car traffic), within the school building (adjacent classrooms and hallways, activity areas, heating/cooling systems), and within the classroom itself (students talking, feet shuffling, noise from moving furniture). These various noise sources contribute to noise levels ranging from 40 to 67 dBA.[1] Such high noise levels result in an unfavorable signal-to-noise (S:N) or speech-to-noise ratio reaching the child's ear. A S:N ratio represents the difference, in decibels, between speech (from the teacher) and the overall ambient noise (noise within the classroom). For example, a S:N ratio of +10 dB means that the teacher's speech is 10 dB more intense than the noise in the classroom. Ideally, a S:N ratio of +20 dB is necessary if a child with hearing loss is to understand speech maximally. Noise surveys in classrooms have shown that S:N ratios typically range from -6 dB to +6 dB, a listening environment that precludes maximal understanding even for normal-hearing children.

Classroom noise is not the only variable that contributes to a difficult listening environment. Reverberation time, a term used to denote the amount of time it takes for sound to decrease by 60 dB after the termination of a signal, also contributes to an adverse acoustic environment. When a teacher talks to the child, some of the speech signal reaches the child's amplification system within just a few milliseconds. The remainder of the signal, however, strikes surrounding areas and reaches the child's ear after the initial sound in the form of reflections. The strength and duration of these reflections are affected by the absorption quality of the surrounding surfaces and the size (volume) of the classroom. If an area has hard walls, ceilings, and floors, the room will have a long reverberation time. In contrast, an acoustically treated room with carpeting, drapes, and an acoustic tile ceiling will have a shorter reverberation time. Generally, as reverberation time increases, the proportion of reflected speech sound reaching the listener increases and speech recognition decreases. In addition, the smaller the room size, the greater the reverberation. Many classrooms for the hearing impaired have reverberation times ranging from a very mild value of 0.2 s to more severe reverberation, with times greater than 1 s.

These factors, noise and reverberation, are known to adversely affect speech recognition. As the noise levels and reverberation times increase, the S:N ratio

---

[1]As noted previously, sound level meters have three weighting networks (A, B, C) that are designed to respond differently to noise frequencies. The A network mainly weighs (filters) the low frequencies below 500 Hz and approximates the response characteristics of the human ear. The federal government recommends the A network for measuring noise levels.

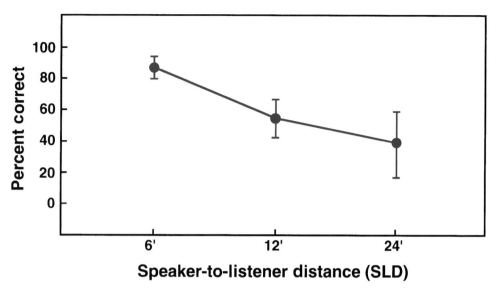

FIGURE 9.6 Typical speech recognition scores for normal-hearing children at different speaker-to-listener distances. At 6 feet, the signal-to-noise ratio is +6 dB and the reverberation time is 0.46 s.

becomes less favorable, and there is a significant breakdown in speech understanding. Further, as the distance between the talker and listener increases, the S:N ratio worsens. Figure 9.6 illustrates this phenomenon.

Children with hearing loss not only experience difficulty understanding speech under difficult listening situations, but they also expend a great deal of effort in attending to the spoken message. Studies have demonstrated that not only does the presence of noise increase learning effort, it even reduces the energy available for performing other cognitive functions. Even young school-age children with very mild forms of hearing loss have reported less energy or were tired more frequently than children with normal hearing. These findings may well be a result of the difficulties these children experience listening under adverse listening conditions. One can speculate that toward the end of a school day, children with hearing loss will be physically and mentally "spent" as a result of focusing so intently on the teacher's speech and on the conversations of other children. This expenditure of effort will no doubt compromise a child's ability to learn in the classroom.

Several types of special educational amplification systems have been designed to overcome the adverse effects of the classroom environment by offering a better S:N ratio (see Vignette 9.7). These system types include hard-wire systems, FM wireless systems, infrared systems, and a system that combines the FM wireless system with a personal hearing aid. More recently, sound-field amplification systems have been developed as yet another option for use in the classroom and

VIGNETTE 9.7 • FURTHER DISCUSSION

Improving the Speech-to-Noise Ratio with an Assistive Listening Device or Classroom System

In this vignette, we will make use of the same "speech audiogram" concept used in Vignette 9.6. The *left-hand panel* below shows the speech audiogram for conversational speech with a background noise (several other people talking) as it has been amplified by a hearing aid. This is the same as the right-hand panel of Vignette 9.6 with the addition of background noise. The level of the noise is indicated by the *heavy dashed line*. The speech and noise levels shown here represent those measured through the hearing aid with the listener in the middle of a living room or classroom full of people at about 1 m from the desired talker.

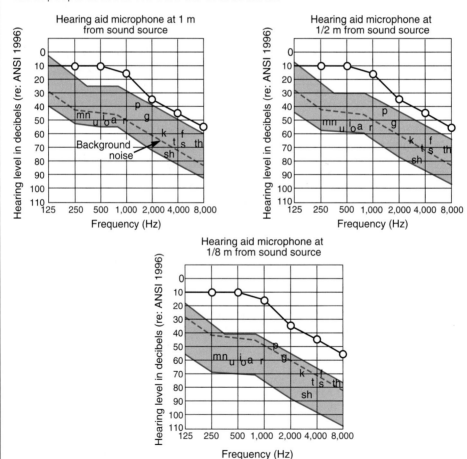

In the *middle panel*, the microphone has been detached from the hearing aid and is now positioned about half a meter from the primary talker. (The hearing aid's microphone really can't be detached. We're just pretending that it is to illustrate the concept behind assistive listening devices.) As the distance to the sound source is halved (from 1 m to a half meter), the sound level increases by 6 dB. Notice that the speech is now 6 dB higher than it was in the *left-hand panel*, whereas the diffuse background noise (*dashed line*) coming from a variety of sources, including reflections from walls and the ceiling, remains unchanged. Thus, the speech-to-noise ratio has improved 6 dB.

In the *right-hand panel*, we have positioned the microphone still closer to the sound source, approximately 1/8 m (4 to 5 inches) from the primary talker's mouth. As a result, the speech level from the talker has increased another 12 dB (two more halvings of the distance), and the speech-to-noise ratio has been improved a total of 18 dB compared with that in the *left-hand panel*.

As noted in Vignette 9.6, the conventional hearing aid does not improve the signal-to-noise ratio but simply amplifies the acoustic signals, speech and noise alike, that arrive at the microphone (*left panel*). By moving the microphone closer to the desired sound source (*middle* and *right panels*), whether a talker or a loudspeaker, the speech signal level is increased while the background noise remains unaffected. The result is an improved speech-to-noise ratio and better communication. This is the primary operational principle behind many assistive listening devices, as well as similar classroom amplification systems.

one that may benefit *all* students in the classroom, not just those with hearing impairment. The concept behind these systems is similar to that described for the assistive listening devices. The microphone is moved closer to the desired sound source, the teacher. A brief description of each of these systems follows.

Hard-Wire System

In this system, a microphone worn by the teacher is wired to an amplifier. Each student then wears headphones or insert-type receivers that are connected to the amplifier by wires so that the teacher and the students are, in effect, "tethered" together (Fig. 9.7, *top*). The primary advantage of a hard-wire system is the high fidelity and high level of output available through earphones. These systems are inexpensive and are simple and easy to operate. The obvious disadvantage is the restricted mobility of both the teacher and students. Hard-wire systems are not very commonplace in classrooms today.

FM Wireless Systems

Most classrooms for the hearing-impaired use either FM devices or a combination of an FM system and a personal hearing aid. A microphone transmitter is worn around the teacher's neck, and a signal is broadcast to an FM receiver worn by the child (Fig. 9.7, *bottom*). Most FM receivers have

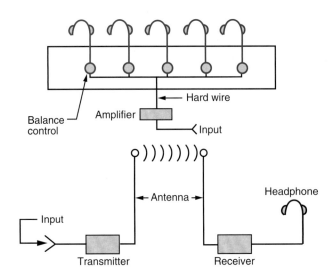

FIGURE 9.7 Two classroom amplification systems. *Top,* hard wire. *Bottom,* FM. The personal hearing aid could replace the headphones shown at *bottom* to produce a dovetailed system.

an environmental microphone so that the child can monitor his or her own voice, the voices of his or her peers, and other environmental sounds. When the environmental microphone is used, however, the S:N ratio is compromised because of the distance between the talker and the microphone. The advantage to this system is the mobility allowed. In other words, the teacher and the students are free to move around the room and the students will continue to receive amplification.

Infrared Systems

Infrared group amplification is seldom used in classroom settings but is used widely as an assistive device in theaters, churches, and other public facilities. As mentioned earlier, the system uses an infrared emitter that transmits the speech signal from the input microphone to individually worn infrared-receiver/audio-amplifier units. It is very similar in design to the FM system shown in Figure 9.7 (*bottom*), except that infrared light waves are used to send the signal from the transmitter to the receiver rather than FM radio waves. Infrared systems, however, are somewhat limited in power output.

Coupling the FM Wireless System to the Child's Ear

With personal FM systems, the teacher wears a microphone/transmitter that broadcasts carrier waves to a receiver worn by the child. A number of options are available for coupling the FM system to the child's ear. A summary of the coupling options that can be used with FM systems is shown in Vignette 9.8.

VIGNETTE 9.8 • CLINICAL APPLICATIONS

Methods of Coupling the FM System to the Child's Ear

Several options exist for coupling the FM system to the ear. One option is to simply combine the FM device to the personal hearing aid. This approach, commonly referred to as dovetailing, is done to take advantage of the benefits of both systems: the improved speech-to-noise ratio offered by the FM system and the custom fitting of the personal hearing aid. One approach for combining the FM system with the personal hearing aid is the incorporation of an FM receiver into an audio boot. When the boot is slipped on to an appropriate hearing aid, FM reception is possible. Some

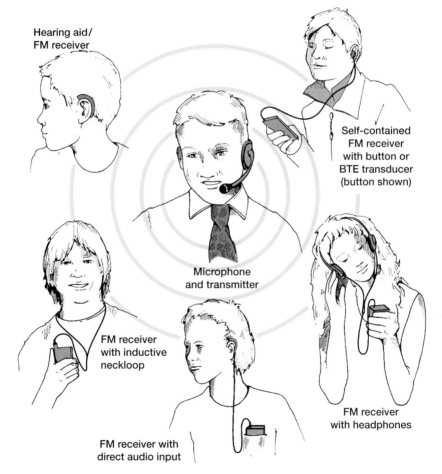

Hearing aid/
FM receiver

Self-contained
FM receiver
with button or
BTE transducer
(button shown)

Microphone
and transmitter

FM receiver
with inductive
neckloop

FM receiver
with headphones

FM receiver with
direct audio input

(Figure adapted from Lewis DE. Classroom amplification. In: Bess FH, ed. *Children with Hearing Impairment: Contemporary Trends*. Nashville, TN: Bill Wilkerson Center Press; 1998.)

boots use an electrical connection from the student-worn receiver to the hearing aid; some manufacturers have developed wireless boots. Another approach to coupling a personal hearing aid to the FM system is via inductive coupling. With this device, the FM signal, which is sometimes mixed with an environmental signal within the student receiver, is converted to an electromagnetic field via a wire loop encircling the child's neck. The personal hearing aid is worn in the telecoil position, thereby inductively coupling a hearing aid to the FM receiver/mini-loop combination. A third approach is the use of a BTE FM receiver, a development brought about through advances in microminiature FM technology. The BTE houses, at ear level, both the FM receiver and the hearing aid circuitry, thus eliminating the need for cords, neckloops, and body-worn receivers. The BTE FM system device looks like a conventional BTE hearing aid. Other techniques for coupling the FM receiver to the child's ear include an FM system receiver with Sony Walkman–type earbuds/headphones or simply a self-contained FM receiver with a button or BTE transducer.

Sound-Field Amplification

Sound-field systems broadcast the signal from the teacher's transmitter via FM transmission to an amplifier connected to a series of loudspeakers placed strategically around the classroom (Fig. 9.8). Often, the loudspeakers are suspended from the ceiling, with at least two loudspeakers in the front and two at the rear of the classroom. The basic idea is that, through the presentation of the teacher's voice from loudspeakers dispersed throughout the classroom, no student is too far from the primary signal (the teacher's voice), and a favorable S:N is maintained throughout the classroom. Thus, the amplified signal is delivered uniformly to *all* students, rather than just those with hearing impairment. This can prove to be of benefit to not just other students with special needs but to normal-hearing

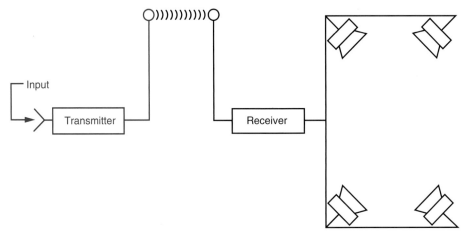

FIGURE 9.8 Diagram of a sound-field amplification system.

children as well. As noted previously, the acoustics in many classrooms are poor and even normal-hearing children may find listening a challenge at times.

Similar to other amplification devices, the sound-field system has limitations— the amount of amplification is limited (8 to 10 dB), and the system amplifies only the teacher's voice, not the voices of other children. Of course, the hearing-impaired child can receive additional benefit from the use of a personal hearing aid in a classroom equipped with sound-field amplification. The low cost of the system and its potential to benefit many students in the classroom, though, make it an attractive alternative for many schools.

A number of other populations known to experience difficulty under classroom-type noise conditions may also receive benefit from sound-field ampli-fication. These populations include young children under the age of 15 years; chil-dren with articulation disorders; children with language disorders; children who are learning disabled, nonnative English speakers; children with central auditory processing deficits; and children with a history of middle ear disease with effusion.

Cochlear Implants

In the 1980s, the cochlear implant emerged as a viable alternative to conven-tional amplification for individuals with profound hearing impairment. Several types of cochlear implants are available commercially today. They all share a common conceptual framework, but differ in its implementation. The cochlear implant is a device that is surgically implanted, with its stimulating electrode array (wire) inserted directly into the cochlea. The implant contains from 1 to 22 channels. Although individuals with the earlier single-channel cochlear implants may still be encountered by the clinician, all contemporary devices make use of multiple electrode arrays. The electrode is used to stimulate the auditory nerve directly with electric current, bypassing the damaged cochlear structures. As in the conventional hearing aid, a microphone is used to convert the acoustic signal into an electrical one. The electrical signal is then amplified and processed in various ways in a separate, body-worn component known as the processor or stimulator. The stimulator is about the size of a body-worn hearing aid or a package of cigarettes. Most recently, however, the stimula-tor and microphone have been combined into one ear-level unit, very similar to a BTE hearing aid. The output of the processor or stimulator is then sent to an external receiver worn behind the ear. This external receiver activates a similar internal receiver implanted surgically just under the skin and behind the ear. The implanted internal receiver converts the received signal into an electrical one and directs it to the electrode array penetrating the cochlea. This electrical signal, when routed to the electrode array, stimulates the remaining healthy auditory nerve fibers of the damaged inner ear. Figure 9.9 illustrates

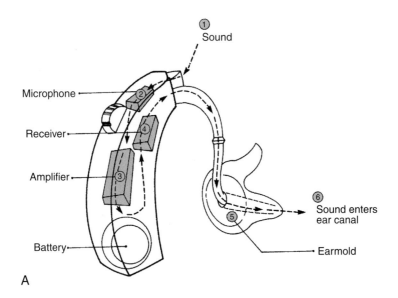

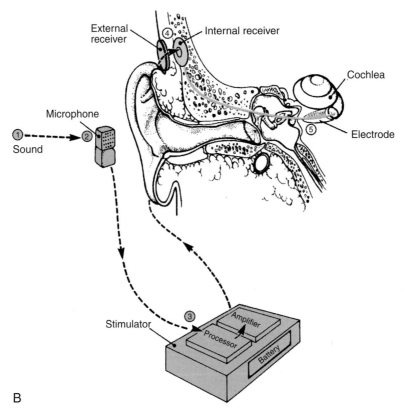

FIGURE 9.9 Illustration of the similarities between conventional BTE hearing aid (*A*) and cochlear implant device (*B*). The components of each system are numbered identically to highlight the similarities.

a typical arrangement for a cochlear implant and compares this device with a conventional hearing aid. As can be seen, these two devices share many features.

As noted, contemporary cochlear implants are multiple-channel devices. The "channels" essentially refer to adjacent bands in the frequency domain analogous to a series of band-pass filters. The sound picked up by the microphone is analyzed and sorted into several frequency-specific packets of information, or channels of information, by the processor. The output of each channel is then routed to a corresponding electrode in the electrode array that is positioned in a specific location along the length of the cochlea. Thus, low-frequency channels are connected to electrodes in the more apical region of the cochlea, whereas high-frequency channels are connected to electrodes in more basal locations. This system is an attempt to restore tonotopic mapping (see Chapter 3) to the damaged cochlea.

For older children and adults, the *ideal* candidates for cochlear implants are those persons who acquired profound bilateral sensorineural hearing loss after acquiring language. Cochlear implants, however, appear to hold even greater promise for profoundly impaired prelingual children under 2 or 3 years of age, although research regarding the comparative benefits of rehabilitative devices in this population is still in progress. Even though the results of clinical trials with these devices have varied markedly between patients, the best performance has been achieved with the multichannel devices implanted at the earliest ages. There are examples of so-called "star" patients who perform remarkably well with the device without any visual cues and do so almost immediately. At a minimum, just about every recipient benefits from the device as an aid to speechreading and by increased awareness of sound. Its primary usefulness as an aid to speechreading seems to lie in making gross cues of timing and voicing available to the patient. Great strides continue to be made in the devices and in the training programs after implantation such that implants are the rehabilitative device of choice for the profoundly impaired, especially if implanted at an early age before the acquisition of language. Benefits of cochlear implantation have also been demonstrated in individuals with severe hearing loss as well, although the superiority of the implant to the hearing aid for severe hearing loss is less well established.

The cochlear implant is intended to be a permanent, long-term solution to an extreme break (profound sensorineural hearing loss) in the communication chain. Compared to the cost of hearing aids, cochlear implants are 40 to 50 times more expensive (at least in terms of initial device purchase). Due to their expense, permanence, and irreversible destruction of any residual sensory structures in the cochlea, it would be beneficial to know the likelihood that a cochlear implant would be successful in a particular person *prior* to implantation. Such predictions are perhaps of greatest value for cochlear implant candidates who are young children who have yet to acquire a language system. This has been an active area of research in recent years, and progress continues to be made in identifying critical factors impacting the successful use of cochlear implants by children. For example, research published in 2003 identified several factors that increased the likelihood for a successful outcome with cochlear implants. Regarding the person receiving the implant, the likelihood of success with cochlear implants was enhanced for those young children who were female, had higher IQs, and were from smaller families with higher socioeconomic status. Of these factors, perhaps the only one that is somewhat surprising is the implant recipient's gender. Smaller families with more money have both the time and financial resources to provide the necessary intensive and extensive follow-up training that is needed. In addition, a higher IQ most likely reflects a better capability of the recipient's brain to make use of this new sensory code. In addition to these characteristics of the child or his or her family, factors associated with the devices themselves and the educational setting of the child were also identified that increased the odds for a successful outcome. Regarding the device, the greater the number of active electrodes, the better the child's performance with the implant. Regarding the educational setting, those who were in auditory-oral classrooms or in regular classrooms with normal-hearing peers performed the best with their cochlear implants. Although this research is still ongoing and only the first few years of longitudinal data have been gathered and analyzed for these children, to date, these data indicate that about 50% of these profoundly hearing-impaired children who were implanted at an early age have achieved language and reading skills at or above their normal-hearing peers.

In the year 2000, there were about 30,000 cochlear implant wearers worldwide and about half of these were children (under the age of 18 years). In 2006, it was estimated that there were 100,000 cochlear implant recipients. By 2010, 219,000 individuals worldwide had received cochlear implants. Clearly, these devices are increasing in popularity and will most likely continue to do so as the technology continues to improve. Just as with hearing aids, the devices have continued to become physically smaller and less conspicuous while concurrently improving the signal-processing technology. Technologies that have proven to be somewhat successful with hearing aids, such as directional microphones to improve speech understanding in noise, are also being investigated with cochlear implants. One current issue under investigation by researchers is the relative benefit of bilateral cochlear implants, or the combination of an implant on one ear and a high-powered hearing aid on the other ear, over a single cochlear implant.

The importance of amplification or cochlear implantation to the hearing-impaired child cannot be overemphasized. The personal hearing aid or cochlear implant and other amplification devices are the primary link many of these children have to an auditory society. If these children are to develop speech and language in a manner somewhat similar to that of the normal-hearing child, everything possible must be done to capitalize on whatever residual hearing exists. Toward this end, the child receives amplification (usually binaural) or cochlear implantation (currently, usually monaural) soon after identification. The audiologist then offers periodic hearing evaluations and modifies the hearing aid fitting(s) or cochlear implant processor as more is learned about the child's hearing sensitivity.

DEVICE MANAGEMENT

The prosthetic device, whether a hearing aid, FM classroom device, or cochlear implant, is one of the most important aspects of rehabilitation for the majority of hearing-impaired individuals. It is essential that every precaution be taken to assure that the device is always in good working order.

For the vast majority of hearing-impaired individuals, the conventional electroacoustic hearing aid is the prosthetic device of choice. Care must be taken to avoid dropping the instrument or exposing the aid to severe environmental conditions, such as excessive moisture or heat. If dampness reaches the microphone or receiver, it can render the unit inoperable. It is also important to check the earmold or canal portion of the device periodically for blockage by cerumen and signs of wear from extended use, such as a cracked earmold or tubing. Perhaps the most common problem that interferes with adequate hearing aid performance is the battery or battery compartment area. Old batteries that have lost their charge, inappropriate battery size, inadequate battery contact, and improper battery placement are all problems that can contribute to a nonworking hearing aid.

Consistent amplification for the young child with hearing impairment is essential. Yet numerous school surveys have revealed that approximately one-half of children's hearing aids do not perform satisfactorily. The most common problems seen among hearing-impaired children are weak batteries, inadequate earmolds, broken cords, bad receivers (sometimes the wrong receiver), and high distortion levels. Even the FM wireless systems are susceptible to faulty performance. Approximately 30% to 50% of these systems have been reported to perform unsatisfactorily in the classroom setting. The solution to inconsistent and inadequate amplification is the implementation of a daily hearing aid check using a form like the one shown in Table 9.1. In addition, the school audiologist must conduct a periodic electroacoustic analysis of every child's hearing aid. Some simple troubleshooting tips for speech-language pathologists working with children wearing hearing aids or cochlear implants in the schools are provided in Vignette 9.9.

9.1

Sample Monitoring Form for a Personal Hearing Aid Worn by a Hearing-Impaired Child

Student _____

Teacher _____ Aid make/model _____

School _____ Serial no. _____

Classroom _____

Electroacoustic check _____ Y _____ N

Date of inspection _____

Overall condition: _____ Satisfactory _____ Marginal _____ Unsatisfactory _____ Missing

Recommendations_____
_____
_____

Examiner _____

Problem Checklist

Item	Inspected? Yes	No	Comments
Battery	_____	_____	_____
Battery compartment	_____	_____	_____
Microphone	_____	_____	_____
Power switch	_____	_____	_____
Gain control	_____	_____	_____
Telephone switch	_____	_____	_____
Tone control	_____	_____	_____
Amplifier	_____	_____	_____
Cord	_____	_____	_____
Receiver	_____	_____	_____
Earmold	_____	_____	_____
Clip/case	_____	_____	_____
Harness	_____	_____	_____
Other	_____	_____	_____
As-worn setting			
Volume control	_____		
Tone control	_____		
Receiver type	_____		

VIGNETTE 9.9 • CLINICAL APPLICATIONS

Simple Troubleshooting Tips for Hearing Aids and Cochlear Implants for the Speech-Language Pathologist

For hearing aids:

- No sound
  - Make sure the aid is turned on.
  - Replace the battery and make sure "+" side is up.
  - If aid has a telecoil ("T") switch, make sure it is in the microphone ("M") position.
  - Use listening device check ("listening stethoscope") to verify function of hearing aid.
  - For a BTE, remove earmold from the earhook of the hearing aid, clean with soapy water, rinse, and dry with air blower; for ITE, use wax loop device to clean receiver tube.
- Whistling/feedback
  - Make sure the earmold is in the ear properly.
  - Check volume control to make sure volume is not too high.
  - For BTE, check earmold to see if clogged with wax and clean as described above; for ITE, use wax loop device to clean receiver tube.
  - Have audiologist or school nurse check child's ear canal for wax.

For cochlear implants:

- Child does not respond to sound during behavioral check.
  - Make sure the processor is turned on.
  - Turn the processor off and then back on.
  - Replace battery (and recharge old battery, if rechargeable).
  - Make sure processor is set to the correct program and settings.
  - Check cables and cords to make sure they are connected properly to the processor. Visually inspect them for twisting, breaks, etc.
  - Use monitor earphones or listening check device to verify microphone function.

(Adapted from Schafer EC, Sweeney M. A sound classroom environment. *ASHA Leader* 2012;14–17.)

SUMMARY

In this chapter, we have reviewed and discussed the more pertinent aspects of amplification, cochlear implantation, and rehabilitation of hearing-impaired children and adults. It was noted that the hearing aid and the cochlear implant are the most important rehabilitative tools we have available to us for the management of the hearing impaired. Numerous types of amplification systems, including personal hearing aids, assistive listening devices, and classroom systems, are available for the habilitation/rehabilitation of hearing-impaired individuals.

CHAPTER REVIEW QUESTIONS

1. Consider two 9-year-old children in a classroom, one of whom has a mild (35-dB HL) flat bilateral sensorineural hearing loss and the other who has a profound (90-dB HL) flat bilateral sensorineural hearing loss. Assume that the hearing loss was present and identified at birth in both children and that optimal early intervention focusing on an auditory-oral approach to rehabilitation followed the identification of hearing loss. What would be the auditory prosthetic device most likely used by each child? Why?
2. For each child in Question 1 above, would it be likely that supplemental auditory prosthetic devices would be used in the classroom? Address this separately for each child and indicate which device(s), if any, would be used by each child in the classroom.
3. Regardless of how you answered Question 1 above, assume for this question that both children have been fit with hearing aids and a two-thirds gain rule was used to set the gain of the hearing aids. How much gain in decibel is needed at each frequency by each child? Assuming that this gain is achieved for each child and there is no limit to output, what would the output of the hearing aids be for each child when a 60-dB SPL input is provided to the hearing aid? For a 90-dB SPL input? Would this cause any problems for the wearer and, if so, how might this be remedied?

REFERENCES AND SUGGESTED READINGS

Bess FH, Gravel JS, Tharpe AM. *Amplification for Children with Auditory Deficits.* Nashville, TN: Bill Wilkerson Center Press; 1996.

Blamey PJ, Sarant JZ, Paatsch LE, et al. Relationships among speech perception, production, language, hearing loss, and age in children with impaired hearing. *J Speech Lang Hear Res* 2001;44:264–285.

Byrne D. Theoretical prescriptive approaches to selecting the gain and frequency response of a hearing aid. *Monogr Contemp Audiol* 1983;4:1–40.

Connor CM. Speech, vocabulary, and the education of children using cochlear implants. Oral or total communication? *J Speech Lang Hear Res* 2000;43:1185–1204.

Connor CM. Examining multiple sources of influence on the reading comprehension skills of children who use cochlear implants. *J Speech Lang Hear Res* 2004;47:509–526.

Dillon H. *Hearing Aids*. 2nd ed. New York, NY: Thieme; 2012.

Geers AE, Moog JS. Predicting spoken language acquisition of profoundly hearing impaired children. *J Speech Hear Dis* 1987;52:84–94.

Geers AE, Brenner C, Davidson L. Factors associated with development of speech perception skills in children implanted by age five. *Ear Hear* 2003;24: 24S–35S.

Geers AE, Nicholas JG, Sedey AL. Language skills of children with early cochlear implantation. *Ear Hear* 2003;24:46S–58S.

Geers AE. Predictors of reading skill development in children with early cochlear implantation. *Ear Hear* 2003;24:59S–68S.

Hawkins D, Yacullo W. The signal-to-noise ratio advantage of binaural hearing aids and directional microphones under different levels of reverberation. *J Speech Hearing Dis* 1984;49:278–286.

High WS, Fairbanks G, Glorig A. Scale for self-assessment of hearing handicap. *J Speech Hear Dis* 1964;17:321–327.

Humes LE, Krull V. Evidence about the effectiveness of hearing aids for adults. In: Wong L, Hickson L, eds. *Evidence-Based Practice in Audiology: Evaluating Interventions for Children and Adults with Hearing Impairment*. Chapter 4. San Diego, CA: Plural, 2012.

Katz J. *Handbook of Clinical Audiology*. 6th ed. Baltimore, MD: Lippincott Williams & Wilkins; 2009.

Giolas TE, Owens E, Lamb SH, et al. Hearing performance inventory. *J Speech Hear Dis* 1979;44:169–195.

Mueller HG, Grimes MA. Hearing aid selection and assessment. In: Alpiner JG, McCarthy PA, eds. *Rehabilitative Audiology: Children and Adults*. 2nd ed. Baltimore, MD: Williams & Wilkins; 1993.

Moeller MP, Brunt MA. Management of preschool hearing-impaired children: A cognitive-linguistic approach. In: Bess FH, ed. *Hearing Impairment in Children*. Parkton, MD: York Press; 1988.

Moeller MP, Carney AE. Assessment and intervention with preschool hearing-impaired children. In: Alpiner JG, McCarthy PA, eds. *Rehabilitative Audiology: Children and Adults*. 2nd ed. Baltimore, MD: Williams & Wilkins; 1993.

Mueller HG, Grimes A. Amplification systems for the hearing impaired. In: Alpiner JF, McCarthy PA, eds. *Rehabilitative Audiology: Children and Adults*. Baltimore, MD: Williams & Wilkins; 1987.

Mueller HG, Hawkins DB, Northern JL. *Probe Microphone Measurements: Hearing Aid Selection and Assessment*. San Diego, CA: Singular; 1992.

Mueller HG, Johnson EE, Carter AS. Hearing aids and assistive devices. In: Schow RL, Nerbonne MA, eds. *Introduction to Audiologic Rehabilitation*. 5th ed. Boston, MA: Allyn and Bacon; 2007.

Northern JL, Downs MP. *Hearing in Children*. 5th ed. Baltimore, MD: Lippincott Williams & Wilkins; 2002.

Pascoe DP. *Hearing Aids. Who Needs Them?* St. Louis, MO: Big Bend Books; 1991.

Ricketts TA, Tharpe AM, DeChicchis AR, et al. Amplification selection for children with hearing impairment. In: Bluestone CD, Alper CM, Arjmand EM, et al., eds. *Pediatric Otolaryngology*. 4th ed. Philadelphia, PA: Harcourt Health Sciences; 2001.

Sanders DA. *Management of Hearing Handicap: Infants to Elderly.* 4th ed. Englewood Cliffs, NJ: Prentice Hall; 1999.

Schow RL, Nerbonne MA, eds. *Introduction to Audiologic Rehabilitation.* 5th ed, Boston, MA: Pearson Education, Inc.; 2007.

Seewald RC, ed. *A Sound Foundation Through Early Amplification.* Chicago, IL: Phonak; 2000.

Seewald RC, Gravel JS, eds. *A Sound Foundation Through Early Amplification*, 2001. Chicago, IL: Phonak; 2002.

Skinner MW. *Hearing Aid Evaluation.* Englewood Cliffs, NJ: Prentice-Hall; 1988.

Studebaker GA, Bess FH, eds. *The Vanderbilt Hearing Aid Report. Monographs in Contemporary Audiology*, Upper Darby, PA: 1982.

Studebaker GA, Bess FH, Beck LB, eds. *The Vanderbilt Hearing Aid Report II.* Parkton, MD: York Press; 1991.

The Pediatric Work Group of the Conference on Amplification for Children With Auditory Deficits. Amplification for infants and children with hearing loss. *Am J Audiol* 1996;5:53–68.

10

Rehabilitation and Habilitation for Individuals with Impaired Hearing

Chapter Objectives

- To appreciate the value of and need for aural rehabilitation or habilitation for individuals with impaired hearing;

- To recognize the differences in the details of the aural rehabilitation process for children versus adults, as well as children who experience impaired hearing before versus after the acquisition of spoken language; and

- To understand the elements of the aural rehabilitation process, including selection, fitting, and maintenance of the auditory prosthetic device; auditory training; speechreading; instruction in effective communication and communication strategies; and counseling.

Key Terms and Definitions

- **Auditory-oral communication:** A communication philosophy that requires the education and rehabilitation of the person with impaired hearing to be entirely based on auditory and spoken communication. Training focuses on optimal use of hearing and speech for communication.

- **Total communication:** A communication philosophy that uses manual communication to supplement, to varying degrees, the auditory-oral communication of the person with impaired hearing.

- **Auditory training:** A variety of sound-based training programs focusing on individual speech sounds, words, or sentences and designed to enhance the perception and understanding of speech by persons with impaired hearing.

- **Speechreading:** Also often referred to as "lipreading"; this is the process whereby the listener uses the visible facial gestures of the talker (not just the talker's lips) during speech production to better understand the spoken message.

As noted, breaks in the communication chain resulting from conductive pathologies are typically remedied via medical intervention, with some exceptions. For those with damage to the sensory structures in the cochlea, however, the damage is permanent and currently not subject to medical remediation. Alternative approaches to repairing the break in the communication chain are required.

Probably the most significant problem experienced by the adult with adult-onset hearing loss is difficulty understanding speech, especially against a background of noise. Individuals with severe or profound sensorineural hearing loss also have trouble hearing speech in quiet and hearing their own speech. The inability to monitor their own speech typically results in speech-production problems as well, making the overall communication process even more difficult. The intent of rehabilitation for the hearing-impaired adult is to restore as much speech-comprehension and speech-production ability as possible. That is, the goal is to circumvent any breaks in the communication chain resulting from an auditory impairment and restore normal or near-normal communication.

For the child with congenital hearing impairment, however, the problem is more complicated because the symbols of our language system have not yet been learned. Vocabulary and the rules of grammatical structure (syntax) of the child's language are being acquired. As noted previously, vocabulary and syntax develop naturally in the typically developing child through repeated exposures to spoken language. For the young child with hearing loss, the emphasis of linguistic remediation is on helping the child to acquire this complex language system and to use language appropriately so that communication skills might be developed. In such cases, the focus is more on habilitation than on rehabilitation. In other words, the objective is not to restore a skill that once existed but to help the child develop a new skill, the ability to communicate orally and auditorily.

As noted in Chapter 9, the central core of any rehabilitation/habilitation program is the use of a prosthetic device that compensates for the individual's hearing loss. The most common such device is the hearing aid, but, in more severe impairments, the cochlear implant, a device that bypasses the damaged cochlea and stimulates the auditory nerve fibers electrically, is becoming more commonplace (see Chapter 9 for more details). Typically, the fitting of the device is the first step in the intervention phase of an aural rehabilitation/habilitation program. This chapter focuses on the provision of treatment that follows the fitting of the prosthetic device. The treatment differs considerably for children and adults. As a result, each is the focus of a separate section of this chapter.

HABILITATION OF THE CHILD WITH HEARING LOSS

Management of the child with hearing loss is a monumental challenge to the clinical audiologist. In learning to understand and produce spoken language, there is no adequate substitute for an intact auditory system. Without normal or near-normal hearing, it is extremely difficult to acquire an adequate oral communication system. Because so much of the language-learning process occurs within the first few years of life, there has been considerable emphasis on early identification and intervention for young hearing-impaired children. The various approaches to early identification were outlined in Chapter 8 and will not be restated here. For the most part, however, the earlier one can identify the hearing loss, preferably during the first few months of life, the sooner intervention can begin and the better the chances for a favorable outcome. As noted in Chapter 8, the Joint Committee on Infant Hearing established ideal timelines of "1-3-6," with screening to detect a possible hearing problem within the 1st month of life, follow-up evaluation of those who failed the screening by 3 months of age, and intervention for treatment by 6 months of age. Generally speaking, hearing-impaired children who exhibit the best spoken language skills and show the most satisfactory progress in school are those who have had the benefit of early identification and intervention. Early intervention is essential to the successful development of speech and language. The intervention must include adequate parent-infant management, wearable amplification or cochlear implants, speech and language training, and development of perceptual and cognitive skills, including listening and literacy skills.

Choosing the Appropriate Communication Mode

An important issue facing audiologists, teachers, and school officials is determining which educational approach is most appropriate for a given hearing-impaired child. Presently, two primary modes of instruction are recommended in the educational system: auditory-oral communication and total communication. The auditory-oral approach places emphasis entirely on the auditory and speech systems for developing receptive and expressive forms of communication, whereas total communication emphasizes a combination of audition, speech, visual, and motor systems (finger spelling and signs) for achieving the same goal. As noted in Chapter 1, the emphasis in this book is on the development of auditory-oral communication. Recent research is somewhat equivocal regarding the superiority of one approach over the other, especially in various areas of language abilities and when giving the child the opportunity to be assessed using oral or oral+sign language. Not surprisingly, however, this same research reveals superior performance of children in auditory-oral environments when either their speech perception abilities or the clarity of their own speech productions has been evaluated. More information about communication modes available for children with impaired hearing can be found in the online supplemental information for this chapter.

Although most would agree that spoken language maximizes the options available to the child, the reality is that not all children are able to learn spoken English. Even in total communication programs, decisions are sometimes made about whether to emphasize spoken language or manual communication. How, then, does one determine which mode of communication is most beneficial?

Two approaches have been proposed for audiologists who must determine, together with parents, teachers, and others on the intervention team, whether a child with hearing loss would be better off in an auditory-oral or a total communication program of instruction. One is the Deafness Management Quotient (DMQ). The DMQ uses a weighted point system (total of 100 points) to quantify a number of factors about the child and the child's environment. These factors include the amount of residual hearing (30 points), central auditory system intactness (30 points), intellectual factors (20 points), family constellation (10 points), and socioeconomic issues (10 points). A child scoring greater than 80 points would be recommended for an auditory-oral program. Unfortunately, it is very difficult to quantify objectively the recommended factors, and more importantly, the DMQ has not been adequately validated. An alternative index, known as the Spoken Language Predictor (SLP), was proposed and validated. Similar to the DMQ, the SLP incorporates five factors considered important to a child's success in an auditory-oral program. The factors are weighted, and a point score (total of 100 points) is derived. The factors include hearing capacity (30 points), language competence (25 points), nonverbal intelligence (20 points), family support (15 points), and speech-communication attitude (10 points). Children with scores of 80 to 100 are judged to have excellent potential for developing spoken language. Not only can the Spoken Language Predictor be of use in deciding on placement, but it can also verify the appropriateness of placement for an older child already enrolled in a program.

Let us now review some of the appropriate management strategies for hearing-impaired children. The approaches to be discussed can accommodate either an auditory-oral or a total communication emphasis.

Parent-Infant Management

The first 3 years of life are critical to a child's general development, especially with respect to communication, and the parents of young handicapped children often lack the specific knowledge and skills necessary to optimize family-infant interactions, which could facilitate the child's communication development. Awareness of this situation has led to the development of parent-infant intervention programs. In addition to espousing early identification and intervention, most parent-oriented programs include family support for parents and members of the child's extended family. Information sharing or exchange, demonstration teaching (in which the family explores a variety of strategies to assist the child in achieving communication), and educational advocacy for the parents are also frequently included. The latter entails helping the parents to become effective consumers of services and knowledgeable child advocates.

An important component of a parent-infant curriculum is audiologic management and amplification or cochlear implantation. Here the emphasis is on helping the child to develop his or her auditory potential. Emphasis is placed on further clarification of the nature of the hearing loss, the selection of amplification, and the development of full-time hearing aid use. Teaching parents the importance of care and maintenance of hearing aids is also an important dimension. Another element of effective parent-infant management is **auditory training**, an organized sequential approach to the development of listening skills. Here, the emphasis is on developing a program of auditory training experiences that will guide the parents through a developmental sequence for their child that parallels the development of auditory perceptual skills in the normal-hearing infant. The hierarchy of skills can be divided into the following levels:

1. Auditory perception of both environmental sounds and the human voice.
2. Awareness of environmental sounds and the human voice as conveyors of information and association of sounds with their physical sources.
3. Development of an auditory-vocal feedback mechanism in which the child monitors his or her own speech.
4. Comprehension of meaning in syllables, words, phrases, and sentences.
5. Increasing verbal comprehension and the emergence of auditory memory and sequencing skills.

The initiation and maintenance of vocal behavior is a major area of the early-intervention program that is critical to young children. Full-time use of hearing aids or cochlear implants is important so that the hearing-impaired child can hear his or her own speech as well as the speech of others. The use of an auditory program to enhance the use of the auditory feedback mechanism is also important. Further, parents are taught to use vocal play interaction techniques that are necessary for the development of prelinguistic speech skills. Parents must also learn to develop strategies that facilitate social and communicative turn taking.

Finally, there are the verbal interaction techniques of language programming. At this point, the focus is on teaching the parent communicative interaction styles, particularly verbal interaction patterns, which enhance the child's acquisition of language. Linguistic development is maximized by training parents to incorporate those principles of adult-child interaction patterns that are reported to occur during the language acquisition of normal children.

Language: Characteristics, Assessment, and Training

As noted in the discussion of the communication chain in Chapter 1, language may be defined as a systematic code used to represent the concepts that designate experience and to facilitate social interaction. Spoken language is the primary means by which humans communicate with one another. Although a comprehensive review of language is beyond the scope of this book, a general knowledge of the dimensions of language is important to the understanding of management issues. Most linguists agree that there are three components of language: form, content, and use. The form of language pertains to the elements of language and the rules for combining those elements. The three aspects of language form include phonology (the sounds or phonemes of the language), syntax (word order rules), and morphology (the internal structure of words). In learning phonology, children acquire the rules for how sounds can be sequenced to formulate words. For example, in English, the /mp/ sequence of phonemes can appear at the end of a word (e.g., jump), but not at the beginning of a word. In learning syntax, children acquire the rules for how words are combined and sequenced to form grammatical sentences. For example, when formulating a question, a subject-noun and an auxiliary verb ("He is…") can be reversed (e.g., Is he eating cookies?), but a subject-noun and main verb ("He eats…") cannot be inverted (e.g., ungrammatical: Eats he cookies?). Lastly, in learning morphology, children acquire the rules for how inflections are added to words (e.g., the plural of cookie is cookies). To learn language, children must process language input (e.g., the talk of their caregiver) and learn the rules to formulate grammatical sentences.

The second component of language is content, also referred to as semantics. Children must learn the meaning of individual words, as well as the meaning of particular phrases (e.g., raining cats and dogs).

The final component of language is pragmatics, or the ability to use language to communicate effectively, for example, how to engage in conversation and how to use language to meet a variety of goals (e.g., seek information, answer questions). The development of language is an extremely complex process, involving the acquisition of skill in each component of language.

Given what we have discussed about language, it is not surprising to learn that children with hearing loss experience great difficulty in learning language. This difficulty increases with increasing hearing loss. Most research dealing with the language characteristics of children with hearing loss has focused on the "form" component because errors in form (phonemes, morphemes, and syntax) are easier to quantify. In addition, the acquisition of form may be more challenging than the acquisition of content and use. Nevertheless, it is important to realize that researchers have documented language-learning difficulties in all aspects of language, form, content, and use for children with hearing loss.

Many commercially available instruments are designed to assist the clinician in the ongoing evaluation of a child's language development. Although formal language tests explore a wide range of language skills, for the most part, they do not adequately evaluate a child's ability to use language in day-to-day situations. Hence, clinicians always need to explore informal nonstandardized tasks to obtain information in areas not covered by the standard diagnostic tools. Language sampling can be an invaluable tool in determining the extent to which hearing loss is affecting the development and the interaction of content, form, and use in the child's language system as the child engages in authentic communication.

A number of approaches have been used in language intervention, most of which have focused on the syntactic forms of language. These approaches can be classified as either analytic or natural methods for teaching language. Analytic methods have concentrated on the form of a child's language, and most techniques categorize the various parts of speech grammatically. These approaches are also characterized by extensive drills and exercises. An example of the analytical method would be drills on grammatical morphemes, such as plural "s" or past-tense "ed" endings. The natural approach, sometimes referred to as the experiential method, holds that language is learned through experiences, not systematic drills and exercises. This content/unit approach emphasizes identifying areas of interest for the child that then serve as the basis for teaching vocabulary in meaningful contexts and practicing spoken and, later, written language.

More recently, language-intervention approaches have begun to consider modern language theory and to develop strategies that attempt to integrate syntactic, pragmatic, and semantic levels. The reader interested in learning more about language-intervention techniques based on current theory for individuals with hearing loss can consult the suggested readings at the end of this chapter.

Speech Production: Characteristics, Assessment, and Training

It was noted earlier that significant hearing losses make it difficult not only to understand speech but also to produce speech. The auditory feedback portion of the communication chain is impaired. Nevertheless, it is the general consensus that many hearing-impaired children, even those with profound losses, can develop speech skills. This is especially true for profoundly impaired children who received early intervention using cochlear implants and were educated in using an auditory-oral approach. Hearing-impaired children manifest a variety of speech-production errors categorized as either segmental (i.e., phonemic and phonetic) or suprasegmental (i.e., related to intonation and prosody). The most common segmental errors include the omission of word final sounds and substitution errors for both consonants and vowels. Suprasegmental errors include inadequate timing, which results in very slow, labored speech and poor control of the fundamental frequency, causing abnormal pitch and distorted intonation. Predictably, as the frequency of errors increases, overall intelligibility decreases and the communication chain is increasingly ineffective.

Assessment of speech production is not as easy as one might predict because many of the assessment tools were designed for normal-hearing children. The evaluation of segmental (vowel, consonant) errors is usually conducted with commonly available picture identification tests. Because most of these tests do not consider the unavoidable problems of testing the child with hearing impairment, it is not unusual for the clinician to develop informal tests that will focus on specific segmental errors frequently seen in this population. Assessment of overall intelligibility of conversational speech is also important for the planning of an intervention program. Some clinicians record spontaneous speech samples, which are then judged by a group of listeners to evaluate a child's intelligibility, including the use of suprasegmental features of spoken language, such as prosody and intonation.

Perhaps the most popular method for teaching speech to the hearing-impaired child is an approach advocated by Daniel Ling. Very briefly, this method focuses on using the child's residual hearing to monitor speech production, as well as to understand the speech of others. The approach to speech acquisition attempts to duplicate the process that normal-hearing children experience. The teaching of speech is carried out primarily at the phonetic and phonologic levels, with emphasis on the phonetic domain. At the phonetic level, there is emphasis on nonsense syllable drills (i.e., /ta, ta, ta/ or /ti, ta, to/). Several stages are proposed in which target behaviors are established using criterion-referenced skills. A child must complete each phase satisfactorily before moving on to the next level. These stages include undifferentiated vocalizations; suprasegmental voice patterns; a range of distinctly different vowel sounds; consonants contrasted in manner of production; consonants contrasted in manner and place of production; consonants contrasted in manner, place, and voicing; and consonant blends. The following additional strategies have been suggested to supplement the Ling approach:

1. Production by imitation—the child produces the target sound using auditory clues only.
2. Production on demand—the child produces the target sound from visual cues.
3. Discrimination—the child selects the speech pattern from a closed set of alternative speech patterns produced by the clinician or model.
4. Self-evaluation—the child evaluates his or her own speech production.

The focus in the preceding paragraphs on habilitation or rehabilitation for children to fix the breakdown in communication due to hearing loss had children with severe or profound hearing loss in mind. It would be incorrect, however, to assume that children with less severe hearing loss do not need aural rehabilitation as well. There is considerable research to demonstrate that children with mild-to-moderate and so-called "minimal" hearing loss experience educational delays and possibly speech-language developmental delays as well. The general approach to aural rehabilitation is the same, but the needs and, therefore, the details of the rehabilitation differ for these children compared to more severely impaired children. Details about the nature of the problems experienced by children with minimal hearing loss or mild-to-moderate hearing loss, as well as appropriate means of intervention, can be found in the online supplemental material for this chapter.

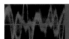 **REHABILITATION OF THE ADULT WITH IMPAIRED HEARING**

The rehabilitation techniques used with the hearing-impaired adult are quite different from the approaches used with children. There are similarities, however. The individual must receive a careful assessment to determine the nature and extent of the problem, amplification plays a major role in the rehabilitation process, and the techniques and strategies used in rehabilitation are determined by the information elicited in the assessment phase. Although cochlear implants can be used by adults with profoundly impaired hearing, the overwhelming majority of adults with hearing impairment have losses that are milder and most appropriately addressed through hearing aids.

Assessment Issues

In the introduction to this chapter, we talked about the importance of the assessment phase and how it is used to establish a rehabilitative program. The assessment phase typically consists of a comprehensive case history, pure-tone audiometry, immittance measurements, speech recognition tests, a communication-specific self-assessment questionnaire, and, occasionally, a measure of speechreading ability. Because we have already reviewed in some detail the basic assessment battery (case history, pure-tone audiometry, immittance measurements, and speech recognition), we will focus here on questionnaires and speechreading skills in the planning of rehabilitation programs.

Assessment with Communication Scales

Communication scales need to be a part of every assessment approach. These scales usually assess how the hearing impairment affects everyday living, that is, the way in which the hearing deficit affects psychosocial, emotional, or vocational performance. Such information can be of value in determining the need for and probable success of amplification, irrespective of the degree of hearing loss and the specific areas in which the rehabilitation should occur. Most scales have focused on communication-specific skills. Examples of questions that could be included in such a scale are "Do you have difficulty hearing when someone speaks in a whisper?" and "Does a hearing problem cause you difficulty when listening to TV or radio?"

The answers to such questions illuminate listening problems. Once the areas of difficulty have been identified, possible solutions can be considered. For example, if the individual reports difficulty only when listening to a television or radio, an assistive listening device might be considered. If, on the other hand, a patient reports difficulty in a variety of listening situations and notes a tendency to withdraw from social activities because of the hearing loss, the individual would be a good candidate for a personal hearing aid. Counseling for this patient and the patient's relatives might also be indicated. Furthermore, the clinician may wish to develop techniques for improving speechreading and auditory training skills in situations that present listening difficulty. Numerous communication scales are available for use, and some of these are illustrated in more detail in the online supplemental material available for this chapter.

Management Strategies with the Hearing-Impaired Adult

Importance of Counseling

Counseling should be a central focus of any management strategy for the adult with hearing loss. In fact, the hearing-impaired adult should receive counseling both before and after the provision of a hearing aid. Counseling is a vital part of the assessment phase because it is during this phase that information about the patient's communication problems is determined. The first component of the counseling process is to explain to the patient, in lay terms, the nature and extent of the hearing loss. If the audiologist believes that the patient can benefit from amplification, counseling is needed to discuss with the patient the value of a hearing aid and what can be expected from it. Possible modification of the patient's motivation and attitudes may also be appropriate at this juncture. The audiologist will have information from the assessment data on the patient's feelings about wearing a hearing aid. Often the patient has no real interest in a hearing aid but is simply responding to the will of a spouse or "significant other." Others have received misleading information about hearing aids from friends or from advertisements. Typically, especially for many older adults with impaired hearing, there is a state of denial that can be difficult to overcome even with counseling. To illustrate, in a 2011 survey of over 2,200 member of the American Association of Retired Persons, 15% of respondents indicated that "I have hearing difficulty but haven't been treated" and another 32% indicated that "My hearing isn't as good as it could be, but I don't think I need to be treated." Thus, for a variety of reasons, there is reluctance among older adults with impaired hearing to seek out treatment, and this form of denial must be dealt with in counseling if there is to be any hope for the successful use of hearing aids. Some patients are concerned about whether the hearing aid will show because of the stigma commonly associated with deafness in the United States (see Vignette 10.1). Under such circumstances, the objective of

VIGNETTE 10.1 • FURTHER DISCUSSION

"The Hearing Aid Effect"

Examine the two top pictures. How would you rate the person on the left on a continuum from bright to dull, from smart to dumb, or from pretty to ugly? How about the person on the right at the top?

Now, examine the two pictures below. How would you rate these two individuals on the same continua listed above?

Notice that the two people pictured in the top set of "photographs" are the same as the two in the bottom set, but the one wearing the hearing aid has changed. When researchers have had large groups of subjects rate their impressions of real photographs similar to these drawings along continua similar to those listed above and have counterbalanced the design so that each person is pictured wearing a hearing aid by the conclusion of the testing, the results indicate that the presence of a hearing aid on the individual in the photo leads to lower ratings on many continua. This negative image associated with the wearing of a hearing aid is called "the hearing aid effect." It has been documented in adults and children alike and is part of the stigma hearing aid wearers must overcome.

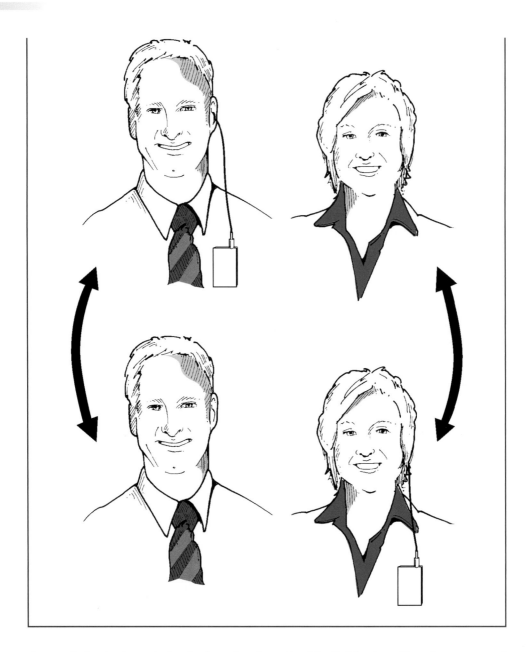

the audiologist is to help the hearing-impaired individual realize that many of the fears or concerns about hearing loss or hearing aids are unwarranted. The individual should be counseled that the use of amplification could help in a variety of listening situations.

Counseling is also sometimes appropriate for relatives and friends who have developed erroneous impressions about hearing loss and amplification. For example, a patient with a high-frequency sensorineural hearing loss will typically experience difficulty in understanding speech. Relatives and friends sometimes interpret this difficulty as a sign of senility, inattention, or even stupidity. It is helpful for the audiologist to counsel relatives and friends about the nature and extent of hearing loss as well as the psychosocial complications associated with a hearing deficit. Reviewing such information with loved ones helps them to understand better and to be more tolerant of the listening difficulties caused by a significant hearing impairment. The audiologist may also choose to offer suggestions for enhancing communication. The significant other can be counseled in the use of deliberate, unhurried speech, good illumination of the speaker's face, and care to ensure that the lips are clearly visible.

Once the hearing aid has been purchased, or just before a purchase, the patient is counseled about the use and care of a hearing aid. The audiologist reviews the manipulation of the various controls, the function of the battery compartment, troubleshooting techniques in cases of malfunction, the proper care of the earmold or shell, and the warranty of the hearing aid. A potential difficulty is that patients often have unrealistic expectations for a hearing aid, especially in the initial stages of use. The audiologist must take care to advise the hearing-impaired patient about the limitations of amplification and to help the individual adjust to very difficult listening situations, such as competing speech or the presence of a competing background noise. Finally, some patients will need special help in the manipulation of hearing aid controls. This is a common problem among the elderly and will be discussed in more detail later in this chapter.

Throughout the entire rehabilitation cycle, counseling is seen as a continuing process. The audiologist spends time listening, advising, and reacting to the needs and concerns of the hearing-impaired individual.

Instruction for Speechreading and Auditory Training

The two primary training aspects of aural rehabilitation for the adult are speechreading and auditory training. Speechreading refers to the ability of a person, any person, to use vision as a supplement to audition when communicating. All persons, regardless of the degree of impairment, can benefit from visual cues. At one time, speechreading was referred to simply as "lipreading." The change in label to "speechreading" has come about in recognition of the fact that more than just the talker's lips provide important visual cues to understanding speech. More recently, some have suggested reserving "speechreading" for the use of visual information during actual speech communication and "lipreading" for use when only the visual stimulus is involved, as in "mouthing the words," but not actually speaking.

Speechreading should be viewed not as a replacement for auditory coding of speech but as an important supplement. With visual information alone, approximately 30% to 40% of a "spoken" message typically can be understood by the average person (the actual level of performance varies depending on a wide variety of factors including the context of the message and numerous factors regarding the visibility of the talker). However, for a given set of conditions, individuals vary widely in this ability.

Acquisition of speechreading skills can take hours of training. There are two basic approaches to speechreading training: analytic and synthetic. Analytic methods begin with training on individual speech sounds and progress to words, phrases, sentences, and continuous discourse, in sequence. The synthetic approach begins training at the phrase or sentence level. The synthetic approach seems to be the one more widely used by audiologists. Training usually begins with simple, commonly encountered questions such as, "What is your name?" or "What time is it?" It then progresses to less frequently encountered statements and continuous discourse.

Auditory training refers to teaching the individual with hearing loss to use his or her hearing as well as possible. The approaches pursued vary with the onset of the hearing loss. Typically, a hierarchy of skills is developed at the phoneme and word level, beginning with detection of the sound or word (can the patient hear anything when the sound is spoken?). The next goal is discrimination of the targeted sound or word (is it the same or different from some other sounds or words?), followed by the development of skills in the identification of the sound or word (which one of several words or sounds was it?). The final goal is often to develop proficiency in the open-set recognition of the speech sound or word (what sound or word was it?). Auditory training is encouraged for all individuals wearing a hearing aid for the first time. It takes time and training to learn to understand speech with a hearing aid. Many individuals with hearing loss have never heard speech or have heard it through the distortion of the hearing loss—in many cases, for a period of several years—before seeking assistance. Fitting the hearing aid or other rehabilitative device will not bring about an instant restoration of normal function. Recent research indicates, for instance, that at least 3 to 6 months may be required for many hearing aid wearers to attain maximum levels of speech-communication performance with their hearing aids. In fact, many patients will probably never perform *completely* as well as a normal-hearing person does, especially under adverse listening conditions all too commonly encountered in everyday communication situations. With continued training, however, they can come much closer to achieving this objective. Auditory training is designed to maximize the use of residual hearing, whereas speechreading is meant to supplement the reduced information received through the auditory system. Extensive training in both areas can result in very effective use of the rehabilitative device chosen for the patient.

LISTENING TRAINING, SPEECH CONSERVATION, AND SPEECH TRACKING

Another role of the audiologist is to help the hearing-impaired patient develop or maintain good listening skills and to assist the patient in maintaining good speech-production skills. Listening training refers to helping the patient to attend better to the spoken message. Some people simply have poor listening skills, and this problem is exacerbated in the presence of a hearing loss. The emphasis in listening training is on teaching the impaired listener to be alert, attentive, and ready to receive the spoken message. Training should focus on eliminating or avoiding distractions, learning to focus on the speaker's main points, attending to nonverbal information, keeping visual contact with the speaker, and mentally preparing oneself to listen to the speaker.

As hearing loss increases, it becomes more difficult for an individual to monitor his or her own speech production. This inability results in faulty speech characterized by poor vocal quality, nasality, segmental errors, and suprasegmental errors. Under such conditions, learning the effective use of kinesthetic (sensation of movement) cues is essential for creating an awareness of the segmental elements of speech. The patient must become physically aware of the kinesthetic qualities of each phonetic element in speech. Auditory training and speechreading can also help in preserving the perception of subtle nuances in the speech message. Techniques for developing an awareness of the rhythm, quality, intonation, and loudness of one's own speech are needed by the hearing impaired. Finally, the importance of listening is critical to this population, and the enhancement of listening skills should be part of any speech-conservation program.

Speech tracking refers to a procedure in which a reader presents connected speech and a listener repeats the message, word for word or syllable for syllable. Both the speaker and the listener participate in the procedure, with the impaired listener attempting to immediately imitate the speaker. The technique has great face validity because the material approximates normal communication more closely than single words do. Tracking ability is measured in terms of the number of words tracked per minute. Rate of speech tracking improves with rehabilitative training (speechreading and/or auditory training) and with the use of amplification or alternative rehabilitation devices. Speech tracking can be used as a tool in aural rehabilitation, especially for measuring the effects of rehabilitation or training.

SPECIAL CONSIDERATIONS FOR THE HEARING-IMPAIRED ELDERLY

We have noted on several occasions throughout this text that a large number of elderly people exhibit significant hearing impairments. Typically, the hearing impairment in the aged is a mild-to-moderate, bilateral, high-frequency sensorineural hearing loss with associated difficulty in understanding conversational speech (see Chapters 6 and 9). The loss usually begins around 50 years of age and progresses with each succeeding decade. In addition, speech understanding difficulties become greater when the listening task is made more difficult. Such hearing loss adversely affects both the functional health status and the psychosocial well-being of the impaired individual. It is generally thought that hearing loss can produce withdrawal, poor self-concept, depression, frustration, irritability, senility, isolation, and loneliness.

Despite the high prevalence of hearing loss among the elderly and the accepted psychosocial complications, the hearing-impaired elderly are not usually referred for audiologic intervention. Frequently, they are not considered candidates for amplification until they reach advanced old age. The reasons for this are not clear. Some elderly persons believe that their hearing loss is simply another unavoidable aspect of the aging process. This feeling lessens the person's felt need to seek rehabilitation or the ability to justify it. This belief, combined with an inadequate knowledge and low expectations of rehabilitative measures, seems to discourage these individuals from seeking assistance. Even those who do seek assistance often fail to use their hearing aids to the fullest. In fact, some stop using their amplification systems soon after purchase.

The special problems of the hearing-impaired elderly require that the audiologist educates physicians and laypersons about the benefits of hearing aids. Audiologists must also recognize the special needs of this population. For example, during the assessment phase, one must determine whether there are any limitations in upper body movement or if arthritis exists. These conditions can interfere with an individual's ability to reach, grasp, or manipulate a hearing aid. Such information is most helpful in deciding on the type of hearing aid to be recommended. For example, a small in-the-canal (ITC) hearing aid with micro controls would be inappropriate for an individual who has arthritis affecting the hands and arms. Another important consideration in the assessment phase is the visual acuity of the patient. Like hearing, vision declines with increasing age. Because visual acuity is important for receiving auditory-visual information, it is prudent for the audiologist to assess the visual abilities of an elderly patient. This can be done simply by posing questions about visual status to the hearing-impaired person. Examples of such questions might include the following:

1. Do you have problems with your vision? If so, what kind?
2. Do you wear eyeglasses? Do they help you to see?
3. Are you able to see my mouth clearly?

Some audiologists actually test for far visual acuity using the well-known Snellen eye chart.

A check of mental status is also appropriate for the elderly population. Many elderly individuals exhibit declines in cognitive function that would reduce the likelihood of successful use of a hearing aid. Formal tests are available to assess mental status. In lieu of these, however, the audiologist can simply pose questions that will offer information about the patient's cognitive functioning (i.e., memory, general knowledge, orientation). Examples for quick screens for dementia in older adults can be questions such as "What day of the week is it?" and "Who is the President of the United States?" If there are problems with mental status, the audiologist will need to work closely with a significant other to assure appropriate use and care of the hearing aid.

Other factors that need to be considered before amplification is recommended to an elderly person include motivation, family support, financial resources, and lifestyle. Special attention is also important for the elderly during the hearing aid orientation program. Greater care is required to explain the various components of a hearing aid. Furthermore, the audiologist should schedule elderly patients for periodic follow-up visits to monitor the patients' progress and to review questions and concerns that they may have about their amplification devices. When considering amplification for this group, one must recognize that they could benefit from many of the assistive listening devices described in Chapter 9. Many of the problems experienced by this group involve use of the telephone, watching television, and understanding speech in group situations, such as church or public auditoriums.

In recent years, a number of aural rehabilitation programs have been developed specifically targeting the older adult with hearing aids. These programs share several features. They are automated, self-paced and easily scored, and typically implemented with a computer or over the Internet. The focus is placed on the primary problem experienced by older adults wearing hearing aids: speech communication in noise, particularly when noise is other people talking in the background. Some of these approaches also focus on the training of cognitive skills, such as memory, that might be important for communication, and some also focus on the comprehension of fast speech. In addition to difficulty understanding speech in noise, another frequent complaint of older adults is that everyone "mumbles" or "talks too fast." Training in the recognition of fast speech, therefore, might help with this difficulty. Currently, several auditory training systems targeting older adults with hearing aids are under development and evaluation. Perhaps, in the future, once this research has been completed, such training systems will be delivered to the patient with the hearing aid as a way to maximize the benefits received from the hearing aids.

To summarize, the hearing-impaired elderly have unique problems and concerns that require the special consideration of the clinician throughout the rehabilitation process. If the clinician attends to these needs and concerns, there is a far greater probability that use of a hearing aid will be successful.

SUMMARY

In this chapter, we have reviewed the treatment provided to children and adults with impaired hearing after the prosthetic device has been fitted. Although the details differ considerably between various approaches and their application to children or adults, the end result is the same: restoration of the function of the normally functioning communication chain. Given that the hearing loss is associated with loss of sensory receptors, whether treated using a hearing aid or a cochlear implant, treatment is required after the fitting of the prosthetic device to optimize the benefits received.

CHAPTER REVIEW QUESTIONS

1. Consider two children with severe bilateral flat sensorineural hearing loss who are otherwise identical, except for the age at which the hearing loss occurred. One child developed the hearing loss at 4 years of age, whereas the hearing loss was present at birth in the other. Assume that the hearing loss was not detected until each child entered school at an age of 5 years. What would be anticipated as likely differences in the communication abilities of these two children when assessed by the clinician at the school?

2. How could the differences observed in the communication skills of the two 5-year-old children with severe hearing loss in Question 1 have been minimized or eliminated?

3. Older adults purchase 2/3 of the hearing aids sold in the United States, yet a majority of those who have purchased hearing aids indicate that they are less than satisfied with them. What factors might contribute to this less than ideal satisfaction, and what steps might be taken to improve satisfaction and benefit from their hearing aids in older adults?

REFERENCES AND SUGGESTED READINGS

Alpiner JG, Schow RL. Rehabilitative evaluation of hearing-impaired adults. In: Alpiner JG, McCarthy PA, eds. *Rehabilitative Audiology: Children and Adults*. 2nd ed. Baltimore, MD: Williams & Wilkins; 1993.

Bess FH, Gravel JS, Tharpe AM. *Amplification for Children with Auditory Deficits*. Nashville, TN: Bill Wilkerson Center Press; 1996.

Bloom L, Lahey M. *Language Development and Language Disorders*. New York, NY: John Wiley & Sons; 1978.

Clark JG, Martin FN. *Effective Counseling in Audiology: Perspectives and Practice*. Englewood Cliffs, NJ: Prentice Hall; 1994.

Fitzgerald MT, Bess FH. Parent/infant training for hearing-impaired children. *Monogr Contemp Audiol* 1982;3:1–24.

Geers AE, Moog JS. Predicting spoken language acquisition of profoundly hearing impaired children. *J Speech Hear Dis* 1987;52:84–94.

High WS, Fairbanks G, Glorig A. Scale for self-assessment of hearing handicap. *J Speech Hear Dis* 1964;17:321–327.

Giolas TE, Owens E, Lamb SH, et al. Hearing performance inventory. *J Speech Hear Dis* 1979;44:169–195.

Katz J. *Handbook of Clinical Audiology.* 6th ed. Baltimore, MD: Lippincott Williams & Wilkins.

Kretschmer RR, Kretschmer LW. Communication/language assessment of the hearing-impaired child. In: Bess FH, ed. *Hearing Impairment in Children.* Parkton, MD: York Press; 1988.

Kurtzer-White E, Luterman D. *Early Childhood Deafness.* Baltimore, MD: York Press; 2001.

Mitchell RE, Karchmer MA. More students in more places. *Am Ann Deaf* 2006;151(2):95–104.

Ling D. *Speech and the Hearing-Impaired Child: Theory and Practice.* Washington, DC: Alexander Graham Bell Association for the Deaf; 1976.

Moeller MP, Brunt MA. Management of preschool hearing-impaired children: A cognitive-linguistic approach. In: Bess FH, ed. *Hearing Impairment in Children.* Parkton, MD: York Press; 1988.

Moeller MP, Carney AE. Assessment and intervention with preschool hearing-impaired children. In: Alpiner JG, McCarthy PA, eds. *Rehabilitative Audiology: Children and Adults.* 2nd ed. Baltimore, MD: Williams & Wilkins; 1993.

Norlin PF, Van Tassell DJ. Linguistic skills of hearing-impaired children. *Monogr Contemp Audiol* 1980;2:1–32.

Sanders DA. *Management of Hearing Handicap: Infants to Elderly.* 4th ed. Englewood Cliffs, NJ: Prentice Hall; 1999.

Schow RL, Nerbonne MA, eds. *Introduction to Audiologic Rehabilitation.* 5th ed. Boston, MA: Pearson Education, Inc.; 2007.

Seewald RC, Gravel JS, eds. *A Sound Foundation Through Early Amplification,* 2001. Chicago, IL: Phonak, 2002.

Acoustic immittance measurements Clinical measurement of the impedance or admittance of the flow of sound energy through the middle ear.

Acoustic neuroma A tumor that affects the eighth/auditory nerve.

Acoustic reflex Reflexive contractions of the middle ear muscles caused by the presentation of a sound stimulus.

Acoustic reflex threshold Lowest possible intensity needed to elicit a middle ear muscle contraction.

Acquired hearing loss Hearing loss obtained sometime after birth.

Acute otitis media Middle ear disease of rapid onset and rapid resolution; characterized by a reddish or yellowish bulging tympanic membrane, obliteration of ossicular landmarks, and conductive hearing loss.

Admittance Ease of flow of energy through a system; reciprocal of impedance.

Afferent Term pertaining to conduction of electrical activity via nerve fibers from peripheral to central locations; ascending nerve fibers.

American Academy of Audiology AAA; professional organization for audiologists.

ANSI American National Standards Institute; organization that develops standards for measuring devices (e.g., audiometers).

American Sign Language ASL; sign language used in the United States. Differs from other forms of manual communication devised to make signs more like the English language.

American Speech–Language–Hearing Association ASHA; professional organization for audiologists and speech-language pathologists.

Anomaly A deviation from normal.

Apex Term used to denote the top or near the top.

Apgar score A common assessment tool for describing the amount of depression exhibited by the infant at birth. Apgar scores consist of five criteria: (a) heart rate, (b) respiratory rate, (c) muscle tone, (d) response to stimulation, and (e) color. The highest possible score is 10.

Articulators Anatomical structures, such as the lips, tongue, and velum (soft palate), which are positioned in various ways by a talker to produce speech sounds.

Assistive listening devices A wide assortment of electronic devices designed as either alternatives to or supplements of other auditory prosthetic devices. Depending on the severity of the hearing loss, common assistive listening devices include wireless systems designed for use while watching television, systems to use while using the telephone, and the use of visual stimulation (e.g., flashing lights) for doorbells, alarm clocks, or other alerting devices.

Atresia Absence or closure of a normal body opening; in hearing, it most often refers to the external acoustic meatus.

Audiogram Graphic representation of a person's hearing. Sound level (in dB) is plotted on the ordinate, and frequency is shown on the abscissa.

Audioscope   Handheld otoscope with a built-in audiometer.

ABR   Auditory brainstem response; a series of five to seven waves in the electrical waveform that appear in the first 10 ms after the presentation of an auditory stimulus such as a click or a tone burst. The ABR is sensitive to dysfunction occurring from the auditory periphery to the upper auditory brainstem portions of the auditory central nervous system.

Auditory central nervous system   Comprises the ascending and descending auditory pathways and centers in the brainstem and cortex.

Auditory cortex   Auditory area of the cerebral cortex located primarily in the region of the temporal lobe.

Auditory periphery   Comprises the outer ear, middle ear, and inner ear, ending at the nerve fibers exiting the inner ear.

Auditory training   A variety of sound-based training programs focusing on individual speech sounds, words, or sentences and designed to enhance the perception and understanding of speech by persons with impaired hearing.

Auditory–oral approach   Method used to teach children with significant hearing loss speech and language; emphasis is on hearing and speechreading with no manual communication.

Auditory-verbal approach   Method used to teach children with significant hearing loss speech and language; emphasis is on listening to and understanding the spoken message via the auditory system with no emphasis on vision for receiving information.

A-weighted scale   A filtering network on the sound-level meter that filters the low frequencies below 500 Hz and approximates the response characteristics of the human ear.

Basal   Term used to denote near the end or base.

Basilar membrane   Membrane in the cochlear duct that supports the organ of Corti.

BOA   Behavioral observation audiometry; evaluation of a child's hearing via observation of responses (e.g., head turn) to sound.

Bilateral   Term used to denote both sides.

Bilirubin   A red bile pigment, sometimes found in urine, that is present in the blood tissues during jaundice.

Binaural   Pertaining to both ears.

BC   Bone conduction; transmission of sound to the inner ear via the skull.

Broadband (white) noise   An acoustic signal that contains energy of equal spectral density (intensity) at all frequencies.

BTE   Behind the ear.

Calibrate   To set the parameters of an instrument such as an audiometer to an accepted standard (e.g., ANSI).

CANS   Central auditory nervous system.

Carhart   Father of the profession of audiology.

Cholesteatoma   Accumulation of debris developed from perforations of the eardrum; sometimes referred to as a pseudo-like tumor.

Chromosome   One of several small rod-shaped bodies, easily stained, that appear in the nucleus of a cell at the time of cell division; they contain the genes, or hereditary factors, and are constant in number in each species.

COM   Chronic otitis media. Otitis media that is slow in its onset, tends to be persistent, and often can produce other complications. The most common symptoms are hearing loss, perforation of the tympanic membrane, and fluid discharge.

Cilium (plural: cilia)   Minute, hair-like structures of sensory cells (inner and outer hair cells) in the cochlea.

Classroom amplification system   An electroacoustic system typically making use of a detached microphone worn by the teacher with the microphone's output sent to personal amplification units worn by members of the class who have impaired hearing.

Cochlea   Auditory portion of the inner ear; sensory organ for hearing.

Cochlear implant   An electronic device that is surgically implanted under the skin behind the ear with electrodes (wires) extending through the middle ear and inserting into the fluid-filled cochlea. The normal transducer function of the inner ear is bypassed, and the nerve fibers exiting the cochlea are stimulated directly by electrical current. These devices currently are reserved for use by individuals with severe or profound amounts of hearing loss who demonstrate little benefit from conventional hearing aids.

Collapsed canal   A canal that collapses as the result of pressure caused by earphone placement.

Communication chain   The sequence of events from the initiation of a thought, idea, or emotion to be communicated by the sender through the reception and interpretation of that message by the receiver. For humans, the message is typically communicated acoustically via speech.

Compression   Technique used to decrease or limit the wide range of sounds in our everyday world to match more closely the dynamic range of listeners with hearing loss.

Computed tomography (CT)   Radiography in which a three-dimensional image of a body structure is constructed by computer from a series of cross-sectional images.

Concha   Depression or bowl-shaped area of the auricle; serves to collect and direct sound to the external auditory meatus.

Congenital   Before birth; usually before the 28th week of gestation.

Contralateral   Pertaining to the opposite side.

Cortex   The outer layer of an organ, such as the cerebrum or cerebellum.

Cytomegalovirus   Congenital viral infection that, in its more severe forms, produces symptoms similar to rubella and may cause hearing loss as well as other abnormalities.

Deaf culture   Beliefs, traditions, customs, and attitudes of a subgroup of the deaf population.

Decibel   The unit of measure used to describe the level or magnitude of a sound wave. The logarithm of the ratio between two sound intensities, powers, or sound pressures.

Deformity   A deviation from the normal shape or size of a specific portion of the body.

Degeneration   Decline as in the nature or function from a former or original state.

Dementia   A breakdown or deterioration in cognitive function.

DNA   Deoxyribonucleic acid; molecules that carry genetic information.

Diagnosis   The process of determining the nature of a disease.

Digital   Numerical representation of a signal especially for use by a computer.

Earmold   Earpiece that is connected to the hearing aid for the purpose of directing sound into the external auditory meatus.

Earphone   A transducer system that converts electrical energy from a signal generator, such as an audiometer, into acoustical energy that is then delivered to the ear.

Educational audiology   A subspecialty in audiology that focuses on providing audiologic services in the schools.

Educational Audiology Association (EAA)   Professional organization for audiologists interested in the provision of audiologic services in the schools.

Effusion   Collection of fluid in the middle ear.

Electroacoustic   Refers to the conversion of acoustic energy to electrical energy, or vice versa, for the purpose of sound generation or measurement.

Electromagnetic field   Field of energy produced by electrical current flowing through a coil or wire.

Emission   Acoustic emissions discharged from the cochlea.

Endogenous   Hereditary forms of hearing impairment; literally means "within the genes."

Endolymph   The fluid contained within the membranous labyrinth of the inner, including the scala media of the cochlea.

Endolymphatic hydrops Ménière disease; buildup of endolymph within the cochlea and vestibular labrynth; typical audiologic findings include vertigo, fullness, and fluctuating sensorineural hearing loss.

ENT Ear, nose, and throat.

Epidemiology Branch of medical science that deals with incidence, distribution, and control of disease in a population.

Epithelium Tissue that forms the surfaces of the body.

Etiology Pertaining to the cause of a disorder or condition.

Exogenous. Acquired forms of hearing impairment; literally means "outside the genes."

Exudate discharge Usually refers to the secretion of fluid from the mucosal lining of the middle ear.

Fetal alcohol syndrome Birth defects that may include facial abnormalities, growth deficiency, mental retardation, and other impairments; caused by the mother's abuse of alcohol during pregnancy.

Filter Pertains to a device that rejects auditory signals at some frequencies while allowing signals at other frequencies to pass.

Fistula A tubular passage way or duct formed by disease, surgery, injury, or congenital defect; usually connects two organs.

Flaccid Weakness—such as a flaccid tympanic membrane.

FM Frequency modulation.

Formant frequencies Regions of prominent energy distribution in a speech sound associated with resonances of the vocal tract.

Frequency The number of complete cycles per second for a vibrating system or other repetitive motion. Expressed in units of Hertz (Hz).

Frequency response The output characteristics of hearing aids or other systems as a function of frequency.

Functional hearing loss Audiometric evidence of hearing loss when there is no organic basis to explain the hearing loss.

Fundamental frequency The harmonic component of a complex wave that has the lowest frequency and commonly the greatest amplitude.

Gain For hearing aids, the difference in dB between the input level of an acoustic signal and the output level.

Gene The biologic unit of heredity, self-reproducing and located in a definite position on a particular chromosome.

Genetic Related to heredity.

Genetic counseling Providing information to families with regard to the probability of an inherited disorder.

Genetics The study of heredity.

Genotype The genetic makeup of an individual.

Geriatric Related to the aging process.

Gestational age Time between mother's last menstrual period and time of baby's birth.

Habilitation Provision of intervention services designed to overcome the handicapping conditions associated with congenital hearing loss.

Hair cells One of the sensory cells in the auditory epithelium of the organ of Corti.

Handicap Conditions that impact on psychosocial function and the consequence of a disability.

Hard of hearing HOH; residual hearing is sufficient to enable successful processing of linguistic information through audition with the use of amplification.

Harmonic A component frequency of a complex wave that is an integral multiple of the fundamental frequency.

Hearing aid A personal electroacoustic device, typically worn in or on the ear of persons with impaired hearing, that primarily serves to amplify sound arriving at the wearer's ear so as to compensate for the wearer's hearing loss.

Hearing aid performance inventory Communication scale that assesses the impact of hearing loss across several dimensions including speech comprehension, signal intensity, response to auditory failure, social effects of hearing loss, and occupational difficulties.

Hearing handicap inventory for the elderly Specific self-report communication scale comprising items dealing with social situational and emotional aspects of hearing loss.

Hearing impairment A generic term indicating disability that may range from slight to complete deafness.

Hearing loss A reduction in the ability to perceive sound; may range from slight to complete deafness.

Hearing sensitivity The ability of the human ear to perceive sound.

Helicotrema Passage that connects the scala tympani and the scala vestibuli at the apex of the cochlea.

Hereditary Genetically transmitted or transmittable from parent to offspring.

Hereditary deafness Genetically transmitted deafness.

Hertz A unit of frequency equal to one cycle per second.

High-risk register Conditions for which children are at greater-than-average risk for hearing impairment.

HINT Hearing in noise test.

Hyperbilirubinemia An abnormally large amount of bilirubin in the circulating blood.

Hypertelorism An abnormal increased distance between two organs or parts.

Hypoxia Depletion of oxygen.

Hz Hertz.

Identification audiometry Typically refers to methods used to screen for hearing loss in a simple, quick, and cost-effective manner.

Idiopathic Pertaining to unknown causation.

Immittance A general term describing measurements made of tympanic membrane impedance, compliance, or admittance.

Impairment Abnormal or reduced function.

Impedance Opposition to the flow of energy through a system; reciprocal of admittance.

Incidence Proportion of a group initially free of a given condition that develops the condition over time.

Inclusion Integration of hearing-impaired children into a regular classroom setting.

Incus The middle bone of the three ossicles in the middle ear; anvil.

Individualized education plan (IEP) Plan developed by a multidisciplinary team for educating children with disabilities including hearing loss; mandated by IDEA 97 and updated on an annual basis.

Individuals with Disabilities Education Act (IDEA) Legislation that insures that children with disabilities over the age of 3 years receive a free and appropriate education and also encourages services for children under 3 years old.

Inertia The tendency of a body to remain in its current state (either motion or rest).

Inner ear The organ of hearing and equilibrium that is located in the temporal bone.

Insertion gain Real ear measurement of the gain of a hearing aid.

Intensive care unit (ICU) Pertains to a separate, designated service area in a hospital that is used for the care and treatment of critically ill patients.

Ipsilateral Typically refers to the same side.

ITC hearing aid In the canal hearing aid.

ITE hearing aid In the ear hearing aid.

Jaundice A yellowish pigmentation of the skin, tissues, and body fluids caused by the deposition of bile pigments.

JND Just noticeable difference.

JCIH Joint Committee on Infant Hearing—organization comprising several different organizations including, but not limited to, the American Academy of Audiology, the American Academy of Otolaryngology, the American Academy of Pediatrics, and the American Speech–Language–Hearing Association.

Kanamycin An ototoxic antibiotic substance consisting of two amino sugars.

Kernicterus A form of jaundice occurring within the newborn; known to be associated with sensorineural hearing loss.

Labyrinth maze In hearing, refers to inner ear.

Labyrinthitis   Inflammation of the labyrinth or inner ear.

Language   The code used by members of the same culture or group to decipher or produce sequences of sounds capable of communicating thoughts, ideas, and actions to other members of the same culture or group.

Larynx   Anatomical structure housing the vocal cords.

Latency   The period of apparent inactivity between the time a stimulus is presented and the moment a response occurs.

Learning disability   Generic term used to denote learning problems in young school-aged children.

Lesion   Wound or injury; area of pathologic change in tissue.

Lexicon   Mental dictionary representing the words known by an individual for a specific language.

Localization   Pertaining to the identification of sound in space (horizontal or vertical plane).

Loudness discomfort level   LDL; the intensity level that causes discomfort for an individual.

Malleus   The largest auditory ossicle; sometimes referred to as the hammer.

Mask   Refers to the ability of one acoustic signal to obscure the presence of another acoustic signal so that it cannot be detected.

Medial   Toward the axis, near the midline.

Ménière disease   Endolymphatic hydrops disease of the membranous inner ear characterized by progressive or fluctuating sensorineural hearing loss, vertigo (dizziness), tinnitus (ringing in ears), and sometimes a fullness sensation.

Meningitis   Inflammation of the meninges caused by bacterial or viral infections causing severe to profound sensorineural hearing loss in some cases (10%).

Meniscus   A crescent-shaped structure.

Microphone   Transducer that converts acoustical energy into electrical energy.

Microtia   A term that implies a small deformed pinna (or auricle).

Mild hearing loss   Hearing loss ranging from 25 to 40 dB HL.

Mixed hearing loss   Type of hearing loss that includes both conductive and sensorineural impairments.

Moderate hearing loss   Hearing loss ranging from 40 to 55 dB HL.

Monaural   Pertaining to one ear.

Montage   Placement configuration of electrodes in electrophysiologic measurements.

Mucus   Viscous secretion of mucous glands.

Mumps   A contagious viral disease occurring mainly in children; symptoms include parotitis, fever, headaches, and sudden profound unilateral sensorineural hearing loss.

Myelin   The fatty sheath or covering of the axon of a neuron.

Myringitis   Inflammation of the tympanic membrane.

Myringotomy   Surgical procedure that involves making an incision in the eardrum to release pressure, remove fluid, and restore hearing sensitivity.

Narrow-band noise   Band of noise limited to a restricted frequency region by filtering.

Nasopharynx   The part of the pharynx (throat) behind and above the soft palate, directly continuous with the nasal passages.

Neomycin   An ototoxic antibiotic, administered orally or locally.

Neonate   Young child—usually during the first 4 weeks.

Nephritis   Inflammation of the kidney.

Nephrotoxic   Toxic to the nephrons of the kidney.

Neuritis   Inflammation of a nerve.

Neuron   Any of the conducting cells of the nervous system; a neuron consists of a cell body, containing the nucleus and the surrounding autoplasm, an axon and a dendrite.

Neurologist   An expert in neurology or in treatment of disorders of the nervous system.

Neurology   Branch of medical science that deals with the nervous system, both normal and in disease.

NICU   Neonatal intensive care unit.

NIHL   Noise-induced hearing loss.

Noise-induced hearing loss   Permanent sensorineural hearing loss as a result of exposure to high noise levels.

Nonorganic hearing loss   See functional hearing loss.

Northwestern Auditory Test Number 6   Common open set monosyllabic word test used in the audiologic assessment to determine word recognition ability at comfortable listening levels.

Occlusion   Blockage or obstruction; typically refers to the ear canal.

Octave   The interval between two sounds with a 2:1 ratio in frequency.

Ohm   Unit of resistance representing opposition to the transference of energy.

Opacification   The development of opacity (imperviousness to light rays), as of the cornea or lens.

Organ of Corti   Sensory organ of hearing located on the basilar membrane.

Ossicles   Refers to the three bones of the middle ear: malleus, incus, and stapes.

Otalgia   Pertaining to the pain in the ear.

Otitis   Inflammation of the ear.

Otitis media   Inflammation of the middle ear space.

Otitis media with effusion   OME; denotes inflammation of the middle ear cleft with a collection of fluid.

Otitis prone   Refers to individual who has a predisposition for middle ear disease.

OTO   Otolaryngology.

Otoacoustic emission (OAE)   Sounds produced by the cochlea; usually evoked by an auditory stimulus but can occur spontaneously; considered an outer hair cell phenomenon.

Otolaryngologist   Physician who specializes in diseases of the ear, nose, and throat.

Otolaryngology   Medical specialty associated with diagnosis and management of diseases of the ear, nose, and larynx.

Otologist   A physician who specializes in diseases of the ear.

Otorrhea   Discharge from the ear.

Otosclerosis   Formation of spongy bone in the labrynthine capsule and the stapes footplate. The most common site of the formation is just in front of the oval window. The disease produces impaired stapedial mobility and a gradual conductive hearing loss. Sometimes referred to as otospongiosis.

Otoscope   Handheld device for visual inspection of the ear canal and eardrum.

Ototoxic   Pertains to toxic effects to the ear.

Outer ear   Pertaining to the auricle, external auditory meatus, and the lateral portion of the tympanic membrane.

Outer hair cells   OHCs; hair cells within the organ of Corti thought to be responsible for frequency resolution and energizing the inner hair cells.

Pascal   The unit of sound pressure, abbreviated Pa.

PB   Phonetically balanced.

Pediatric audiologist   Audiologist who specializes in the assessment and management of young children.

Perforation   Small hole; typically refers to perforation of the tympanic membrane.

Perilymph   The fluid contained within the space separating the membranous from the osseous labrynth of the inner ear, including the scala vestibuli and scala tympani of the cochlea.

Perinatal   Pertains to a condition that occurs in the period shortly before or after birth (from 8 weeks before birth to 4 weeks after).

Periosteum   Specialized connective tissue covering all bones of the body, consisting of a dense, fibrous outer layer and a more delicate inner layer capable of forming bone.

Peripheral   Toward the outward surface or port.

Petrous   Denoting or pertaining to the hard, dense portion of the temporal bone containing the internal auditory organs.

Pneumatic otoscope Handheld instrument used to examine visually the external acoustic meatus and the tympanic membrane. A pneumatic bulb connected to the otoscope allows the examiner to vary air pressure in the canal while examining the mobility of the eardrum.

Postnatal A condition acquired later in life.

Potential Electric tension or pressure; electric activity in a muscle or nerve cell during activity.

Prenatal Something that occurs to the fetus before birth.

Presbycusis Hearing loss due to the aging process.

Prevalence The number of cases of hearing impairment in a given population at a given point in time.

Psychogenic hearing loss See functional hearing loss.

Pure-tone audiometry The measurement of hearing thresholds for pure tones of various frequencies using standardized equipment and procedures.

Pure-tone average PTA; average of hearing thresholds at 500 Hz, 1,000 Hz, and 2,000 Hz.

Real-ear aided response REAR; real ear measurement, with a probe-tube microphone, of the SPL as a function of frequency with the hearing aid in place and turned on.

Real-ear insertion gain REIG; probe microphone measurement of the difference between the unaided response and the real-ear aided response. REIG = REAR – REUR.

Real-ear unaided response REUR; real ear measurement, with a probe-tube microphone, of the SPL as a function of frequency in the ear canal without the hearing aid in place.

Recessive hereditary sensorineural hearing loss Form of hereditary deafness; both parents of a child with hearing loss are clinically normal—appearance of the trait requires that the individual possess two similar abnormal genes, one from each parent. The recessive genes account for the transmission of hearing loss; can skip several generations.

Recruitment Refers to an abnormally fast growth of loudness with increasing sound intensity in an ear with sensorineural hearing loss once threshold has been exceeded.

Reflex An involuntary, relatively invariable adaptive response to a stimulus.

Rehabilitation Management strategies used to restore function following insult or injury.

Renal Term that refers to the kidney.

Residual hearing Refers to hearing that remains in individuals with hearing impairment.

Resonance A frequency region for which the maximum transference of energy through a system occurs.

Reticular lamina Net-like layer extending over the surface of the organ of Corti.

Retinitis Inflammation of the retina.

Retrocochlear Refers to beyond the cochlea, especially nerve fibers along the auditory pathways from the internal auditory meatus to the cortex.

Reverberation Persistence of sound within an enclosed space following its termination.

Rubella German measles; a mild viral infection characterized by a pinkish rash that occurs first on the face before spreading to other parts of the body. If contracted during pregnancy, especially during the first trimester, abnormalities of the fetus can result, producing mental retardation, hearing loss, visual complications, and mild heart problems.

Sagittal plane A vertical plane through the longitudinal axis dividing the body into left and right portions.

Scala A subdivision of the cavity of the cochlea.

Scala media Middle cavity within the cochlea; filled with endolymph and contains the organ of Corti.

Scala tympani   Perilymph-filled cavity below the scala media. Includes the round window.

Scala vestibuli   Perilymph-filled cavity above the scala media. Includes the oval window.

Screening   A program designed to expediently and reliably identify those likely to have a disorder within the general population. More definitive follow-up testing is typically required to confirm (or refute) the findings of the screening.

Semantics   The meaning(s) associated with the words of a language.

Sensation level   SL; refers to the level of a signal (dB) above one's threshold.

Sensitivity   Proportion of truly hearing impaired persons in a screened population correctly identified by a screening test.

Serous   A clear fluid free of debris and bacteria.

Serous otitis media   Inflammation of the middle ear with a collection of clear, thin fluid.

Sickle cell anemia   Hereditary disease of the blood that occurs almost exclusively in blacks.

SNR (or S:N)   Signal-to-noise ratio; usually refers to the relative difference in dB between the signal (usually speech) and (ambient) noise.

SOAE   Spontaneous otoacoustic emission.

Sound field   An area (usually a room) into which sound is introduced (usually by a loudspeaker).

Sound pressure level   SPL; magnitude of sound relative to a reference pressure (0.00002 Pa).

Sound wave   A disturbance created in a medium, such as air, by a source of vibration.

Specificity   Proportion of truly normal hearing persons in a screened population correctly identified by a screening test.

Spectrum   Display of a sound's amplitude (amplitude spectrum) or phase (phase spectrum) as a function of frequency. Plural form is spectra.

Speech audiometry   The measurement of speech recognition threshold (SRT) in decibels and measures of the ability to understand speech when it is many decibels above this threshold.

Speechreading   Also often referred to as "lipreading," this is the process whereby the listener uses the visible facial gestures of the talker (not just the talker's lips) during speech production to better understand the spoken message.

Speech reception threshold   SRT; threshold for speech using spondaic words; the sound level representing the lowest sound level at which speech can be heard 50% of the time.

Spiral ganglion   Group of nerve cell bodies located in the modiolus of the cochlea, from which nerve fibers extend into the spiral organ.

Spondee   Two-syllable words (e.g., baseball, cowboy).

Stapes   The innermost ossicle of the middle ear (stirrup).

Stigmata   Findings or landmarks indicative of a specific disorder.

Streptomycin   Ototoxic antibiotic.

Suppurative   Pus or fluid often found in acute otitis media; characterized by white blood cells, cellular debris, and many bacteria.

Symmetrical hearing loss   Hearing loss that is essentially equivalent in both ears.

Synapse   Region of contact between processes of two adjacent neurons where a nervous impulse is transmitted from one neuron to another.

Syndrome   A group of symptoms that are characteristic of a specific condition or disease.

Syntax   The rules of a language used to string words together into meaningful phrases or sentences. The grammar of a language.

Tactile   Pertaining to touch.

Tangible Reinforcement Operant Conditioning Audiometry   TROCA; reinforcement technique for difficult-to-test children;

the child receives reinforcement (candy, cereal, toys) for the correct identification of a signal.

Tectorial membrane Membrane that projects like a roof over the organ of Corti; the edge of the outer hair cells are embedded within the tectorial membrane.

Temporary threshold shift (TTS) Temporary elevation of an auditory threshold after exposure to noise. Frequently used to predict the potential danger of a noise environment.

TC Total communication; intervention approach that incorporates a combination of auditory/oral and manual communication techniques.

TEOAE Transient evoked otoacoustic emission; echo emitted by the cochlea in response to a transient stimulus.

Threshold Softest level at which a stimulus or change in a stimulus can be detected.

Time compression Process whereby speech is recorded and then played back in less time than the original recording; commonly expressed as a percentage. For example, speech that originally was recorded in 1 second and played back in 1/2 second would be 50% time-compressed.

Tinnitus Sensation of ringing in the ear.

TM Tympanic membrane.

Tonotopic The orderly mapping of sound frequency to anatomical place or location in the auditory system, beginning in the cochlea and proceeding through the auditory portions of the cortex.

TORCH Acronym used to categorize major infections that may be contracted in utero; *T*oxoplasmosis, *O*ther, *R*ubella, *C*ytomegalovirus, and *H*erpes simplex. Syphilis has been added to the list to form the acronym STORCH.

Total communication A manual communication system that is taught to supplement, to varying degrees, the auditory-oral communication of the person with impaired hearing.

Toxoplasmosis Organism that is transmitted to the child via the placenta. Infection is typically contracted by eating uncooked meat or making contact with the feces of cats. Possible cause of hearing loss.

Transducer A device or system that converts one form or energy to another.

Treacher Collins syndrome Craniofacial anomaly characterized by poorly developed cheek bones, antimongoloid slant of the eyes, microtia, atresia, and micronathia.

Tympanogram Graphic representation of middle ear immittance as a function of air pressure presented to the ear canal.

Uncomfortable loudness level Level (in dB) at which audio signals (pure tones, noise, or speech) become uncomfortably loud.

Unilateral Refers to one side as in unilateral hearing loss.

Usher syndrome Usher syndrome is a genetic disorder with symptoms of hearing loss and an eye disorder called retinitis pigmentosa.

Utero Pertaining to the uterus; the womb.

Vertigo Dizziness; an illusionary sensation of movement such as spinning or whirling.

Vibrotactile Denotes the detection of vibrations via touch.

Viscosity The property of fluid that resists change in the shape or arrangement of its element during flow.

Visual reinforcement audiometry VRA; audiologic technique for testing the hearing of young children; a head turn in response to an auditory stimulus is rewarded with a flashing lighted toy or a computerized animated character (e.g., Sponge Bob).

Vocal cords Cartilaginous structures within the larynx that vibrate when air from the lungs is forced through them. The vibration of the vocal cords is the primary determiner of the pitch of a talker's voice.

Vocal tract   The air-filled cavity between the vocal cords and the lips (or nostrils). Changes in the shape of the vocal tract, primarily via movement of the tongue and velum, change the resonant frequencies of the tract and alter the speech sound produced.

Waardenburg syndrome   A group of genetic conditions that can cause hearing loss and changes in coloring (pigmentation) of the hair, skin, and eyes.

Waveform   Display of an acoustic (or electrical) signal with amplitude along the y-axis and time along the x-axis.

Word recognition   Ability to recognize (repeat) monosyllabic words spoken by the clinician when presented well above threshold; typically expressed as percent correct.

(Note: Page numbers followed by "v" indicates vignette; those followed by "f" indicates figure; those followed by "t" indicates table.)